# Advances in Cosmetic Dermatology

# Advances in Cosmetic Dermatology

Edited by **Emily Howling**

hayle medical

New York

Published by Hayle Medical,
30 West, 37th Street, Suite 612,
New York, NY 10018, USA
www.haylemedical.com

**Advances in Cosmetic Dermatology**
Edited by Emily Howling

International Standard Book Number: 978-1-63241-413-7 (Hardback)

The publisher's policy is to use permanent paper from mills that operate a sustainable forestry policy. Furthermore, the publisher ensures that the text paper and cover boards used have met acceptable environmental accreditation standards.

**Trademark Notice:** Registered trademark of products or corporate names are used only for explanation and identification without intent to infringe.

Printed in the United States of America.

# Contents

# Preface

Every book is initially just a concept; it takes months of research and hard work to give it the final shape in which the readers receive it. In its early stages, this book also went through rigorous reviewing. The notable contributions made by experts from across the globe were first molded into patterned chapters and then arranged in a sensibly sequential manner to bring out the best results.

Dermatology is the branch of medicine that is mainly concerned with diagnosing and treating diseases related to skin, hair and nails. Cosmetic dermatology is the sub-branch of dermatology that completely focuses on beautifying a person by using medicines and surgical processes such as blepharoplasty, facelifts and liposuction. This book contains exclusive researches on a variety of topics such as plastic surgery, rejuvenation, laser treatment, cosmetic chemistry, skin physiology, acne treatment, hair conservation and restoration, aesthetic treatments, etc. The various studies that are constantly contributing towards advancing technologies and evolution of this field are examined in detail. This book is an essential guide for dermatologists, cosmetologists, academicians and those who wish to pursue this discipline further.

It has been my immense pleasure to be a part of this project and to contribute my years of learning in such a meaningful form. I would like to take this opportunity to thank all the people who have been associated with the completion of this book at any step.

**Editor**

# Epidemiological and Clinical Aspects of Acne in the Dermatology Department of the Teaching Hospital of Parakou (Benin)

Hugues Adégbidi[1*], Christiane Koudoukpo[2], Félix Atadokpèdé[1],
Florencia do Ango-Padonou[1], Hubert G. Yédomon[1]

[1]Faculté des Sciences de la Santé de Cotonou, Université d'Abomey-Calavi, Cotonou, Bénin
[2]Faculté de Médecine de Parakou, Université de Parakou, Parakou, Bénin
Email: *adegbidih@yahoo.fr

## Abstract

Introduction: Acne is an affection that concerns 80% of young people in the world with a significant impact on their quality of life. The purpose of this study was to determine the epidemiological and clinical aspects of the acne in the Dermatology Department of the Teaching Hospital of Parakou (THP). Patients and Methods: We achieved a cross sectional study carrying on 167 files collected on a 20-month period in the Dermatology Department of the THP. Results: The prevalence of the acne was 31.21%. Female subjects represented 69.46%. Vulgaris acne was the most prevailing clinical form (47.30%). A peak of frequency was noted in the age bracket of 21 - 25 years in the 2 sexes. The lesions were mainly located on the face (82.63%). Some factors influencing the eruption have been evoked by the patients notably: foods, cosmetics products and stress respectively to 41.00%, 33.33% and 25.67%. Conclusion: Our study allowed confirming the female ascendancy of acne. Besides, the adults are more represented, precisely women because of depigmenting practice. It seems in favor of an influence of the food in the intervening of the acne. Vulgaris acne was the predominant clinical form as described in literature.

## Keywords

Acne, Epidemiology, Foods

## 1. Introduction

The term "acne", in accordance with the recommendations of the terminology commission, designates follicles

---

*Corresponding author.

damages that occur to adolescence and that are bound to the seborrhea and the formation of comedons. It is an affection that concerns 80% of young people in the world with the significant impact on their quality of life [1] [2]. Moreover a genetic predisposition, some factors seem to have a link with acne occuring as alimentation and premenstrual period. No study confirms that link nowadays but patients used to talk about them. After 12 months of work in a new dermatology department and because acne is the most frequent reason of consultation in dermatology department [3] [4], we considered this study. Its purpose was to determine the epidemiological and clinical aspects of the acne and search if there was a link between its occurrence, and food and premenstrual period in the dermatology department of the Teaching Hospital of Parakou (THP).

## 2. Patients and Methods

The study took place in the Dermatology Department of the THP. Any patient seen in consultation in the service has a medical file. This medical file includes the civil status, clinical, paraclinical, therapeutic and evolutive data. We achieved a cross sectional study carrying on 167 files collected on a 20-month period: from February 1, 2009 to September 30, 2010. The study has been made from the medical files, and concerned all patients with acne diagnosis during the period of study and after obtaining the informed consent. Acnenosological classification has been made into 4 types: vulgaris acne (**Picture 1**), inflammatory acne (**Picture 2**), nodular acne (**Picture 3**) formerly named nodulocystic [5] and cosmetic acne (**Picture 4**). The variables: sex, age, profession, the clinical variants and the location of damages have been studied. The data have been collected on a card of investigation, their treatments and analyses facts with the help of the software Ear info. The data were collected in a anonymous way and an enlightened consent was give by the patients. The medical ethic committee of the hospital gave it authorization. Chi 2 test was used for proportions comparison and a value of p < 0.05 is statistically significative.

## 3. Results

1) Epidemiological aspects

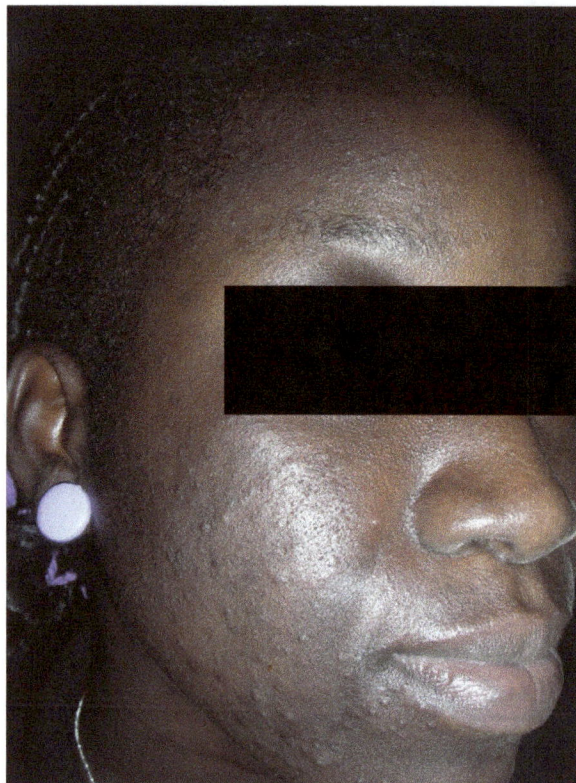

**Picture 1.** Vulgaris acne.

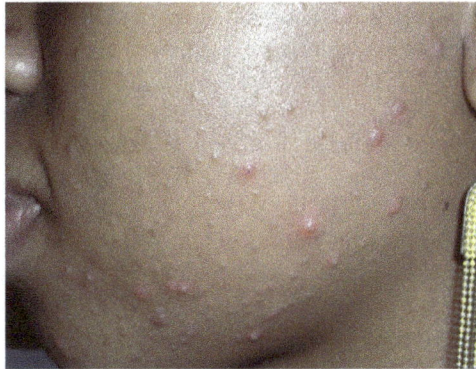

**Picture 2.** Inflammatory acne.

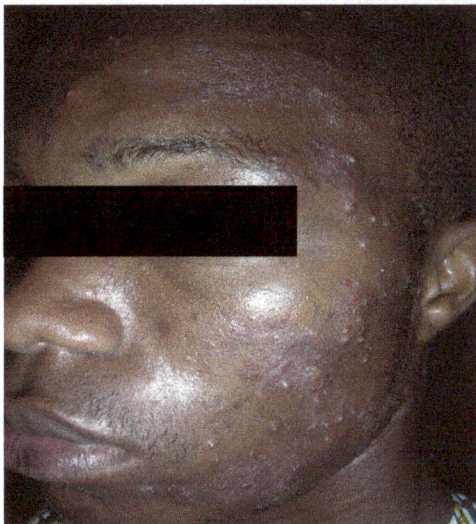

**Picture 3.** Nodular acne.

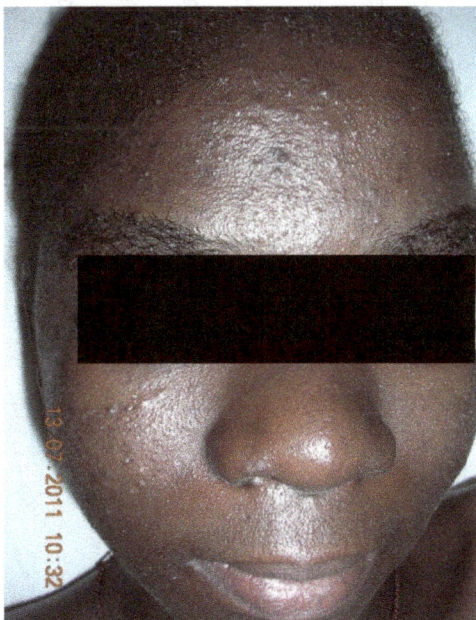

**Picture 4.** Cosmetical acne.

For 535 cases of skin diseases registered during the period of study, 167 cases of acne have been kept either a prevalence of 31.21%. On the 167 cases of acne registered, 116 are females (9.46%) against 51 either (30.54%) for males. The sex M/F ratio was therefore of 0.44. On the 116 females, 112 were pubescent and 4 were non pubescent.

**Figure 1** shows the distribution of the acne according to the sex and the age groups.

One hundred and six cases of 167 (63.47%) had a family history of acne. The students and the pupils constituted respectively 61.68% and 19.76% of the size, and the other 18.56% were represented by teachers, secretaries, nurses, policemen, storekeepers and the craftsmen.

The notion of previous medicinal hold in the beginning of the symptoms has not been signaled at any of the patients. Some factors influencing the eruption have been evoked by the patients notably: foods, cosmetics products and stress respectively to 41.00%, 33.33% and 25.67%. The periods have been revealed like factors coming with the regular aggravation of the acne at 93 of our 112 pubescent patients (74.11%).

2) Clinical Aspects

a) Distribution of the acne according to clinical forms

Vulgaris acne was the most prevailing clinical form in our study (**Figure 2**).

b) Distribution of the acne according to the location of damages

Acne damages had distributed themselves differently on the reached location: 82.63% to the face, 22.95% to the shoulders, 17.36% to the necklines and 6.58% to the back (**Table 1**). Let's note that several locations were often reached at the same patient.

c) Distribution of the clinical forms of acne according to the location of damages.

## 4. Discussion

1) Epidemiological aspects

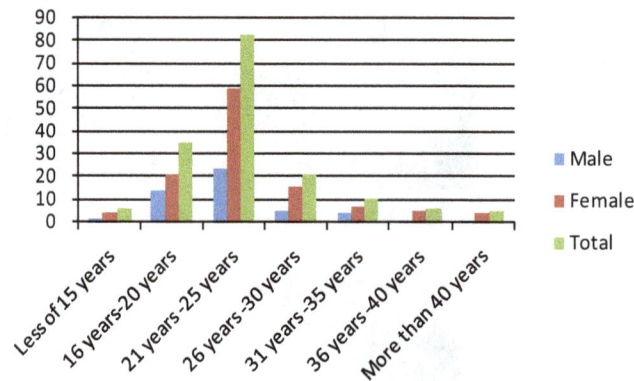

**Figure 1.** Distribution of the acne according to the sex and the age groups.

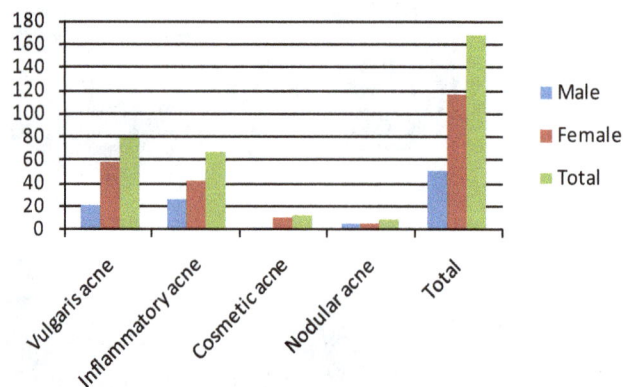

**Figure 2.** Distribution of the acne according the clinical forms.

**Table 1.** Repartition of acne localizations.

| Clinical forms | Face | Shoulders | Necklines | Back |
|---|---|---|---|---|
| Retentional acne | 74 (53.62%) | 5 (13.51%) | 10 (34.48%) | 2 (18.18%) |
| Infflammatory acne | 35 (25.36%) | 17 (45.95%) | 9 (31.04%) | 6 (54.55%) |
| Cosmetical ane | 18 (13.05%) | 6 (16.22%) | 4 (13.79%) | 2 (18.18%) |
| Nodular acne | 11 (7.97%) | 9 (24.32%) | 6 (20.69%) | 1 (9.09%) |
| Total | 138 (100.00%) | 37 (100.00%) | 29 (100.00%) | 11 (100.00%) |

NB: Some patients had several localizations.

Acne constitutes the most frequent reason of consultation in dermatology department [3]. It represents 15 to 20% of the consultations [6]. In a study published in 2005 by Onayemi et al. in Nigeria [4], it represents the third reason of consultation after the infectious and allergic dermatosis. Its prevalence in our study is 31.21%. It is widely superior to the one described in the literature [6] [7]. The female subjects represented 69.46% against 30.54% of male subjects in our study. Kane et al. in Senegal, then Mseddi et al. in Morocco had similar results respectively 62.43% and 75% against 37.57% and 25% [1] [3].

A peak of frequency was noted in the age bracket of 21 - 25 years in the 2 sexes. What goes against the data of the literature which gives evidence that acne disappears at the majority of subjects between 18 and 25 years [7]. This peak of frequency in this age bracket 21 - 25 years is understandable on one hand by a bigger attendance of the center by this age bracket represented especially by the students and the pupils, facilitated by the closeness of the hospital with a secondary school and Parakou University; and on the other hand by the existence of some factors contributing acne eruption. The study of contributing factors showed that the food has been signaled by 41% of our patients as influencing their acne eruption, constituting the first contributing factor. The incriminated foods are: chocolate, peanut, butter, mayonnaise and milk. The use of cosmetics in particular depigmenting and fat occlusive ones was noted in 33.33% of our patients and constituted the second contributing factor after food. This use of cosmetics in particular depigmenting ones containing corticoids induces numerous dermatosis of which acne constitutes the first and third reason of consultation in dermatology according respectively to Gathse and Mahé [8] [9]. Few clinical trials were realized on the role of food in occurrence of acne. The published works are former and obligatorily lacking [10] [11]. Their results go to the sense of an absence of link between food and acne, what it is now admitted by dermatological community. A recent epidemiological study based on reviews data of the "children's nurses Heath Study II" cohort shows a correlation between the consummate quantity of milk and the presence of severe acne during the adolescence on 47,355 American women [12].

Of our 112 pubescent patients, 71.41% experiment a regular worsening of acne in the second half of the menstrual cycle. The physiopathology of this premenstrual exacerbation is not clear but would be in connection with the physiological progestational phase [13]. Progesterone is metabolized in androsteron before it elimination during the premenstrual period.

Sixty three, forty-seven percent of our patients had a brother or a sister or their direct parents affected by acne. These results suit to those of Daniel et al. who in a comparative study found that 68% patients had a brother or a sister affected by acne against 57% without acne [14].

2) Clinical Aspects

Vulgaris acne was the most represented in our study 47.30% this suits to literature data with higher percentages going from 72.80% to 79.73% according respectively to Mseddi and Poli [3] [15]. Daniel et al. also indicated the ascendancy of vulgaris acne in metropolitan France [14]. It was more frequent in females than males in our study contrary to Daniel et al. study. In the same way inflammatory acne was more noted in females than males in Kane et al. study [1], but Daniel et al. in France [14] observed more raised about males suffering inflammatory acne than females. Nodular acne was more noted also in females than males, what does not suit to literature data reporting an ascendancy of the inflammatory forms and nodular forms in males [7]. The cosmetic acne due to fat occlusive and depigmenting creams was present in 7.19% of our patients and the greater part was female. This depigmenting practice is reported by several authors as cause of cosmetic acne [8] [9].

In our study, 82.63% of damages were located on the face. This preferential location was also reported in literature with percentages varying from 86.37% to 95.50% according to respectively Mseddi and Poli [3] [15]. This fact was also reported in literature in which acne is mainly located on face, particularly on nose, cheeks and forehead [7] [14]. In inflammatory acne, damages were also to the face but especially to the back and to the shoulders.

## 5. Conclusion

Our study allowed confirming the female ascendancy of acne. Besides, the adults are more represented, precisely women because of depigmenting practice. It seems in favor of an influence of the food in the intervening of the acne. Vulgaris acne was the predominant clinical form as described in literature.

## References

[1]   Kane, A., Niang, S.O., Diagne, A.C., Ly, F. and Ndiaye, B. (2007) Epidemiological, Clinical and Therapeutical Aspects of Acne at Dakar. *Nouvelles Dermatolologiques*, **26**, 39-41.

[2]   Dréno, B. (2010) What Are the News in Acne? *Annales de Dermatologie et de Vénéréologie*, **137**, S49-S51. http://dx.doi.org/10.1016/S0151-9638(10)70024-7

[3]   Mseddi, M., Abdelmaksou, D.W., Borgi, N., Elloumi, Y., Daoud, L., Souissi, A., Tutki, H. and Zahaf, A. (2005) Epidemiological and Clinical Aspects of Acne in School Children. *Medecine du Magreb*. No. 124, 53-55.

[4]   Onayemi, O., Isezu, S.A. and Njoku, C.H. (2005) Prevalence of Different Skin Conditions in an out Patients' Setting in North. Western Nigeria. *International Journal of Dermatology*, **44**, 7-11. http://dx.doi.org/10.1111/j.1365-4632.2004.02298.x

[5]   Humbert, P. (2003) Severe Forms of Acne. *Annales de Dermatologie et de Vénéréologie*, **130**, 117-120.

[6]   Auffret, N. (2003) What Are the News in Acne Physiopathology? *Annales de Dermatologie et de Vénéréologie*, **130**, 101-106.

[7]   Revuz, J. (2003) Youngest Polymorphic Acne and Adult Acne. *Annales de Dermatologie et de Vénéréologie*, **130**, 113-116.

[8]   Gathse, A., Obengui and Ibara, J.R. (2005) Motifs of Consultation Linked to Bleaching in 104 Women at Brazzaville, Congo. *Bulletin de la Société de Pathologie Exotique*, **98**, 387-389.

[9]   Mahé, A., Kéita, S. and Bobin, P. (1994) Dermatological Complications of the Using of Bleaching Products at Bamako (Mali). *Annales de Dermatologie et de Vénéréologie*, **121**, 46-51.

[10]  Magin, P., Pond, D., Smith, W. and Watson, A. (2005) A Systematic Review of the Evidence for "Myths and Misconceptions" in Acne Management Diet Face-Washing and Sunlight. *Family Practice*, **22**, 62-70. http://dx.doi.org/10.1093/fampra/cmh715

[11]  Puzenat, E., Riou-Gotta, M.O., Messick, R. and Humbert, P. (2010) Facial Dermatosis: Acne, Rosacea, Seborrhoeic Dermatitis. *Revue du Praticien*, **60**, 849-755.

[12]  Adebamowo, C.A., Spiegelman, D., Danby, W., Frazier, L., Wiellett, W.C. and Holmes, M.D. (2005) High School Dietary Dairy Intake and Teenage Acne. *Journal of the American Academy of Dermatology*, **52**, 207-214. http://dx.doi.org/10.1016/j.jaad.2004.08.007

[13]  Stoll, S., Shalita, A.R., Webster, G.F., Kaplan, R., Danesh, S. and Penstein, A. (2001) The Effect of the Menstrual Cycle on Acne. *Journal of the American Academy of Dermatology*, **45**, 957-960. http://dx.doi.org/10.1067/mjd.2001.117382

[14]  Daniel, F., Dreno, B., Poli, F., Auffret, N., Beylot, C., Bodokh, I., *et al.* (2000) Descriptive Epidemiology of Acne in Metropolitan France School Children in Autumn 1996. *Annales de Dermatologie et de Vénéréologie*, **127**, 273-278.

[15]  Poli, F., Dreno, B. and Verschoore, M. (2001) An Epidemiological Study of Acne in Female Adults: Results of a Survey Conducted in France. *Journal of the European Academy of Dermatology and Venereology*, **15**, 541-546. http://dx.doi.org/10.1046/j.1468-3083.2001.00357.x

# 2

# The Effects of a Hyaluronan Lotion with a Molecular Weight of around 50 - 110 kDa on the Aged Atrophic Skin

Asako Ito

Ookuma Hospital, Nagoya, Japan
Email: info@tclinic.jp

## Abstract

Background: Hyaluronic acids act upon keratinocytes via CD44 receptors and regulate proliferation and differentiation. Some cosmetic hyaluronan lotions manufactured based upon the fact are nowadays available. Aims: To evaluate a cosmetic hyaluronan lotion (Dr. Fukaya's skin repair lotion or Hyaluprotect) from the viewpoint of anti-aging effects and to consider its mechanism. Patients/Methods: In ten healthy volunteers at the age over 60, immunohistochemical research of the biopsied skin was performed before and after the application of the hyaluronan lotion for two weeks. Results: Expression of PCNA in the lower epidermis increased in 8 of 10 subjects. Filaggrin expression of the upper epidermis increased in 6 subjects. $11\beta$HSD1 decreased in 5 subjects and $11\beta$HSD2 increased in 5 subjects. Conclusions: The proliferative and differentiative effects of the hyaluronan lotion upon keratinocytes were confirmed immunohistologically. There is a possibility that hyaluronic acids work through the regulation of corticosteroids by $11\beta$HSD1 and $11\beta$HSD2.

## Keywords

Hyaluronic Acid, Anti-Aging, PCNA, Filaggrin, $11\beta$HSD1, $11\beta$HSD2, Atrophic Skin

## 1. Introduction

Hyaluronic acids have been proved to be important stimulants onto keratinocytes via CD44 receptors. Kaya [1] reported that intermediate sized HA fragments (HAFi) of 50 kDa to 400 kDa were effective in recovering the epidermal atrophy due to aging in patients over 60 years old. Barnes [2] added the knowledge that HAFi can compete with the epidermal atrophy due to corticosteroids. Bourguignon [3] revealed that hyaluronic acids of around 27 kDa in molecular weight have the effect of cell proliferation while 700 - 1000 kDa HAs increase filaggrin in the upper epidermis. The effects of HAs seem to be different according to their molecular weights.

As the above articles interested the developers of skin care materials, there appeared such products that aim at anti-aging effects grounded on them. Dr. Fukaya's skin repair lotion (Japanese product name is Hyaluprotect) is one of them. The lotion is made of FCH-SU of Kikkoman Biochemifa Co. as a principal ingradient which is HA originated from the product of streptococcus zooepidemicus and its main molecular weight is published as 50 - 110 kDa. The other components of the lotion involve 0.3% of phenoxyethanol as a conservative, 0.0012% of iodopropynyl butylcarbamate as an anti-fungal agent and 0.0094% of hydroxypropyl beta cyclodextrin as a solubilizing agent.

The author evaluated its efficacy to the epidermal atrophy due to aging by immunohistochemical study before and two weeks after application of the lotion to the neck in aged volunteers over 60 years old.

## 2. Materials & Methods

Ten healthy aged volunteers were enrolled in the study under the written informed consent. The admission by an ethical committee was obtained beforehand. All patients were over 60 years old and the average age was 73.2. Two were male while eight were female. The neck skin was biopsied by 1.5 mm trepan and application of the lotion two times per day followed. After two weeks the second biopsy was undertaken from the neck skin. The specimen were fixed by 20% formaldehyde solution immediately and submitted to paraffin embedding procedure. Enzyme labelled immunohistochemical staining was performed using anti-PCNA, filaggrin, 11$\beta$HSD1 and 11$\beta$HSD2 antibodies. The manufacturers and dilution rate of primary antibodies are as follows. PCNA; Neo-Markers: ×1000, filaggrin; Abcam: ×100, 11$\beta$HSD1; Santa Cruz Biotechnology: ×200 and 11$\beta$HSD2; Santa Cruz Biotechnology: ×400. All paired specimen were stained at a time for avoiding technical variance of color densities. As the study aims to compare the findings before and after application of the lotion, the results were simplified using mathematical symbols of <,> and =. Namely, before < after means the expression of the targeted antigen has increased.

As a supplementary examination to detect the distribution of molecular weight of the lotion, agarose gel electrophoresis was performed together with various kinds of cosmetic materials of hyaluronic acids.

## 3. Results

In 8 of 10 subjects, PCNA positive cells increased. Filaggrin expression increased in 6 subjects. 11$\beta$HSD2 increased in 5 and decreased in only one subject while 11$\beta$HSD1 decreased in 5 subjects. All the results are in the **Table 1** and photographs of two subjects (cases 1 and 2) are in the **Figure 1** and **Figure 2** for the purpose of presenting examples. In case 1, PCNA-positive nuclei increased in number (a), filaggrin increased in the corneal layer (b), 11$\beta$HSD1 didn't change (c) and 11$\beta$HSD2 increased especially at the basal layer (d). In case 2, PCNA-positive nuclei increased in number (a), filaggrin increased in the corneal layer and upper of the keratinocytes (estimated granular layer) (b), 11$\beta$HSD1 and 11$\beta$HSD2 didn't change ((c), (d)).

**Table 1.** The result of comparison of the findings before and after application of HA lotion is shown.

| Case | Age | Sex | PCNA | Filaggrin | 11$\beta$HSD1 | 11$\beta$HSD2 |
|------|-----|-----|------|-----------|---------------|---------------|
| 1 | 84 | M | < | < | = | < |
| 2 | 79 | F | < | < | = | = |
| 3 | 77 | F | = | = | > | < |
| 4 | 76 | F | < | = | > | = |
| 5 | 76 | M | < | < | = | > |
| 6 | 75 | F | < | < | = | < |
| 7 | 70 | F | = | < | = | < |
| 8 | 69 | F | < | = | > | = |
| 9 | 65 | F | < | < | > | < |
| 10 | 61 | F | < | = | > | = |

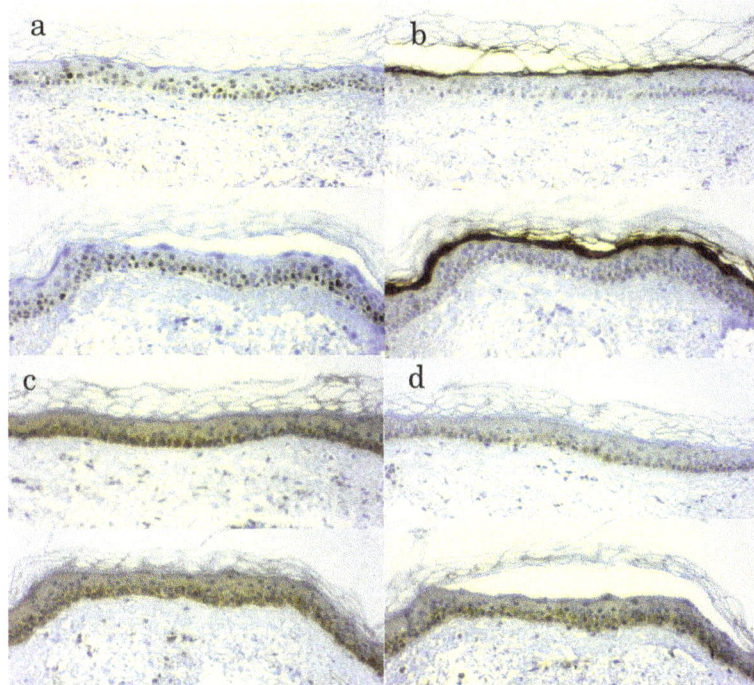

**Figure 1.** Immunohistochemical staining before (upper) and after (lower) application of HA lotion in the case 1. (a) PCNA, (b) filaggrin, (c) 11$\beta$HSD1, (d) 11$\beta$HSD2. In PCNA, filaggrin and 11$\beta$HSD2 the staining intensity increased after the application of HA lotion.

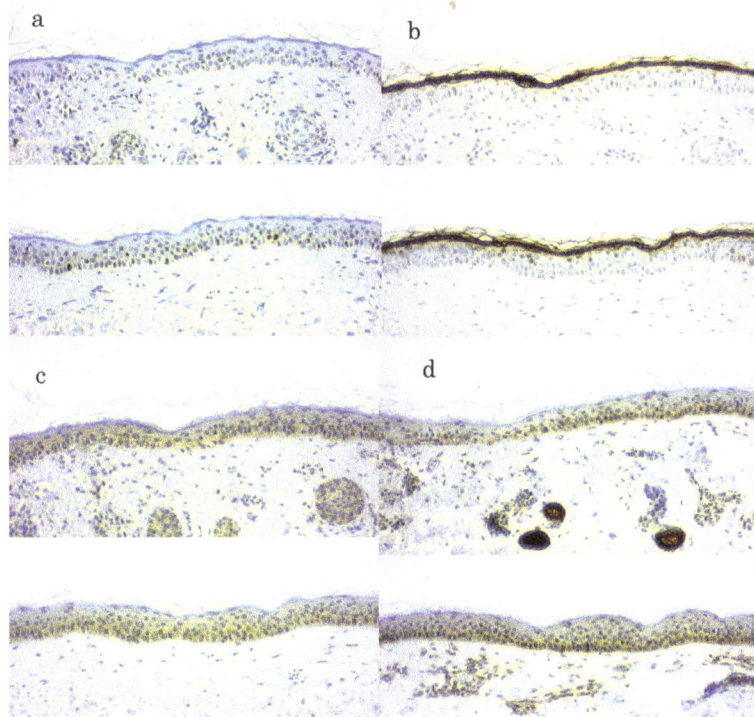

**Figure 2.** Immunohistochemical staining before (upper) and after (lower) application of HA lotion in the case 2 is shown. (a) PCNA, (b) filaggrin, (c) 11$\beta$HSD1, (d) 11$\beta$HSD2. Note that filaggrin is expressed not only in the corneal layer but also in the upper keratinocytes in the lower photo of (b).

## 4. Discussion

PCNA (proliferative cell nuclear antigen) is a marker of activity of cell division and proliferation. Kaya [1] and Bourguignon [3] also demonstrated PCNA expression increases in keratinocytes by application of intermediate or small sized HAs. The result in the study coincides with their results.

Filaggrin expression on the upper epidermis or the corneal layer was also reported by Bourguignon by application of larger molecular sized HAs. The result in the study also agrees with Bourguignon's though the molecular size seems to be much smaller. Kaya's or Bourguignon's HAs were strictly fractionated according to molecular size while the hyaluronic acid lotion in the study is for the commercial use and the molecular size ranges rather wider (**Figure 3**). So the effect of filaggrin expression can be due to the same mechanism as Bourguignon's by its inclusion of the larger sized HAs.

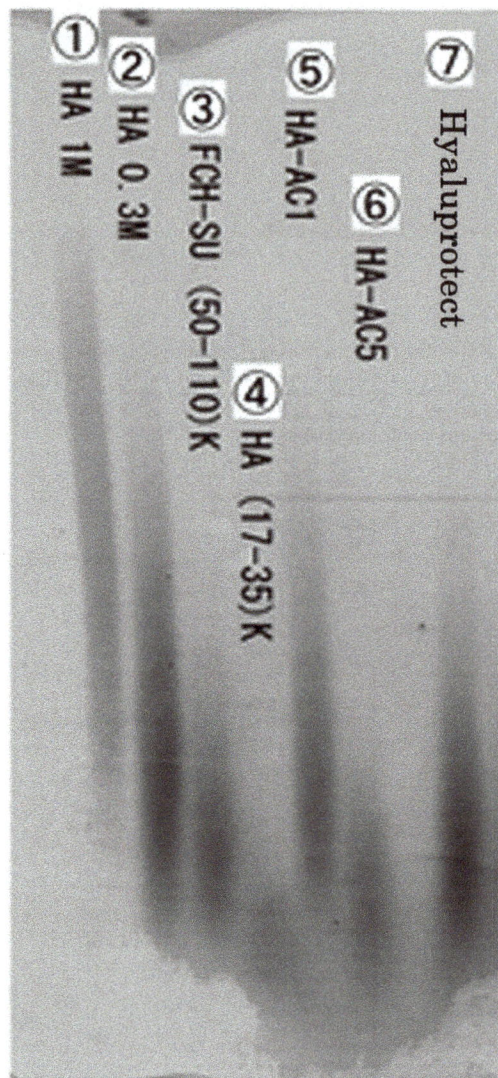

**Figure 3.** Electrophoresis of various cosmetic hyaluronic acid materials and products is shown. 1 (HA 1M); a material with a main peak at 1000 kDa, 2 (HA, 0.3 M); a material with a main peak at 300 kDa, 3 (FCH-SU (50 - 110) k); The raw material used in the product examined in the study with the peak range at 50 - 110 kDa, 5 (HA-AC1) and 6 (HA-AC5); Other products for cosmetic use, 7 (Hyalupurotect): the product examined in the study. Note that upper portion of No. 7 coincides with the peak in No. 1 though the density is weaker. As the experiment is complementary one, molecular weight markers were substituted by 1-4.

Keratinocytes have been recently revealed to produce corticosteroids by themselves [4]. The synthesis of corticosteroids is balanced by two isozymes of 11$\beta$HSD1 and 11$\beta$HSD2. The former converts inactive cortisone into active cortisol and the latter reverses them. It is well known that corticosteroids fall the epidermis into atrophy as a side effect. So there is a possibility that hyaluronic acids increase the PCNA positive keratinocytes by suppressing 11$\beta$HSD1 or accelerating 11$\beta$HSD2.

As a result in the study, 11$\beta$HSD1 suppression or 11$\beta$HSD2 acceleration was observed in 9 of 10 subjects. It suggests the possibility that proliferation of keratinocyte due to HAs is controlled by the density of cortisol in the epidermis. Further study at the level of RNA expression of the two enzymes in keratinocytes is desirable by using cultured cells. It is the limitation of the study using biopsied specimen.

Dahl [5] reported that HAs of around 100 kDa temporarily increases in the amniotic fluid of the 16th weeks of pregnancy. The period coincides with the time of epidermis formation of stratifying. Ghazi [6] reported 100 - 300 kDa HAs have the ability of improvement of wound injury. Pandey [7] reported 40 - 400 kDa HA activates NF-$\kappa$B mediated gene expression and its peak activity was observed in 137 kDa. These findings suggest HA of the range has the possibility of becoming an anti-atrophic or anti-aging agent. HAs have long been regarded as the simple moisturizer that retains water on the surface of the skin in the field of cosmetology. However there are farther functions beyond it [8] [9]. It is very reasonable and natural if the aged atrophic skin can be rejuvenated by hyaluronic acids in the amniotic fluid at the period when the embryo's skin is constructed.

## Disclosure

The author reports no conflicts of interest except accepting Dr. Fukaya's skin repair lotion only for the study from Dr. Mototsugu Fukaya. The immunohistochemical staining was performed at Morphotechnology Co. (Sapporo, Japan) and the expenses were also born by him.

## References

[1]  Kaya, G., Tran, C., Sorg, O., *et al.* (2006) Hyaluronate Fragments Reverse Skin Atrophy by a CD44-Dependent Mechanism. *PLoS Medicine*, **3**, 2291-2303. http://dx.doi.org/10.1371/journal.pmed.0030493

[2]  Barnes, L., Ino, F., Jaunin, F., Saurat, J.H. and Kaya, G. (2012) Inhibition of Putative Hyalurosome Platform in Keratinocytes as a Mechanism for Corticosteroid-Induced Epidermal Atrophy. *Journal of Investigative Dermatology*, **133**, 1017-1026. http://dx.doi.org/10.1038/jid.2012.439

[3]  Bourguignon, L.Y., Wong, G., Xia, W., *et al.* (2013) Selective Matrix (Hyaluronan) Interaction with CD44 and RhoGTPase Signaling Promotes Keratinocyte Functions and Overcomes Age-Related Epidermal Dysfunction. *Journal of Dermatological Science*, **72**, 32-44. http://dx.doi.org/10.1016/j.jdermsci.2013.05.003

[4]  Cirillo, N. and Prime, S.S. (2011) Keratinocytes Synthesize and Activate Cortisol. *Journal of Cellular Biochemistry*, **112**, 1499-1505. http://dx.doi.org/10.1002/jcb.23081

[5]  Dahl, L.B., Kimpton, W.G., Cahill, R.N., Brown, T.J. and Fraser, R.E. (1989) The Origin and Fate of Hyaluronan in Amniotic Fluid. *Journal of Developmental Physiology*, **12**, 209-218.

[6]  Ghazi, K., Deng-Pichon, U., Warnet, J.M. and Rat, P. (2012) Hyaluronan Fragments Improve Wound Healing on *in Vitro* Cutaneous Model through P2X7 Purinoreceptor Basal Activation: Role of Molecular Weight. *PLoS One*, **7**, Article ID: e48351. http://dx.doi.org/10.1371/journal.pone.0048351

[7]  Pandey, M.S., Baggenstoss, B.A., Washburn, J., Harris, E.N. and Weigel, P.H. (2013) The Hyaluronan Receptor for Endocytosis (HARE) Activates NF-$\kappa$B Mediated Gene Expression in Response to 40 - 400 kDa, but Not Smaller or Larger, Hyaluronan. *Journal of Biological Chemistry*, **288**, 14068-14079. http://dx.doi.org/10.1074/jbc.M112.442889

[8]  Maytin, E.V., Chung, H.H. and Seetharaman, V.M. (2004) Hyaluronan Participates in the Epidermal Response to Disruption of the Permeability Barrier *in Vivo*. *American Journal of Pathology*, **165**, 1331-1341. http://dx.doi.org/10.1016/S0002-9440(10)63391-3

[9]  Nyman, E., Huss, F., Nyman, T., Junker, J. and Kratz, G. (2013) Hyaluronic Acid, an Important Factor in the Wound Healing Properties of Amniotic Fluid: *In Vitro* Studies of Re-Epithelialisation in Human Skin Wounds. *Journal of Plastic Surgery and Hand Surgery*, **47**, 89-92. http://dx.doi.org/10.3109/2000656X.2012.733169

## Abbreviations

PCNA: proliferative cell nuclear antigen
HSD: hydroxysteroid dehydrogenase
HA: Hyaluronic acid
HAFi: intermediate sized hyaluronic acid fragments

# 3

# Antioxidant Activity of Cosmetic Formulations Based on Novel Extracts from Seeds of Brazilian *Araucaria angustifolia* (Bertoll) Kuntze

**Gabriela Sprada Tavares da Mota[1,2], Angela Bonjorno Arantes[1], Gianni Sacchetti[3], Antonella Spagnoletti[3], Paola Ziosi[2], Emanuela Scalambra[3], Silvia Vertuani[2,3], Stefano Manfredini[2,3]**

[1]School of Health and Biosciences, Pontifícia Universidade Católica do Paraná, Curitiba, Brasil
[2]Ambrosialab, University of Ferrara, Ferrara, Italy
[3]Department of Life Sciences and Biotechnology, School of Pharmacy and Health Products, University of Ferrara, Ferrara, Italy
Email: mv9@unife.it

## Abstract

The process of oxidation, due to free radicals, is the cause of major concern for human health. In particular damages related to the skin have great relevance; therefore, many antioxidants based products are developed and marketed with the intention to counteract the action of free radicals. The seed of *Araucaria angustifolia* is a rich source of antioxidants due to the presence of bioflavonoids to counteract free radicals damages. In this study, two extracts, one from the seed external teguments (shell) and the other from the inner seed pulp (endosperm and embryo) were obtained in order to evaluate possible applications to the dermo-cosmetic field. In parallel the following different methods were employed to characterize both the extracts and to determine their antioxidant capacity: HPTLC, ABTS and DPPH, ORAC and PLC. The qualitative analysis showed that both extracts have the antioxidant activity, but the quantitative evaluation revealed a more promising bioactivity from the shell than from the pulp. Therefore, it was evaluated the potential skin application of different cosmetic formulations, based on the presence of seed shell extract (W/O emulsion, O/W emulsion and gel). The best result was achieved with the W/O emulsion.

## Keywords

*Araucaria angustifolia*, Sustainability, Seed Alcoholic Extracts, Antioxidant Activity,

**Characterization, HPTLC, ORAC, PCL**

## 1. Introduction

During the last few years, an increasing amount of evidences have been accumulated on the involvement of free radicals and other oxidative species as major responsible for aging and related degenerative processes, among them, cancer, cataract, brain and cardiovascular diseases [1]-[4].

The skin antioxidant system has an extensive area exposed to the environment to protect and, as a consequence, highly exposed to the exogenous radical attack, which makes the defense system be constantly challenged. Consequently, the cosmetology has a significant role in the prevention and attenuation the cutaneous aging through the study of substances with effective antioxidant activity, to be incorporated on cosmetic products for daily care [5].

Plants are known to be important sources of functional substances. Most of them with antioxidant capacity related to innate defense system of the specie against biological (for e.g. phytopathogens) and physical (for e.g. UV radiation) factors which always causes the generation of free radicals. Moreover, plant species from geographical areas such those Amazonian, are often qualitatively and quantitatively more rich in antioxidant compounds most probably because the important biodiversity which characterizes these regions strongly forced the evolutionary process to diversify the secondary metabolism of the plants.

Different plant extracts, when applied in animal models or in cell culture, are capable of neutralizing the free radical reactivity, and decreasing the cellular injuries. These compounds are the polyphenols, and among them, flavonoids are probably those more known, studied and promising active compounds [6] [7].

The present investigation has been carried out on *Araucaria angustifolia*, a tree belonging to Araucariaceae family, also commonly known as the Paraná-Pine tree or Brazilian pine (Portuguese: pinheiro-do-paraná or pinheirobrasileiro). Its female strobilus consisting of seeds, "pinhão", (the edible part of *A. angustifolia*) and bracts (non-developed seeds), has a long history of use as a food in Southeast of Brazil, like flour in regional dishes or baked. Although the common names in various languages refer to the species as a "pine" because of its similarity with the real *Pinus* species, it is instead more properly an evergreen tree growing to 40 m (130 ft) tall and 1 m (3 ft 3 in) diameter at breast height. The leaves are thick, tough and scale like, triangular, 3 - 6 centimetres (1.2 - 2.4 in) long, 5 - 10 millimetres (0.2 - 0.4 in) broad at the base, and with razor-sharp edges and tip. They persist 10 to 15 years, and spread all over the tree, but not on the trunk and older branches. Under a systematic point of view, it is related to *Araucaria araucana* that lives further southwest in South America, differing in the narrower leaves. The main isolated flavonoids belong to the class of the biflavonoids: amentoflavone, monomethylamentoflavone, di-O-methyl amentoflavone, ginkgetin, tri-O-methyl amentoflavone, tetra-O-methyl amentoflavone, that differ by the number and position of the methoxyl group. The biflavonoids found in *A. angustifolia* act like free radicals scavengers and show an efficient protection against oxidative damage, demonstrating to be an excellent option to the use of antioxidants and photoprotectives [8] [9].

The flavonoids are found in the secondary metabolism of the plants and they are characterized for having antibacterial properties, anticarcinogenic, anti-inflammatory, among others [10]. According to Yamaguchi [8], the flavonoids, not only show antioxidant and antiaging properties, but also protect the skin from the UV solar radiation. Thus, the objective of this work was to characterize and evaluate alcoholic extracts obtained from the pine tree seeds and to explore their possible applications as antioxidant in cosmetic, trying to further valorize, under a functional point of view, this Brazilian plant species with an ancient story of traditional uses [8] [9]. Finally, valorization of local plants through the development of NTFP (non timber forest products) contributes to supporting biodiversity and sustainable use of natural resources.

## 2. Materials and Methods

Seeds from the *Araucaria angustifolia* were collected in July 2009, in Curitiba/Paraná and delivered to the University of Ferrara/Italy where they were stored at −20°C until the preparation of the extracts. The plant material to be investigated was dried at room temperature and the seeds were separated in pulps (endosperm and embryo) and shells (external teguments). The shells were pulverized in a mill rotor (Variable-Speed Rotor Mill PULVERISETTE 14, Fritsch GmbH, 55743 Idar-Oberstein, Germany), while the pulps were grinded on a hand grail. The samples were stored at 4°C with controlled humidity. The extracts were prepared macerating 20 g of the crushed material with 100 ml of methanol for 20 minutes under sonication. The choice of methanol was due, after several attempts, to its polarity and capability of extracting flavonoids and biflavonoids [10]. The material was then filtered in a Büchner filter and evaporated under vacuum; part of the sample was re-suspended at a 10 mg/ml concentration in methanol and processed as described below.

## 2.1. Quantitative Analysis of the Main Chemical Constituents by HPTLC and Spectrophotometry

Fifty microliters (10 mg/mL) of each sample extract (pulp and shell) of *A. angustifolia* were solubilized in methanol and analyzed using High Performance thin layer plates (HPTLC) eluted in two steps with different mobile phases: the first using ethyl acetate, formic acid, acetic acid and water (100:11:11:26 v/v/v/v) to elute total flavonoid, and the second one using chloroform, acetone and formic acid (75:16.5:8.5 v/v/v) for biflavonoid. The plates were then treated with NP/PEG reagent, NP 1.0% in methanol, followed by a solution of PEG 4000 5.0% in ethanol [11]. The quantitative assays were performed in triplicate, and the results were expressed by the average of the data achieved followed by the coefficient of variation. Plants phenolic compounds are classified in many categories, such as simple phenols, phenolic acids, coumarines, flavonoids, stilbenes, condensed and hydrolysable tannins, lignans and lignins [12]. The total polyphenols determination has been accomplished according to the method proposed by Folin and Denis in 1912 and successively modified by Folin and Ciocalteu in 1927. The total phenols were determined at 765 nm through a calibration curve of gallic acid, being the result expressed in equivalent of gallic acid [13]. The analysis of the total flavonoids was accomplished mixing 1 mg/ml of the extract suspension with 1 ml of solution at 2% of $AlCl_3$ in methanol. The spectrophotometer was previously restarted with methanol and a calibration curve was obtained using hyperoside as reference. After 10 minutes at room temperature, the absorbance of the samples was measured at 394 nm. For the quantitative determination of flavonoids the calibration curve was prepared with a solution of hyperoside (range 0 - 60 μg/ml and the results were expressed as milligram hyperoside equivalents (HE) per gram of samples, *i.e.* oils and methanol macerate (mg HE/g). For determination of total proanthocyanidins, the phenolic compounds known also as condensed tannins, the method described by Porter *et al.* [14] was used. 2.4 of butanol/HCl (95:5 v/v) was added to 1 mg/ml of extract suspension, plus 80 μL of 2% solution of $NH_4Fe(SO_4)_2$. The mixture was placed at 95°C for 40 minutes. The spectrophotometer (Thermo Spectronic Helios, Cambridge, UK) was previously restarted with methanol to avoid solvent interference. The total proanthocyanidins levels are expressed as cyanidinchloride, therefore, a calibration curve was prepared with an appropriate set of cyanidin chloride concentrations. Absorbance of samples and control was taken at 550 nm leading to total proanthocyanidins determination in *A. angustifolia* seed samples extracts.

## 2.2. Evaluation of Antioxidant Activity

### 2.2.1. Spectrophotometric Method

The evaluation was based on the capacity of the *A. angustifolia* seed extracts to reduce the free radicals ABTS and DPPH, generated *in vitro*. The inactivation of these free radicals represents the total antioxidant capacity of the extracts [15] [16].

**DPPH.** The method is based on the reduction of the DPPH radical [17]. The samples were prepared by mixing 100 μL of each extract with a methanol solution of DPPH $1 \times 10^{-4}$ M kept under mixing at a speed of 200 rpm in the dark. The absorbance of the reaction mixture was read in a spectrophotometer (at 517 nm) after 30 min incubation. Methanol (1 ml) was used as control. The percentage of free radical scavenging effect [18] was calculated as follows: $\% \text{ inhibition} = 1 - \dfrac{AA}{AB} * 100.$ where AA represents the absorbance of DPPH with the extracts and AB represents the absorbance of DPPH without the extracts; was all the data are expressed as $IC_{50}$.

**ABTS.** The ABTS radical was obtained by a 2 mM solution of ABTS (0.011 g/10mL water) keeping the mixture in the dark for 16 hours. Before the analysis the spectrophotometer was set at 734 nm with a phosphate buffer (PBS) 5 nM at pH 7.4. Different dilutions have been prepared for both extracts in a concentration range of 5 - 200 μL/mL in methanol. The samples have been prepared by mixing 10 μL of each dilution with 990 μL of ABTS, while 10 μL of methanol sample was used as blank. A measure of the absorbance has been made of each sample 1 min after the addition of the radical. The inhibition percentage of the radical ABTS has been calculated with the following equation:  $\% \ \text{inhibition} = 1 - \dfrac{AA}{AB} * 100.$  Where AA is the absorbance of ABTS with the extract and AB is the absorbance of ABTS without the extract and was expressed as $IC_{50}$.

### 2.2.2. Oxygen Radical Absorbance Capacity Using Fluorescein as a Fluorescent Probe (ORAC-FL)

The ORAC assay was carried out on a Fluoroskan FL® ascent (Thermo Fisher Scientific, Inc. Waltham, MA, USA) with fluorescent filters (excitation wavelength: 485 nm; emission filter: 538 nm), following the procedure by Hong, Guohua & Ronald properly adapted as reported in a previous work [19]. Briefly, in the final assay mixture (0.2 mL total volume), fluorescein sodium salt (85 nM) was used as a target of free radical with 2,2'-azobis (2-amidinopropane) dihydrochloride (AAPH) as a peroxyl radical generator. Trolox®, a water-soluble analogue of vitamin E, was used as a standard control: a calibration curve was carried out with 10, 20, 30, 40, 50 µM solution. The tested compounds were dissolved in PBS and prepared immediately before the experiments. The fluorescence measurements, carried out at 37°C, were recorded at 5 min intervals up 30 min after the addition of AAPH. The ORAC values, calculated as difference of the areas under the quenching curves of fluoresceine between the blank and the sample, were expressed as Trolox® equivalents (TE) (µmol TE/g) pH = 7.4. All the experiments were performed in three replicates.

### 2.2.3. Photochemiluminescence (PCL)

In the aim to fully evaluate the antioxidant capacity of the extracts, another experimental protocol, based on photochemiluminescence (PCL) was performed. The method allows evaluating the activity of the extract of *A. angustifolia* through the setting up of a calibration curve with a reference antioxidant, thus expressing the values obtained as µmol of Trolox® per gram of extract. The analysis has been made using Photochem® and following the method described by Lewin and Popov [20] and conducted according to the protocol provided by Analytik Jena, Jena, Germany. The concentration of the added extract solution was such that the generated luminescence during the 180 s sampling interval fell within the limits of the standard curve. The extracts were centrifuged (5 min at 16,000 g) prior to analysis. The antioxidant assay was carried out in triplicate for each sample, and 20 µL of the diluted extract (1:40, v/v) in HPLC-grade methanol was sufficient to correspond to the standard curve.

### 2.2.4. HPTLC Method Using 2,2'-Azinobis-(3-Ethylbenzothiazoline-6-Sulfonate) (ABTS) Radical Assay, Diphenylpicrylhydrazyl (DPPH) Radical Assay

To evaluate the antioxidant activity of the compounds that characterizes the extract, rehearsals have been made with the radicals ABTS and DPPH on chromatography plates coated with a high performance silica gel. The objective was to evaluate the capacity of the extract of discoloring the solutions of ABTS and DPPH, which presented, respectively, the colors green and purple. This methodology involves the preparation and the elution of two plates, that are then derivatized, one with a watery solution of ABTS and the other one with an ethanolic solution of DPPH, following properly modified procedures reported by Rossi *et al.* [13]. The activity of the eluted extract was immediately monitored both after the derivatization and 24 hours, for verifying those bands most involved in antioxidant capacity together with the presence of less abundant biomolecules with slower reactivity and/or with a delayed appearance of stains.

## 2.3. Preparation of the Cosmetic Formulations

The final goal of the investigation was to find application, as antioxidant, of Brazilian *Araucaria angustifolia* seed extracts—*i.e.* from external teguments (shell), and from endosperm and embryo (pulp)—in cosmetic products. The target would be that of verifying if the samples derived from the seeds, when incorporated to the formulations, will exert anti-aging and moisturizing properties in view of their antioxidant capacity expressed as crude extracts.

### 2.3.1. Composition of the O/W Emulsion

The compounds on phase A (oil phase) and phase B (water phase) have been heated in separated containers, at 70°C. The oily phase has been incorporated to the watery phase under mechanic agitation and it has been cooled with a cold bath at a temperature below 40°C, and then, phase C has been added. At the end, the pH has been adjusted to 6.0 (**Tables 1-3**).

**Table 1.** Composition of the O/W emulsion.

| Composition (INCI) | Function | Amount (%) |
|---|---|---|
| **Phase A** | | |
| Glyceryl stearate (and) ceteareth-20 (and) ceteareth-12 (and) ceteayl alcohol (and) cetyl palmitate | Base self emulsifying | 8.00 |
| Cetylstearyl alcohol | Emollient/hickener | 1.50 |
| Hydrogenated polyisobutene | Emollient/emulsifier | 3.50 |
| Hydrogenated polydecene | Emollient | 2.00 |
| Decyl oleate | Emollient | 1.50 |
| Cyclopentasiloxane | Emollient | 2.00 |
| Dimethicone | Defoamer/emollient | 0.50 |
| Phenoxyethanol (and) butylparaben (and) propylparaben (and) isobutylparaben | Preservative | 0.50 |
| **Phase B** | | |
| Aqua | Vehicle | 66.40 |
| Disodium EDTA | Chelating | 0.10 |
| Glycerin | Moist | 3.00 |
| **Phase C** | | |
| Ethyl alcohol | Denaturant/solvent | 10.00 |
| Powder extract of the *A. angustifolia* | Active principle | 1.00 |
| Sodium hydroxide/citric acid | pH corrector | q.s pH 6 |

**Table 2.** Composition of the W/O emulsion.

| Composition (INCI) | Function | Quantity (%) |
|---|---|---|
| **Phase A** | | |
| PEG-30 dipolyhydroxysteara | Emulsifier | 1.50 |
| Hydrogenated polydecene | Emollient | 8.00 |
| Cetearyl isononanoate | Emollient | 8.00 |
| Decyl oleate | Emollient | 2.00 |
| **Phase B** | | |
| Aqua | Vehicle | 68.50 |
| Phenoxyethanol (and) methylparaben (and) ethylparaben (and) butylparaben (and) propylparaben (and) isobutylparaben | Preservative | 0.50 |
| Magnesium sulfate | Viscosity modifier | 0.50 |
| **Phase C** | | |
| Ethyl alcohol | Solvent/preservative | 10.00 |
| Powder extract of the *A. angustifolia* | Active principle | 1.00 |

**Table 3.** Composition of the nonionic gel.

| Composition (INCI) | Function | Quantity (%) |
|---|---|---|
| **Phase A** | | |
| Aqua | Vehicle | 84.00 |
| Hydroxyethylcellulose | Emulsion stabilizer, viscosity controller | 1.00 |
| Pentylene glycol | Antimicrobial, solvent, improves water resistance | 5.00 |
| **Phase B** | | |
| Ethyl alcohol | Denaturant/solvent | 9.00 |
| Powder extract of the *A. angustifolia* | Active principle | 1.00 |

### 2.3.2. Composition of the W/O Emulsion

The compounds from phase A and phase B have been separately weighted and warmed at 70°C. Phase B has been slowly added into A and homogenized by a mixer. The compound has been cooled until it hits 40°C, and then, phase C was added. Finally, the final pH was adjusted to 6.0.

### 2.3.3. Composition of the Nonionic Gel

The water has been heated at 60°C, hydroxyethylcellulose and the pentylene glycol were added under mixing. Phase B was added over phase A. The pH was checked and corrected until approximately 5.5 - 6.

## 2.4. Evaluation of the Antioxidant Activity of the Finished Cosmetic Formulations

After the preparation of the three cosmetic formulations, the evaluation of the antioxidant activity of these final compositions was conducted as previously described by PCL in Section 2.2.3 [21]. The analysis has been made to compare the three different formulations with the cosmetic bases and, then, establish which one has the highest antioxidant power. For the analysis of the emulsion bases, both O/W and W/O, a quantity of sample of about 370 mg has been accurately weighted, dissolved in 10 mL of a mixture of ethanol/ether/hexane (1:1:1 v/v/v), and it has been sonicated for 20 seconds at 60% and centrifuged for 10 seconds. For the analysis, 300 μL of both mixtures have been used. For the cosmetic formulations with the *Araucaria angustifolia* extracts, about 200 mg of product has been accurately weighted, dissolved in 10 mL of the same previous mixture, treated with ultrasounds during 20 seconds and centrifuged for 10 seconds. An amount of 25 μL of each sample was used for analysis.

## 3. Results and Discussions

Seeds of Brazilian *Araucaria angustifolia* were processed to obtain fresh plant material, 55.33 g of shell and 122.77 g of pulp, were extracted by ultrasound-assisted maceration. The dry weighted extraction yields were 1.7044 g for the shell and 0.9818 g for pulp samples, corresponding to 8.5% and 4.91%, respectively.

### 3.1. Qualitative Analysis of the Main Chemical Constituents by HPTLC

At first a preliminary qualitative evaluation of the methanol extracts (pulp and shell), was lead by chromatography on high performance silica gel thin layer (HPTLC), the plates were sprayed with NP/PEG reagent (diphenylboryloxyethylamine 1.0% in methanol, followed by a solution of polyethylene glycol 4000 (5.0% in ethanol) and the orange stain revealed the presence of flavonoids (polyphenols compounds, and proanthocyanidins). This result supported the continuation of the studies (**Figure 1** and **Figure 2**).

### 3.2. Quantitative Determination of the Active Principles

The quantitative data were obtained coupling HPTLC and spectrophotometric evidences (see Section 2.1), the amounts of flavonoids resulted visibly higher in the methanol extract of the shell, **Figure 3**, of *A. angustifolia* than in those of the pulp, **Figure 4** and **Figure 5**.

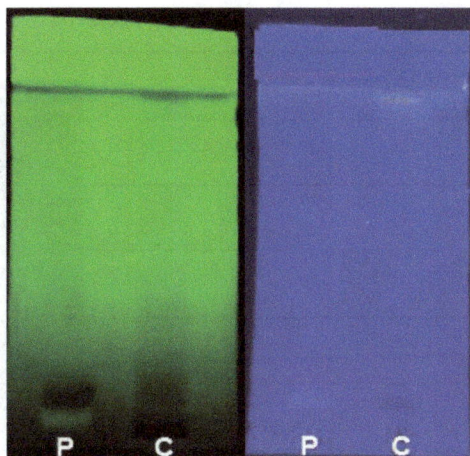

**Figure 1.** CCD plates sprayed by NP/PEG 400 and visualized under ultraviolet light, first at $\lambda$ = 254 nm and after at $\lambda$ = 366 nm. P: methanolic extract of the pulp shell of the *A. angustifolia*. Mobile phase: ethyl acetate/formic acid/acetic acid/water (100:11:11:26 v/v/v/v).

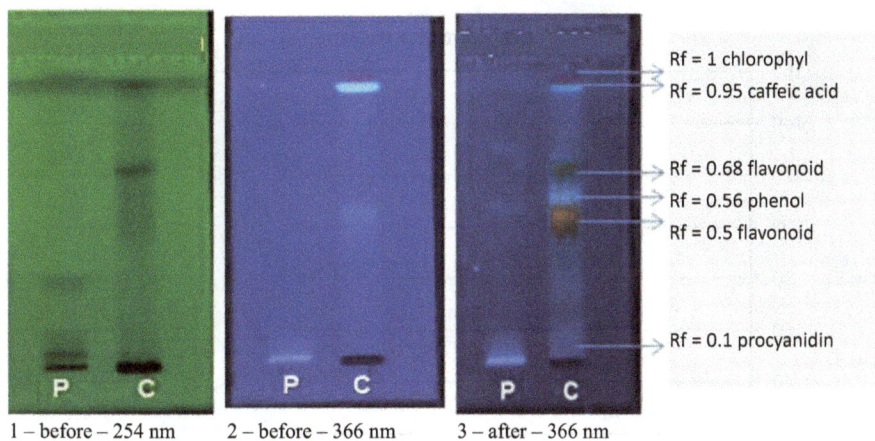

1 – before – 254 nm    2 – before – 366 nm    3 – after – 366 nm

**Figure 2.** CCD plates sprayed with NP/PEG 400 and visualized under ultraviolet light, initially (1) in $\lambda$ = 254 nm, lately (2) at $\lambda$ = 366, and after 24 hours. P: methanolic extract of the pulp of *A. angustifolia*; C: methanolic extract of the shell of *A. angustifolia*. Mobile phase: chloroform/acetone/formic acid (75:16.5:8.5 v/v/v).

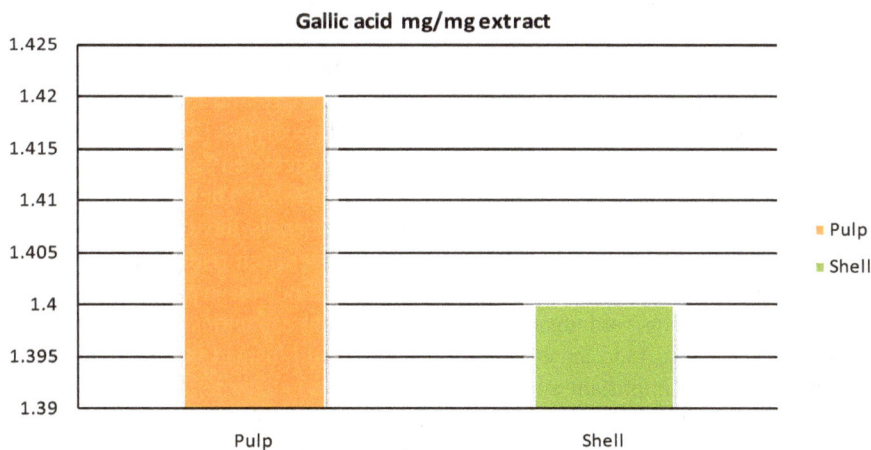

**Figure 3.** The total polyphenols expressed in mg gallic acid/mg extract, of the methanolic extract of the pulp and shell of *A. angustifolia*.

**Hyperoside mg/mg extract**

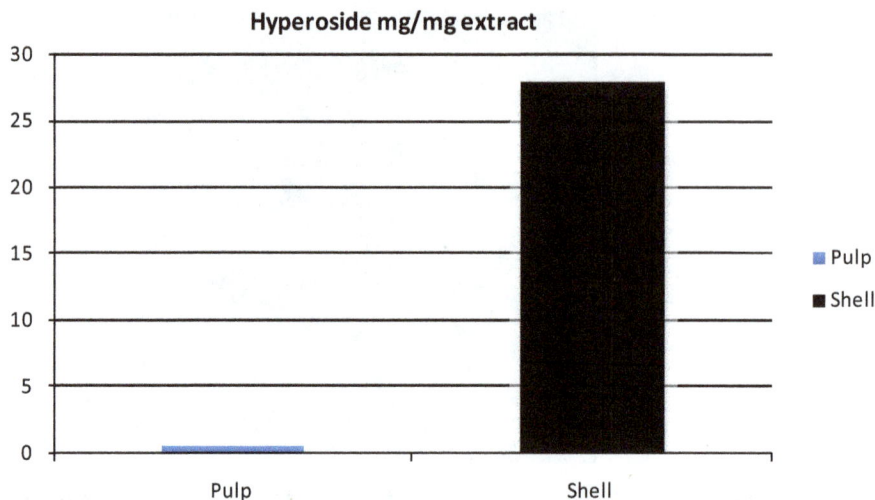

**Figure 4.** The total flavonoids values expressed in mg hyperoside/mg, pulp and shell of *A. angustifolia.*

**cyanidine chlorohydrate mg/mg extract**

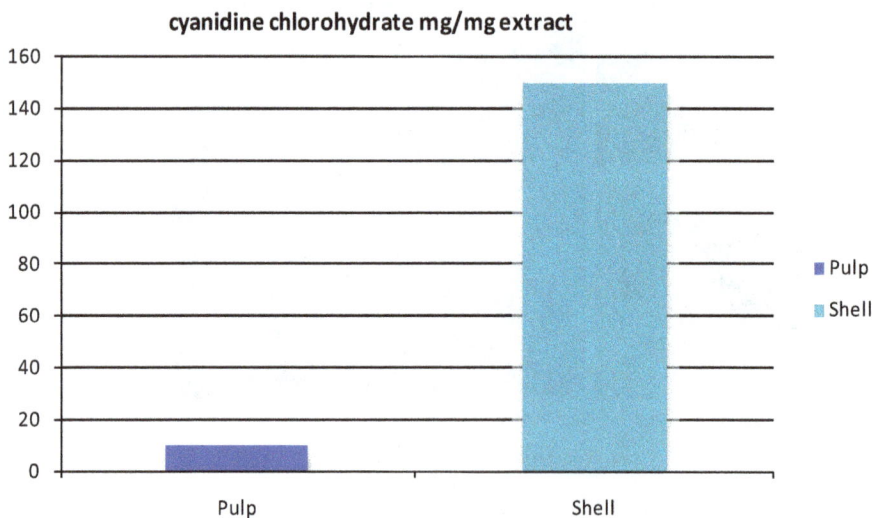

**Figure 5.** The total proanthocyanidins values expressed in mg cyaniding chloride/mg extract, methanolic extract of the pulp and shell of *A. angustifolia.*

In general, the plant secondary metabolites content in seeds parts is a debated argument since the related literature reports different evidences with regard to the many species and the different compounds investigated for their occurrence in embryos, endosperm and teguments [21] ecotypes [22]. However, for what concerns in particular phenolic and polyphenol compounds, they are often detected in the highest amounts in the seed teguments as confirmed by the data here achieved for *A. angustifolia*. Their occurrence in the external part of the seeds supports the general opinion that phenols and polyphenols have a key role in defense mechanisms in plants. Moreover, phenols and polyphenols in teguments give often rise to seed coat color which is reputed an important aspect for dissemination of the plant species [23]. Since these polyphenols are however known to have also important health benefits for humans (for e.g. antioxidant capacities) the seed teguments—often rejected as waste plant material in agro-food industrial processing—could instead represent an important renewable source of these compounds with important applications, as for e.g. as cosmetic ingredients. In light of these considerations, the results achieved about quantitative determination of polyphenols compounds, flavonoids, proanthocyanidinsin *Araucaria angustifolia*seed teguments support the above stated use. In a world economy in which the role of wastes achieve more and more importance in designing food processing of natural raw materials, these results further confirm the added value of sustainable development approaches.

## 3.3. Antioxidant Activity on HPTLC Using Radicals 2,2'-Azinobis (ABTS) and 2,2-Diphnyl-1-Pycril-Hydrazile (DPPH)

The pictures show the antioxidant activity, displayed by the bands, which corresponds to the main compounds of the seeds extracts, expressed by HP-TLC-bio-autography, using DPPH and ABTS as testing radicals [15]. It resulted clearly evident the most interesting efficacy of the eluted shell extract with both the assays, where a diffused discoloration along all the eluted bands is representative of the antioxidant capacity of the different phenolic compounds (flavonoids, phenols, procyanidins). Only a weak activity has been displayed by pulp extracts probably due to the capacity of the detected procyanidins to reduce ABTS radical. After 24 hours, no other reducing reactions were detected on plated through discoloring bands, indicating that there are no other substances with antioxidant activity against DPPH and ABTS. Moreover, these results are also self-explaining the long capacity of the compounds in neutralizing the oxidant agent.

## 3.4. Antioxidant Activity by Spectrophotometric Method

Through linear regression analysis between the oxidation inhibition percentage and the sample concentration, different equations and angular coefficients have been obtained for each extract and for the standard substance (Trolox®), allowing to calculate the concentration in μg/mL necessary to inhibit the radical oxidation 50% (IC$_{50}$), where low values of IC$_{50}$ correspond to a high antioxidant activity [24]. Therefore, from these data, see **Figure 7**, it is evident that both analyzed samples exhibit a higher antioxidant activity than the potent Trolox® used as positive control with a slightly prevalent efficacy of the shell extract than that of pulp (**Figure 6**).

## 3.5. Antioxidant Activity by ORAC-FL Method

The ORAC method was used to evaluate the antioxidant activity of the extracts against the free radicals generated by AAPH. The methanol extract from the pulp showed 332.6 ± 25.6 μmol TE/g, while the methanol extract from the shell was 2197.9 ± 169 μmol TE/g; indicating a much better antioxidant activity in the extract from the shell of *A. angustifolia* confirming the evidences acquired with the previous strategies.

## 3.6. Antioxidant Activity by PCL Method

This method has been used for evaluating the antioxidant capacity of the extracts and cosmetic formulations including them. The methanol extract from the pulp was 90.6 ± 2.0 μmol T/g, while the one from the shell was 1569.8 ± 47.3 μmol T/g. Also through this instrumental procedure, the antioxidant capacity of both the extracts from seeds of Brazilian *A. angustifolia* resulted different with a more interesting efficacy of those from shell than that from pulp.

There is no universal system able to provide information about the "real" antioxidant capacity of a molecule or a mixture. Each method is descriptive of a particular limited behavior, thus a panel of methods, with complementary mechanism is needed. A comparative evaluation of antioxidant efficacy is difficult to perform because the activity depends on the substrate, the reaction medium, the oxidation conditions, interfacial phenomena and

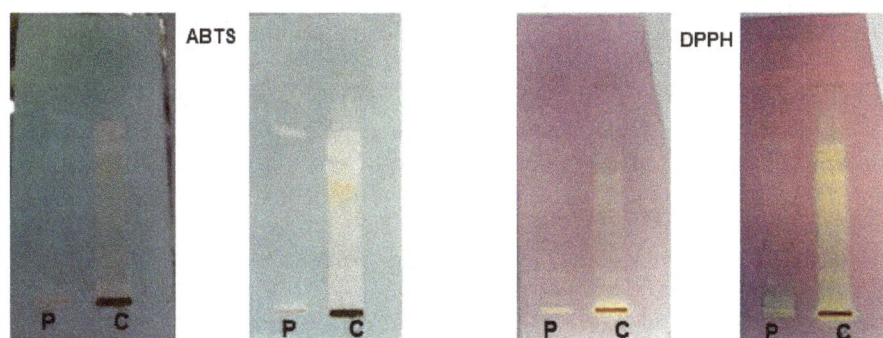

**Figure 6.** Antioxidant activity revealed with the radical, respectively, ABTS and DPPH, right after their addition and 24 hours later. P: methanolic extract from the pulp of *A. angustifolia*; C: methanolic extract from the shell of *A. angustifolia*.

the antioxidant partitioning properties between phases [25]. Two main mechanism are believed involved in antioxidant capacity assays:

The first is an "assessment of antioxidant efficacy in relation to free radical species". This category includes different reaction mechanisms models such as:

    1) Hydrogen atoms transfer reactions model (HAT) based on the transfer of hydrogen atoms;

    2) Single electron transfer reactions model (SET) based on the transfer of a single electron;

    3) Hydrogen-electron transfer reactions model combining the two mechanisms HAT and SET.

This category is useful to describe the properties of a molecule or raw material.

The second category is an "assessment of antioxidant efficacy using biological significant markers and significant substrates". This category involves the determination of antioxidant efficacy via evaluation of the protection against damaging effects on a biological substrate, produced by reactive species of oxygen (ROS) or related nitrogen oxide species (RNOS). Typically, when reacting with lipids, lipoproteins, DNA etc.

In this work we have taken into consideration models based on the first mechanisms. The HAT reaction, *i.e.* ORAC, is a key step promoting radical chain reactions and thus measure the capacity of inhibits propagation of oxidation (*i.e.* oxidation of fats). Among models based on SET mechanisms, we have selected ABTS, PCL and DPPH. SET based assays are useful to assess the capability of an antioxidant to reduce a specific oxidant. About the most well known ORAC and DPPH assays it must be underlined that they are not strictly related to a compound's efficacy against ROS and consequently not strictly related to the antioxidant activity, but rather to describe the property of a raw material (molecule, food, etc.). On the other hand, PCL and ABTS are more suited to evaluate the capability of an ingredient or mixture to be effective against an oxidative stressor.

### 3.7. Evaluation of the Antioxidant Activity of Cosmetic Formulations

Previous studies conduced by us have demonstrated [26] that the type of formulation, *i.e.*, W/O, O/W, W/O/W, gel, etc., the final pH or storage conditions and the cosmetic base could influence the expression of a functional ingredient's antioxidant capacity. Therefore, in case of ingredients claimed for antioxidant activity, we believe necessary to evaluate, at least, the real ability, in relation with the other ingredients and excipients, to confer antioxidant capacity to the finished formulation. Therefore, three different cosmetic formulations were prepared using the shell extracts. The antioxidant capacity was then checked and compared with the corresponding cosmetic bases as the reference sample. As demonstrated by our previous study, the PCL method can provide evaluation of the cosmetic formula as well as the raw ingredients thus consenting effective comparison. As expected, all bases displayed a much lower potency as compared to those containing *A. angustifolia* extracts. Furthermore, the formulation W/O and gel showed the higher antioxidant activity (4.41 ± 0.07 µmol T/g and 4.0 ± 0.07 µmol T/g) followed by O/W emulsion (3.5941 ± 0.172 µmol T/g), as shown in the graphics (**Figure 7**, **Figure 8**). Such potencies are compatible with a potential efficacy on skin.

## 4. Conclusion

The determination of polyphenols compounds, flavonoids, proanthocyanidins content in *A. angustifolia* seed parts pointed out their highest abundance in the teguments. In any case, the quantitative determination in the *A. angustifolia* seed teguments of these important antioxidants supports the possible use of these plant materials as renewable source of active molecules for cosmetic products. In fact, the methanolic extracts obtained from the shell (external teguments) and pulp (endosperm and embryo) of Brazilian *Araucaria angustifolia* seeds have both shown the presence of molecules that have the capacity of trapping free radicals (for e.g. polyphenols compounds, flavonoids, proanthocyanidins). The overall antioxidant capacity of the shell extracts resulted always higher than that of the pulp with all the assays performed, *i.e.* DPPH, ABTS, ORAC, and the higher values were even better than the Trolox® (synthetic vitamin E analog used as reference), suggesting an interesting applicative perspective in cosmetic and nutritional fields, where the search for natural antioxidant has been increasing in the last few years. In the light of these results, the potential cosmetic application was explored through the incorporation of the methanolic extract from the shell in three different cosmetic formulations (gel, O/W, W/O). The data collected strongly support the suggestion to valorize the Brazilian *A. angustifolia* seeds—shell in particular—as source of antioxidant biomolecules for formulation of antiaging cosmetic products. Further studies are currently ongoing in order to confirm antioxidant activity on volunteers.

**IC50 mg/ml**

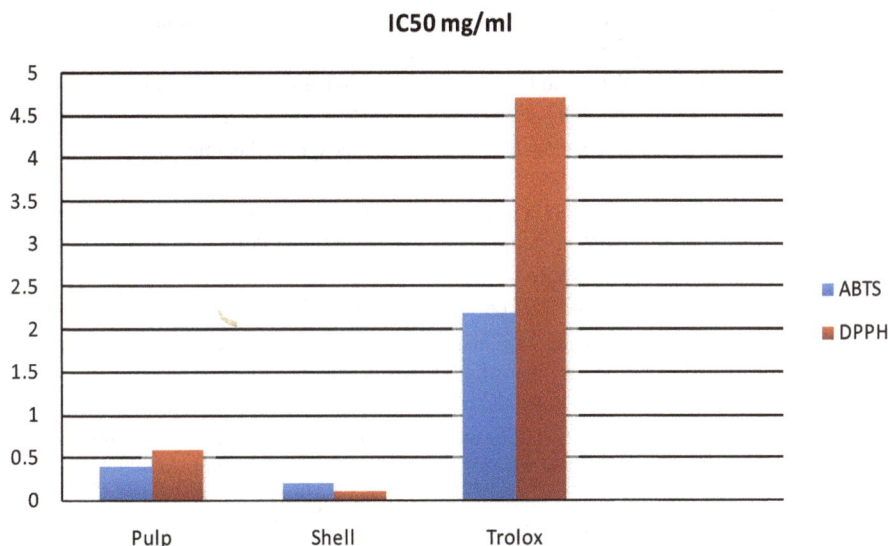

**Figure 7.** Antioxidant activity, expressed as IC50 of the extracts, evaluated by the DPPH and ABTS methods, compared to the standard substance (Trolox®).

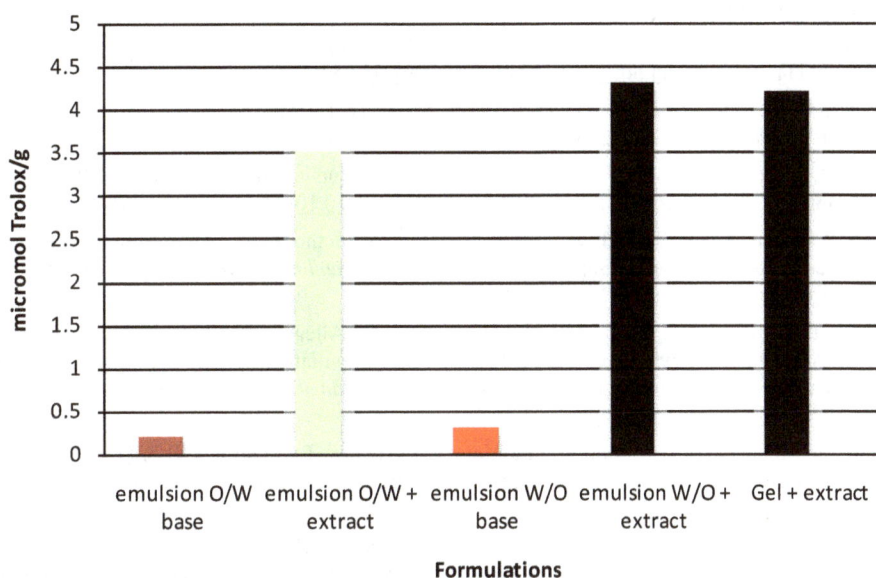

**Figure 8.** Antioxidant activity of cosmetic formulations containing the methanolic extract from the shell, compared the base formulations, expressed in μmol Trolox/g.

## Acknowledgements

We thank the Ministry of Education and Research (PRIN, Grant 20105YY2HL_006) and Ambrosialab for financial support. Prof. Gianfranco Franz, International Master Course Eco-polis, for the kind full collaboration in Curitiba. Elisa Durini, Alberto Casolari and Immacolata Maresca are gratefully acknowledged for technical assistance.

## References

[1]    Atoui, A.K., Mansouri, A., Boskou, G. and Kefalas, P. (2005) Tea and Herbal Infusions: Their Antioxidant Activity and Phenolic Profile. *Food Chemistry*, **89**, 27-36. http://dx.doi.org/10.1016/j.foodchem.2004.01.075

[2]    Barreiros, A.L.B.S., David, J.M. and David, J.P. (2006) Estresseoxidativo: Relação entre geração de espéciesreativas e defesa do organismo. *Química Nova*, **29**, 113-123. http://dx.doi.org/10.1590/S0100-40422006000100021

[3]   Halliwell, B. (1994) Free Radicals and Antioxidants: A Personal View. *Nutrition Reviews*, **52**, 253-265. http://dx.doi.org/10.1111/j.1753-4887.1994.tb01453.x

[4]   Pompella, A. (1997) Biochemistry and Histochemistry of Oxidant Stress and Lipid Peroxidation. *International Journal of Vitamin and Nutrition Research*, **67**, 289-297.

[5]   Magalhães, J. (2000) O uso de cosméticosatravés dos tempos, envelhecimentocutâneo. In: Rubio, Ed., *Cosmetologia*: *Com questões de avaliação*, Rio de Janeiro, 33-42.

[6]   F'Guyer, S., Afaq, F. and Mukhtar, H. (2003) Photochemoprevention of Skin Cancer by Botanical Agents. *Photodermatology, Photoimmunology & Photomedicine*, **19**, 56-72. http://dx.doi.org/10.1034/j.1600-0781.2003.00019.x

[7]   Nikolic, K.M. (2006) Theoretical Study of Phenolic Antioxidants Properties in Reaction with Oxygen-Centered Radicals. *Journal of Molecular Structure*: *THEOCHEM*, **774**, 95-105. http://dx.doi.org/10.1016/j.theochem.2006.07.017

[8]   Yamaguchi, L.F., Vassão, D.G., Kato, M.J. and Mascio, P. (2005) Biflavonoids from Brazilian Pine *Araucaria angustifolia* as Potentials Protective Agents against DNA Damage and Lipoperoxidation. *Phytochemistry*, **66**, 2238-2247. http://dx.doi.org/10.1016/j.phytochem.2004.11.014

[9]   Michelon, F., Branco, C.S., Calloni, C., Giazzon, I., Agostini, F., Spada, P.K.W. and Salvador, M. (2012) *Araucaria angustifolia*: A Potential Nutraceutical with Antioxidant and Antimutagenic Activities. *Current Nutrition & Food Science*, **8**, 155-159. http://dx.doi.org/10.2174/157340112802651103

[10]  Middleton, E. and Kandaswami, C. (1986) The Impact of Plant Flavonoids on Mammalian Biology: Implications for Immunity, Inflammation and Cancer. In: Harbone, J.B., Ed., *The Flavonoids*: *Advances in Research since* 1986, Chapman & Hall, London, 619-652.

[11]  Wagner, H. and Bladt, S. (2001) Plant Drugs Analisis, a Thin Layer Chromatography. 2nd Edition, Springer-Verlag Berlin, Heidelberg, New York.

[12]  Shahidi, F. and Nazck, M. (2004) Extration and Analysis of Phenolics in Food Review. *Journal of Chromatography A*, **1054**, 95-111. http://dx.doi.org/10.1016/j.chroma.2004.08.059

[13]  Singleton, V.L. and Rossi, J.A. (1965) Colorimetry of Total Phenolics with Phosphomolibdic-Phosphotungstic Acid Reagent. *American Journal of Enology and Viticulture*, **16**, 144-158.

[14]  Porter, L.J., Hrstich, L.N. and Chan, B.C. (1985) The Conversion of Procyanidis and Prodelphinidins to Cyanidin and Delphinine. *Phytochemistry*, **25**, 223-230. http://dx.doi.org/10.1016/S0031-9422(00)94533-3

[15]  Prior, R.L., Wu, X. and Schaich, K. (2005) Standardized Methods for the Determination of Antioxidant Capacity and Phenolics in Food and Dietary Supplements. *Journal of Agricultural and Food Chemistry*, **53**, 4290-4302. http://dx.doi.org/10.1021/jf0502698

[16]  Butera, D., Tesoriere, L., Di Gaudio, F., Bongiorno, A., Allegra, M., Pintaudi, A.M., Kohen, R. and Livrea, M.A. (2002) Antioxidant Activities of Sicilian Prickly Pear (Opuntiaficusindica) Fruit Extracts and Reducing Properties of Its Betalains: Betanin and Indicaxanthin. *Journal of Agricultural and Food Chemistry*, **50**, 6895-6901. http://dx.doi.org/10.1021/jf025696p

[17]  Wang, M., Rangarajan, M., Shao, Y., La Voie, E.J., Huang, T.C. and Ho, C.T. (1998) Antioxidative Phenolic Compounds from Sage (*Salvia officinalis*). *Journal of Agriculture and Food Chemistry*, **46**, 4869-4873. http://dx.doi.org/10.1021/jf980614b

[18]  Moure, A., Franco, D., Sineiro, J., Dominguez, H., Núñez, M.J. and Lema, J.M. (2000) Evaluation of Extracts from Gevuinaavellana Hulls as Antioxidants. *Journal of Agriculture and Food Chemistry*, **48**, 3890-3897. http://dx.doi.org/10.1021/jf000048w

[19]  Baldisserotto, A., Malisardi, G., Scalambra, E., Andreotti, E., Romagnoli, C., Vicentini, C.B., Manfredini, S. and Vertuani, S. (2012) Synthesis, Antioxidant and Antimicrobial Activity of a New Phloridzin Derivative for Dermo-Cosmetic Applications. *Molecules*, **17**, 13275-13289. http://dx.doi.org/10.3390/molecules171113275

[20]  Lewin, G. and Popov, I. (1994) Photochemiluminescent Detection of Antiradical Activity III: A Simple Assay of Ascorbate in Blood Plasma. *Journal of Biochemical and Biophysical Methods*, **28**, 277-282. http://dx.doi.org/10.1016/0165-022X(94)90003-5

[21]  Giovanni, D., Bonetti, A., Minelli, M., Marotti, I., Catizone, P. and Mazzanti, A. (2006) Content of Flavonols in Italian Bean (*Phaseolus vulgaris* L.). *Food Chemistry*, **99**, 105-114. http://dx.doi.org/10.1016/j.foodchem.2005.07.028

[22]  Bruni, R., Medici, A., Guerrini, A., Scalia, S., Poli, F., Romagnoli, C., Muzzoli, M. and Sacchetti, G. (2002) Tocopherol, Fatty Acids and Sterol Distributions in Wild Ecuadorian *Theobroma subincanum* (Sterculiaceae) Seeds. *Food Chemistry*, **77**, 337-341. http://dx.doi.org/10.1016/S0308-8146(01)00357-0

[23]  Loginov, M., Boussetta, N., Lebovka, N. and Vorobiev, E. (2013) Separation of Polyphenols and Proteins from Flaxseed Hull Extracts by Coagulation and Ultrafiltration. *Journal of Membrane Science*, **442**, 177-186. http://dx.doi.org/10.1016/j.memsci.2013.04.036

[24] Stocks, J., Gutteridge, J.M.C., Sharp, R.J. and Dormandy, T.L. (1974) The Inhibition of Lipid Autoxidation by Human Serum and Its Relationship to Serum Proteins and Crtocopherol. *Clinical Science & Molecular Medicine*, **47**, 223-233.

[25] Litescu, S.C., Eremia, S. and Radu, G.L. (2010) Methods for the Determination of Antioxidant Capacity in Food and Raw Materials. *Advances in Experimental Medicine and Biology*, **698**, 241-249. http://dx.doi.org/10.1007/978-1-4419-7347-4_18

[26] Ziosi, P., Manfredini, S., Vertuani, S., Ruscetta, V., Sacchetti, G., Radice, M. and Bruni, R. (2010) Evaluating Essential Oils in Cosmetics: Antioxidant Capacity and Functionality. *Cosmetic & Toiletries*, **125**, 6.

# 4

# Production of Citric Acid from Corncobs with Its Biological Evaluation

Ahmed Ashour[1,2], Saleh El-Sharkawy[2,3], Mohamed Amer[2], Amani Marzouk[2], Ahmed Zaki[2], Asuka Kishikawa[1], Momiji Ohzono[4], Ryuichiro Kondo[1], Kuniyoshi Shimizu[1*]

[1]Department of Agro-Environmental Sciences, Faculty of Agriculture, Kyushu University, Fukuoka, Japan
[2]Department of Pharmacognosy, Faculty of Pharmacy, Mansoura University, Mansoura, Egypt
[3]Department of Pharmacognosy, Faculty of Pharmacy, Delta University for Science and Technology, Mansoura, Egypt
[4]Zenshin Incorporated, Chikushino City, Japan
Email: *shimizu@agr.kyushu-u.ac.jp

## Abstract

Corncobs could serve as a substrate for citric acid production using solid state fermentation technique. The culture optimization concerning substrate concentration, culture duration, pH, temperature and substrate hydrolysis was carried out for maximum productivity of citric acid. Under the optimized conditions, 48.4 g of citric acid was produced from 1 kg dry corncobs. Biological evaluation was carried out for citric acid such as melanin synthesis inhibitory, anti-allergy, anti-bacterial, and hyaluronic acid production activities. The results showed that citric acid has potent melanin inhibitory activity, good inhibition for $\beta$-hexosaminidase release and potent stimulatory effect for the production of hyaluronic acid. These activities (melanin synthesis inhibitory, anti-allergy and hyaluronic acid productive activities) of citric acid have been reported for the first time.

## Keywords

Corncobs, Citric Acid, Fermentation, Melanin, Allergy, Hyaluronic Acid

## 1. Introduction

The vast development in industry, agriculture and the human civilization resulted in intensive production of a huge amount of agro-industrial wastes. In Egypt, a large amount of corncobs are produced every year and no effective methods are being used for its utilization. The accumulation of this waste causes a serious environmental

*Corresponding author.

disposal problem represented in the fermentation of such wastes, their degradation products, psychological hazards and other related health problems [1] which increase the burden on the national economy.

Corncobs are an important by-product of the sweet corn processing industry in Egypt, where they represent about 15% of total corn production.

The amount of corncobs produced was estimated to be about 54,424 tons in 2008 (according to data obtained from the Directorate of Agriculture, Egypt). Worldwide, these large amounts are either used as animal feed or are returned to the harvested field [2].

Corncobs are rich in cellulose and hemicellulose that has been used as a cheap source of raw material for production of soluble sugars and other value-added products by enzymatic and microbial fermentation processes [3].

Citric acid is one of the world's largest tonnages of fermentation products. It has a wide variety of application due to high solubility, low toxicity and palatability in the food and beverage industry (70%), in pharmaceuticals (12%) and in other industrial applications (18%) [4]. It is produced commercially by submerged fermentation of sucrose or molasses based medium [5]. Recently, there have been an increasing number of reports on the use of solid state fermentation (SSF) processes as an alternative to submerged fermentation [6]. This is because of lower energy requirements, higher product yields, little risk of bacterial contamination, less waste water generation and environmental concerns concerning the disposal of solid waste [7].

## 2. Material and Methods

### 2.1. Agro-Waste Material

Corncobs were obtained on August 2008 by Prof. Dr. Ahmed Nader, Agronomy Department, Faculty of Agriculture, Mansoura University, from plants grown in a field at the university campus.

Corncobs type was identified as *Zea mays* hybrid individual 3080. They were milled to a particle size of 1.25 μm. A voucher specimen (No. 1536) was deposited at the Department of Pharmacognosy, Faculty of Pharmacy, Mansoura University.

### 2.2. Biotransformation

#### 2.2.1. Microorganisms

*Aspergillus niger* ATCC 10549, *Aspergillus alliaceus* UI 315, *Aspergillus flavipes* ATCC 11013, *Aspergillus flavipes* ATCC 16795, *Congronella butleri* ATCC 22822, *Rhodotorula rubra* ATCC 20129, *Fusarium oxysporum* ATCC 7601 and *Debaryomyces polymorphus* ATCC 20280.

The strains were maintained on potato dextrose agar (PDA) slants at 4°C and sub-cultured at intervals from 1 to 2 months [8].

#### 2.2.2. Methods

Experiments were conducted in 250 mL flasks, each containing 10 g powdered corncobs with 50 mL water adjusted to pH 7.4.

All flasks containing corncobs were sterilized at 121°C for 15 min, cooled and inoculated with test organisms, all experiments were done in duplicates.

All flasks were incubated at 30°C and the production of acidic conditions was monitored by means of pH paper where a sample was pipetted every day for 30 days, the flask which converted the color of the paper to the red color indicated acidic medium produced by the microorganism in this flask. The results of this screening are shown in **Table 1**.

The liquid medium, which showed acidic condition, was further subjected to HPLC using reversed column C18 to determine the type of acid produced by comparing the retention time of acid produced with the library of retention times.

Citric acid was determined by HPLC (series 200 HPLC, Perkin Elmer, USA) under the following conditions: RP-18 column (inertsil ODS-3, Shimadzu 5 μm, 25 cm × 0.5 cm i.d.).

Separation was achieved using phosphate buffer, pH 2.1 as mobile phase at flow rate 1 mL/min for 30 min. Eluting peaks were monitored by UV detector at 210 nm.

It was concluded that *A. niger* ATCC 10549 produce citric and oxalic acids while all other tested organisms produced only oxalic acid so *A. niger* ATCC 10549 was selected for further study.

**Table 1.** Results of screening of different microorganisms for production of acidic medium from corncobs[*].

| Microorganism | Result |
|---|---|
| *Aspergillus niger* ATCC 10549 | + |
| *Aspergillus alliaceus* UI 315 | -- |
| *Aspergillus flavipes* ATCC 11013 | -- |
| *Aspergillus flavipes* ATCC 16795 | -- |
| *Congronella butleri* ATCC 22822 | + |
| *Rhodotorula rubra* ATCC 20129 | + |
| *Fusarium oxysporum* ATCC 7601 | + |
| *Debaryomyces polymorphus* ATCC 20280 | + |

[*]+: acidic medium, --: non acidic medium.

### 2.2.3. Culture Optimization

1) Optimization of concentration of the spores for citric acid production. Concentration of the spores of the highest citric acid producing organism (*A. niger* ATCC 10549) was adjusted to $9.6 \times 10^6$ spores/mL and used in each experiment.

2) Culture incubation period: 6, 8, 10, 12, 14 and 16 days.

3) Substrates concentration: conical flasks (250 mL) containing 50 mL of water supplemented with 3, 6, 9, 12, 15, 20, 30 g corncobs to obtain a substrate concentration 6%, 12%, 18%, 24%, 30%, 40% and 60%, respectively.

4) Initial pH values of 3, 5, 5.5, 6, 6.5, 7 and 8 were adjusted by 1 N HCl and 1 N NaOH.

5) Temperature: 5°C, 15°C, 24°C, 30°C, 37°C and 42°C.

Quantitative analysis of citric acid was done conducting the acetic anhydride and pyridine method of Marier and Boulet [9]. It should be noted that no other organic acid such as oxalic acid was interfering with quantitative data of citric acid.

### 2.2.4. Standard Curve of Citric Acid [9]

Appropriate dilutions (50 - 300 µg/mL) were made from the stock solution of citric acid (5 mg/mL). One millitre of each dilution followed by 1.30 mL of pyridine was added into individual test tubes and swirled. Acetic anhydride (5.70 mL) was then added into each tube. These samples were placed in a water bath at 32°C for 30 min. A blank was run in parallel replacing 1 mL of the sample with distilled water. The intensity of yellow color obtained was measured at 405 nm. A calibration curve was drawn taking the citric acid concentration at X-axis and optical density at Y-axis.

### 2.2.5. Estimation of Citric Acid in the Culture Filtrate

The diluted culture filtrate (1 mL) was treated as mentioned above, blank test was carried out parallel with the sample using 1 mL distilled water instead of culture filtrate.

### 2.3. B16 Melanoma Cell Line Assay

This assay was performed as described previously [10]. The cells were placed in two 24-well plastic culture plates (one plate for determining melanin and the other for cell viability) at a density of $1 \times 10^5$ cells/well and incubated for 24 h in media prior to being treated with the samples. After 24 h, the media were replaced with 998 µL of fresh media and 2 µL of the test sample at concentrations of 6.25, 12.5, 25, 50, 100, and 200 mg/mL (n = 3). At the same time, a negative control (2 µL DMSO) and a positive control (2 µL DMSO with arbutin at a concentration of 50 mg/mL) were tested. The cells were incubated for an additional 48 h, and then the medium was replaced with fresh medium containing each sample. After 24 h, the remaining adherent cells were assayed. To determine the melanin content (for one plate) after removing the medium and washing the cells with PBS, the cell pellet was dissolved in 1.0 mL of 1 N NaOH. After being kept in the dark overnight, the crude cell extracts were assayed by using a microplate reader at 405 nm to determine the melanin content. The results from the cells treated with the test samples were analyzed as a percentage of the results from the control culture. Cell viability was determined by an MTT assay, which provides a quantitative measure of the number of viable cells by determining the amount of formazan crystals produced by metabolic activity in treated versus control cells. For the other well plate, 50 μL of MTT reagent in PBS (5 mg/mL) was added to each well. The plates were incubated in a humidified atmosphere of 5% of $CO_2$ at 37°C for 4 h. After the medium was removed, 1.0 mL iso-propyl alcohol (containing 0.04 N HCl) was added, and the absorbance was measured at 570 nm after cells were kept in the dark overnight.

## 2.4. RBL-2H3 Cell Line Assay

RBL-2H3 cells are the tumor analog of mast cells, which after being sensitized with mouse monoclonal IgE or ionophore A23187 respond by releasing inflammatory mediators such as $\beta$-hexosaminidase [11]. As a result, the sample is considered to have anti-allergic activity if it can inhibit mast cells degranulation and produce a significant reduction in $\beta$-hexosaminidase release. Firstly, we performed a cell viability assay (using MTT) to ensure that the activity of the sample at the used concentration was related to the inhibition of histamine release rather than to the cytotoxicity of the RBL-2H3 cells. The cell viability assay was done as follows: RBL-2H3 cells (100 μL, $1 \times 10^5$ cells/well) were cultured with EMEM in a 96-well plate for 24 h. Then samples (1 μL/well; DMSO 1 μL as control) were added. After 24 h incubation in a $CO_2$ incubator at 37°C, MTT (10 μL, 5 mg/mL in PBS) was added to each well, and the plate was incubated for another 4 h. The medium was then removed, acid iso-propanol (100 μL, containing 0.04 N HCl) reagent was added to each well, the plate was incubated overnight at room temperature, and the absorbance was read at 570 nm using a microplate reader.

The anti-allergy assay was determined as previously described [12] with minor modification, as follows: RBL-2H3 cells ($1 \times 10^6$ cells/well) were inoculated with EMEM in a 96-well plate for 48 h, then EMEM medium was replaced by tyroid buffer [100 μL, 130 mM NaCl, 5 mM KCl, 1.4 mM $CaCl_2$, 1 mM $MgCl_2 \cdot 6H_2O$, 10 mM HEPES (4-(2-hydroxyethyl)-1-piperazineethanesulfonic acid), 5.6 mM glucose, 0.1% BSA, pH 7.2/well], sample (1 μL/well) was added, and the plate was incubated for 30 min in $CO_2$ incubator at 37°C. A23187 (10 μg/mL, 2 μL/well) was added after removal of the sample and the addition of new tyroid buffer (100 μL/well). After 30 min incubation, 50 μL from each well was collected and transferred to another 96-well plate. An equal volume of substrate solution (1 mM), p-nitrophenyl-N-acetyl-$\beta$-glucosaminide was added to each well, and the plate was left at room temperature on the shaker for 1 h. Finally, the reaction was terminated by adding 100 μL of stopping buffer ($Na_2CO_3$, 100 mM, pH = 10), and the absorbance was measured at 405 nm using a microplate reader. The statistical difference between the control and each sample was determined by student's t-test.

## 2.5. Antibacterial Assay

This assay was determined as described previously [13] with little modification. Briefly, a single colony of the test strain (*Escherichia coli* and *Staphylococcus aureus*) was taken and added to 5 mL of NB medium. This medium was incubated at 37°C ± 1°C, 120 rpm for 20 h. It was then added to bacterial suspension to prepare a bacterial concentration at $10^5$ CFU/mL. The bacterial solution was used for the following antibacterial assay. In each well of a 96-well plate, 133.5 μL of NB medium, 15 μL of bacteria suspension, and 1.5 μL of DMSO were added with or without each sample. Also, sorbic acid (400 μg/mL) was used as a positive control. The plate was incubated at 37°C ± 1°C, 1160 rpm for 18 h. Finally, bacterial growth was measured by a micro-plate reader (630 nm). The statistical difference between the control and each sample was determined by student's t-test. The MIC (minimum inhibitory concentration) was the lowest concentration of the test extract that completely prevented growth until 18 h.

Also the activity of citric acid was tested against *Propionibacterium acnes* using the same procedure as above except the use of GAM broth instead of N. broth, bacterial concentration at $10^1$ CFU/mL and finally plate was incubated at 37°C ± 1°C, 1160 rpm for 24 h. Also benzalkonoium chloride was used as positive control in case of *P. acne*.

## 2.6. Hyaluronic Acid (HA) ELISA Assay

Scientific studies have shown that HA improves skin hydration, stimulates production of collagen in skin, works as an antioxidant and free radical scavenger, maintains skin elasticity, cushions joints and nerve tissues, has an antibacterial and anti-inflammatory activity and maintains the fluid in the eye tissues, which may help to protect against numerous possible eye concerns [14].

Citric acid was tested for the effect of the production of HA by the use of HA ELISA assay using Biotech Trading Partners (Encinitas, California) according to manufacture's instruction.

This kit is an enzyme-linked binding protein assay that uses a capture molecule known as hyaluronic acid binding protein (HABP). After growing of the fibroblast cells, they are incubated in HABP-coated micro well plate. Properly samples and HA reference solution are added to this plate, allowing HA present to react with the immobilized binding protein. After removal of unbound molecules by washing, HABP conjugated with horseradish peroxidase (HRP) solution is added to the microwells to form complexes with bound HA. Following another washing step, a chromogenic substrate of tetramethylbenzidine and hydrogen peroxide is added to develop a colored reaction. The intensity of the color is measured in optical density units with a spectrophotometer at 450 nm. The higher the intensity of the color, the higher ability of the sample to produce hyaluronic acid.

## 3. Results and Discussion

### 3.1. Biotransformation

#### 3.1.1. Effect of Time
**Table 2** shows the time course of citric acid production from corncobs, it was concluded that *A. niger* ATCC 10549 produces the highest amount of citric acid on 8th day.

#### 3.1.2. Effect of Temperature and pH
As shown in **Table 3** and **Table 4**, temperature and pH were found to have a profound influence on fungal production of citric acid from corncobs. *A. niger* ATCC 10549 produce the highest amount of citric acid at 30°C and pH 3.

#### 3.1.3. Effect of Substrate Concentration
The effect of substrate concentration on citric acid production was illustrated in **Table 5**. As corncobs concentration was increased from 6% to 24%, the yield of citric acid by *A. niger* ATCC 10549 was increased from 56.6 to 459.6 µg/mL. Corncobs concentration above this value decreases the yield of citric acid. The reduction of

**Table 2.** Production of citric acid from corncobs using *A. niger* ATCC 10549.

| Time | Concentration (µg/mL) (mean ± SD, n = 2) |
|---|---|
| 6 days | 263.5 ± 5.93 |
| 8 days | 295.0 ± 3.81 |
| 10 days | 273.5 ± 2.17 |
| 12 days | 243.5 ± 2.17 |
| 14 days | 195.8 ± 2.12 |
| 16 days | 113.5 ± 5.44 |

**Table 3.** Result of the effect of temperature on citric acid production.

| Temperature °C | Concentration (µg/mL) (mean ± SD, n = 2) |
|---|---|
| 5 | 101.2 ± 39.17 |
| 15 | 135.8 ± 8.76 |
| 24 | 221.2 ± 50.06 |
| 30 | 443.5 ± 6.50 |
| 37 | 284.3 ± 27.22 |
| 42 | 92.7 ± 16.33 |

**Table 4.** Result of different initial pH values on citric acid production.

| pH value | Concentration (µg/mL) (mean ± SD, n = 2) |
|----------|------------------------------------------|
| 3 | 458.2 ± 6.50 |
| 5 | 270.5 ± 88.65 |
| 5.5 | 302.0 ± 1.62 |
| 6 | 275.0 ± 3.30 |
| 6.5 | 272.0 ± 12.42 |
| 7 | 382.0 ± 55.48 |
| 8 | 342.7 ± 39.16 |

**Table 5.** Result of the effect of corncobs concentration in the culture filtrate on citric acid production.

| Concentration of corncob in water (%, w/v) | Concentration of citric acid (µg/mL) (mean ± SD, n = 2) |
|--------------------------------------------|---------------------------------------------------------|
| 6 | 56.6 ± 8.65 |
| 12 | 176.61 ± 40.24 |
| 18 | 327.3 ± 3.26 |
| 24 | 459.6 ± 2.17 |
| 30 | 137.3 ± 14.14 |
| 40 | 143.5 ± 19.57 |
| 60 | 142.7 ± 6.52 |

citric acid yield at high substrate concentration could be due to decrease in water content in the medium as has been observed for sucrose hydrolysis at very high concentration by yeast beta-fructofuranosidase.

## 3.2. B16 Melenoma Cell Line Assay

An important concept when selecting bioactive compounds that modulates skin pigmentation that for obvious reasons, they should have minimal effects on cell proliferation and/or toxicity. Taking into consideration about the cytotoxicity to cell lines, the most active concentration of citric acid exhibiting melanin synthesis inhibition (~33%) and at the same time with moderate cytotoxicity (16%) was 200 µg/mL, followed by concentration 100 µg/mL (20% inhibition) with low cytotoxicity (10% cytotoxicity). Citric acids at concentrations of lower than 100 µg/mL have no melanin inhibition effect. Results are shown in **Figure 1**.

## 3.3. RBL-2H3 Cell Line Assay

The highest inhibition of $\beta$-hexosaminidase release was recorded at both concentration of 1000 µg/mL and 500 µg/mL (82% in A23187 assay). However, citric acid showed high toxicity (75%) at 1000 µg/mL compared to those at 500 µg/mL which showed lower cytotoxicity (29%). Citric acid at 250 µg/mL showed 45% inhibition of $\beta$-hexosaminidase release without cytotoxicity. Results are shown in **Figure 2**.

## 3.4. Antibacterial Assay

From the results, it was shown that citric acid completely inhibit the growth of *S. aureus*, *E. coli* and *P. acne* with MIC = 25, 50 and 200 µg/mL, respectively. Results are shown in **Figure 3**.

## 3.5. Hyaluronic Acid (HA) Production Assay in Fibroblast

It was found that citric acid at both tested concentration have a very good stimulating effect for the production of hyaluronic acid more than *N*-acetyl glucosamine (NAcG) which is used as positive control and at the same time they showed no cytotoxic to the cell. Results are shown in **Figure 4**.

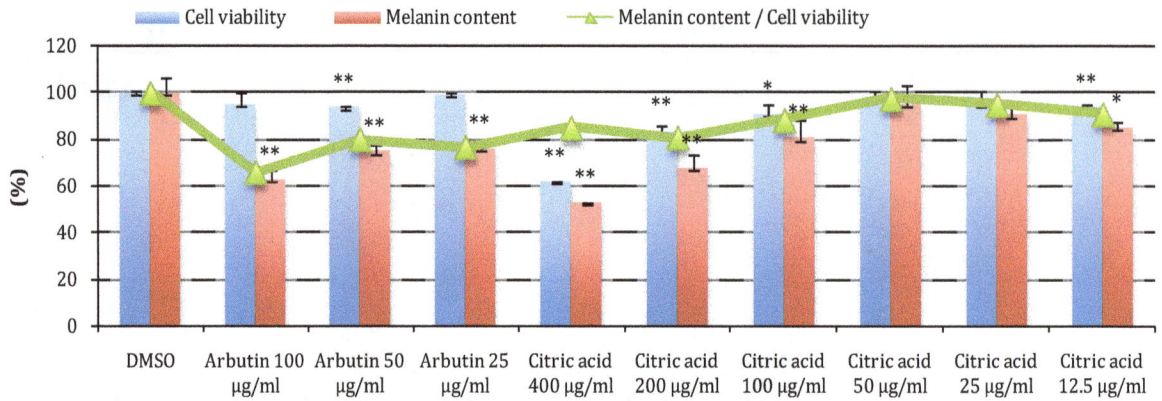

**Figure 1.** Effect of citric acid on melanin formation in B16 melenoma cell. The values are represented as the mean ± standard deviation (SD), n = 3. Significant difference from the control value and each compound was determined by student's t-test: $^*P < 0.05$, $^{**}P < 0.01$.

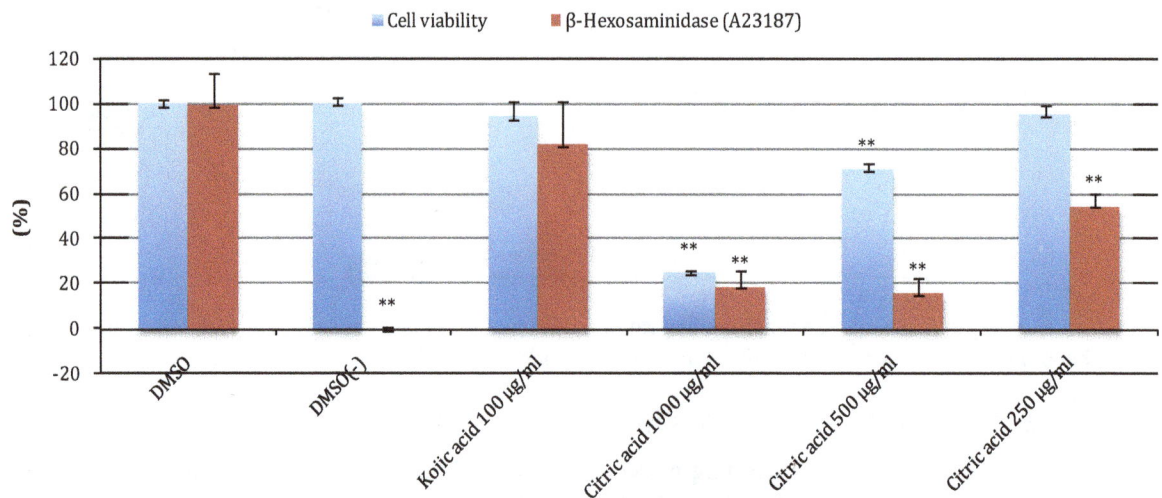

**Figure 2.** Cell viability and effects of various citric acid concentrations on ionophore A23187-stimulated $\beta$-hexosaminidase release from RBL-2H3 basophilic leukemia cells, DMSO group represent the wells with addition of A23187. DMSO (−) represent the wells without addition of A23187. All the values are the mean ± SD (n = 5). $^*$Significant difference from the control group ($P < 0.01$).

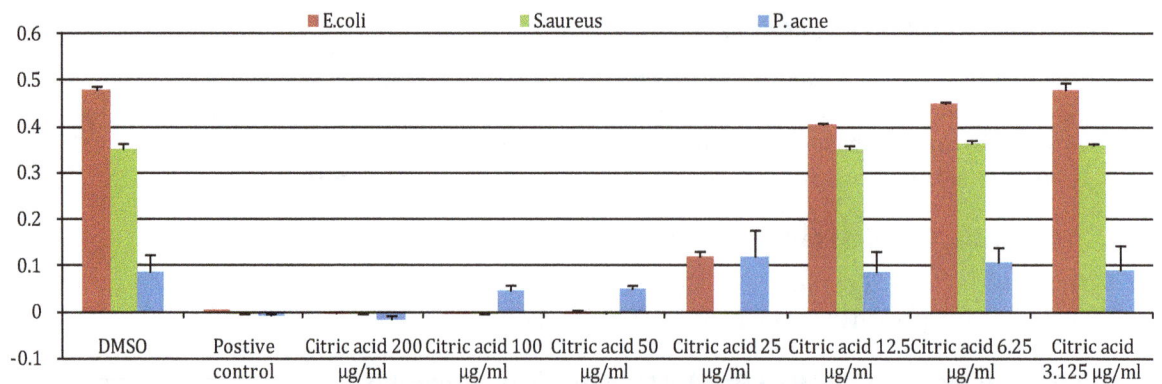

**Figure 3.** Anti-bacterial activity against *E. coli*, *S. aureus* and *P. acne*. The values are represented as the mean ± standard deviation (SD), n = 3. Final concentrations; 400 μg/mL for sorbic acid (*E. coli*, *S. aureus*) and benzalkonium chloride (*P. acne*). Significant difference between 1% DMSO and each concentration was determined by student's t-test: $^*P < 0.05$, $^{**}P < 0.01$.

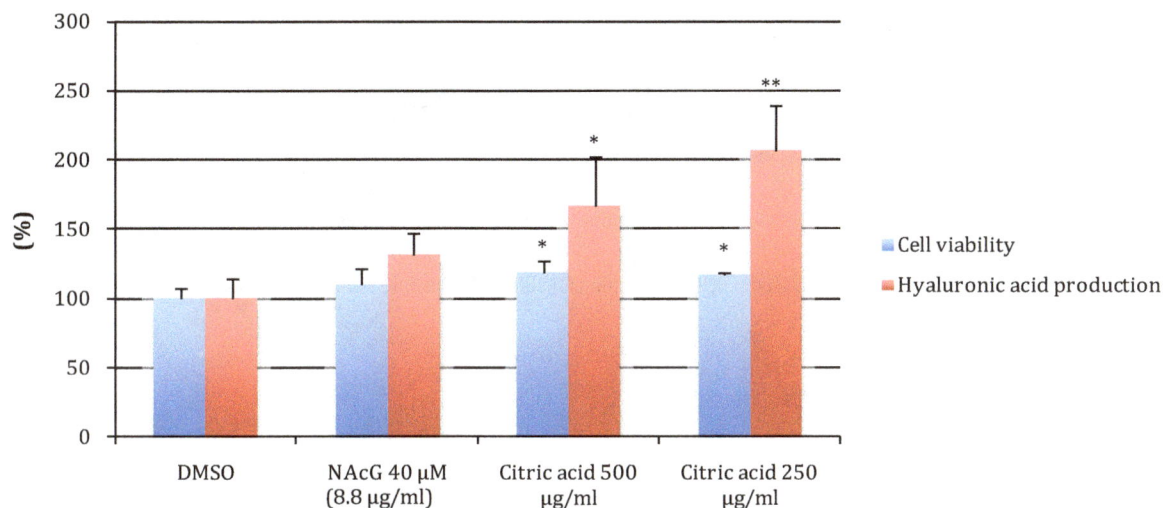

**Figure 4.** Effect of citric acid on the production of hyaluronic acid. The values are represented as the mean ± standard deviation (SD), n = 3. Significant difference between 1% DMSO and each concentration was determined by student's t-test: [*]$P <$ 0.05, [**]$P < 0.01$.

## 4. Conclusions

The present work investigates the feasibility of using corncobs as substrates for production of citric acid.

Under the optimal conditions, the fermenting organism was capable of producing 48.4 g citric acid per kg dry matter of corncobs after 8 days of fermentation. The biological experiment for citric acid indicated that citric acid has interesting biological activities. Previous results showed that the most common use of citric acid as a preservative for its antibacterial effect. However in this study other important biological activities such as melanin inhibition activity, anti-allergy activity and stimulation of hyaluronic acid production were done here for the first time. To the best of our knowledge that citric acid was proved to have interesting result in these biological experiments.

## References

[1]    Diomi, M., Elisavet, K. and Paul, C. (2008) Fungal Multienzyme Production on Industrial By-Products of the Citrus-Processing Industry. *Bioresource Technology*, **99**, 2373-2383. http://dx.doi.org/10.1016/j.biortech.2007.05.018

[2]    Inglett, G.E. (1970) Corn: Culture, Processing and Products. AVI Publishing Co., Waetport.

[3]    Barl, B., Biliaderis, C., Murray, E. and MacGregor, A. (1991) Combined Chemical and Enzymic Treatments of Corn Husk Lignocellulosics. *Journal of Science of Food Agriculture*, **56**, 195-214. http://dx.doi.org/10.1002/jsfa.2740560209

[4]    Prescott, S.C. and Dunn, C.G. (1982) Citric Acid. In: *Industrial Microbiology*, 4th Edition, AVI Pub. Co. INC., Westport, 709-747.

[5]    Kapoor, K., Chaudhary, K. and Tauro, P. (1982) Citric Acid. In: Reed, G., Ed., *Precott and Dunn's Industrial Microbiology*, 4th Edition, The AVI Publishing Co., Westport.

[6]    Hang, Y. and Woodams, E. (1998) Production of Citric Acid from Corncobs by *Aspergillus niger*. *Bioresource Technology*, **65**, 251-253. http://dx.doi.org/10.1016/S0960-8524(98)00015-7

[7]    Doelle, H.W., Mitchell, D.R. and Rolz, C.E. (1992) Solid Substrate Cultivation. Elsevier Applied Science, London, 7-16.

[8]    Sankpal, N.V., Joshi, A.P. and Kulkarni, B.D. (2001) Citric Acid Production by *Aspergillus niger* Immobilized on Cellulose Microfibrils: Influence of Morphology and Fermenter Conditions on Productivity. *Process Biochemistry*, **36**, 1129-1139. http://dx.doi.org/10.1016/S0032-9592(01)00155-8

[9]    Marier, J. and Boulet, M. (1958) Direct Determination of Citric Acid in Milk with an Improved Pyridine-Acetic Anhydride Method. *Journal of Dairy Science*, **41**, 1683. http://dx.doi.org/10.3168/jds.S0022-0302(58)91152-4

[10]  Arung, E., Shimizu, K. and Kondo, R. (2007) Structure-Activity Relationship of Prenyl-Substituted Polyphenols from *Artocarpus heterophyllusas* Inhibitors of Melanin Biosynthesis in Cultured Melanoma Cells. *Chemistry & Biodiversity*,

**4**, 2166-2171. http://dx.doi.org/10.1002/cbdv.200790173

[11] Ikawati, Z., Wahyuono, S. and Maeyama, K. (2001) Screening of Several Indonesian Medicinal Plants for Their Inhibitory Effect on Histamine Release from RBL-2H3 Cells. *Journal of Ethnopharmacology*, **75**, 249-256. http://dx.doi.org/10.1016/S0378-8741(01)00201-X

[12] Yun, S., Kang, M., Park, J. and Nam, S. (2010) Comparison of Anti-Allergenic Activities of Various Polyphenols in Cell Assays. *Applied Biological Chemistry*, **53**, 139-146. http://dx.doi.org/10.3839/jabc.2010.026

[13] Tatli, İ. and Akdemir, Z. (2005) Antimicrobial and Antimalarial Activities of Secondary Metabolites from Some Turkish *Verbascum* Species. *Fabad Journal of Pharmceutical Sciences*, **30**, 84-92.

[14] Necas, J., Bartosikova, L., Brauner, P. and Kolar J. (2005) Hyaluronic Acid (Hyaluronan): A Review. *Veterinarni Medicina*, **53**, 397-411.

# 5

# Adipose Derived Stem Cells and Growth Factors Applied on Hair Transplantation. Follow-Up of Clinical Outcome

Federica Zanzottera[1*], Emilio Lavezzari[1], Letizia Trovato[2], Alessandro Icardi[2], Antonio Graziano[2]

[1]Hair Transplantation Surgery, Studio Dr. Lavezzari, Como, Italy
[2]HBW Srl, Torino, Italy
Email: *federica.zanzottera@hotmail.it

## Abstract

Different studies show the need of immature adipose cell to induce the proliferation of bulge stem cells in order to kick off the anagen phase of hair cycle. Furthermore, the adipose derived stem cell, adipose progenitors, and growth factors secreted by mature adipocytes can help the wound healing and the vascular neogenesis. Nowadays, it is not known any protocol of tissue regeneration applied to hair transplantation, especially if aimed to the reconstruction of the main vascular network for the engraftment of transplanted hair and the healing process. The aim of the work is to investigate how the application of autologous cellular suspension obtained by Rigenera system, mechanical fragmentation procedure which allows to obtain a physiological saline solution consisting of a heterogeneous pool of cells rich in adipose derived mesenchymalstem cells and growth factors, helps the wound healing and engraftment of the transplanted hair. During hair restoration surgery, the adipose tissue recovered from the discard of follicular slicing, was processed using the Rigenera system. The obtained cell suspension was applied in the area of hair transplantation, increasing the natural background of adipocyte lineage and raising the amount of growth factors. In addition, the cellular suspension was applied to the suture on the occipital region. The cell population was characterized by FACS. The monthly evaluation of hair transplantation follow-up with photos and the patient's impressions demonstrates that there is a faster healing of the micro-wound and a continuous growth of the transplanted hair even two months after the procedure, with a shortening of the dormant phase. In conclusion, this new approach aims to integrate regenerative medicine and hair restoration surgery in order to improve the outcome for the patient. It would be wonderful to continue this research to elaborate on the molecular cause behind this satisfying clinical.

---

*Corresponding author.

## Keywords

**Stem Cell, ADSC, Hair Transplantations, Regenerative Medicine, Hypoderm Hair Transplantations**

## 1. Background

The field of hair transplantations has made countless step forward and now it is possible to obtain results not even imagine thirsty years ago.

In the last ten years, we have witnessed the rise of regenerative medicine applied at many surgical disciplines aiming to increase the results and reduce the pain of patients. Nowadays, except for Platelet Rich Plasma (PRP), it is not known any protocol of tissue regeneration applied to hair transplantation, especially if aimed to the reconstruction of the main vascular network for the engraftment of transplanted hair and the healing process.

A number of researches underline the existence of cells in the adult body capable of repairing and regenerating damaged tissues.

Adipose tissue is a multifunctional organ that contains various cellular types, such as mature adipocytes and the stromal vascular fractions (SVF), which consists of endothelial cells, pericytes, fibroblasts, pre-adipocytes and mesenchymal stem cells, called Adipose Derived Stem Cells (ADSC) (**Figure 1**). These pluripotent cells with their secretome mediate different skin regenerative effects, such as wound healing, antioxidant protection and antiwrinkling [1]. Autologous ADSC have been applied for several regenerative treatments such as widespread traumatic calvarial bone defects [2], breast augmentations [3], fistulas in patients with Crohn's disease [4] and for wound healing in treatment of chronic ulcers [2].

Festa [5] shows the need for immature adipocytes to promote the proliferation of bulge stem cells. Sumikawa [6] shows the potential of leptine and adipokine as an inducer of anagen phase. Furthermore, growth factors stimulate hair growth in both *ex vivo* and *in vivo* animal model [7] [8].

It is clear that the adipocyte lineage is critical to tissue regeneration and hair growth.

## 2. Aim

The aim of this work is to evaluate how a pool of cells consisting of ADSC, pericytes, endoteliocytes, preadipocytes and their secretome can improve the hair transplantation outcome, helping wound healing and follicular units' engraftment.

## 3. Methods

### 3.1. Subjects

Three patients, subjected to hair restoration surgery with the application of adipose derived stem cells and growth factors, were monitored after 5 days, 2 weeks and 1 month. The selection of the patients was casual and based on their availability.

### 3.2. Cellular Suspension Obtainment

During hair restoration surgery, a strip of scalp form the occipital region is cut and sliced to isolate the follicular units. Below the dermis there are hypodermis and adipose tissue that had been discarded in the past. These tissues were processed using Rigenera system.

Rigenera device is a safe standardized sample preparation system, for the automated mechanical disaggregation of cells population. This mechanical fragmentation, allows extracting from tissue only smallest cells that represents the progenitor cells responsible of the tissue formation. In addition, this system is able to cut, without crash, the single extracellular matrix constituents, which play an important role in reducing inflammatory process and so help the healing of tissue. **Figure 2** states all steps to obtain a cell suspension.

## 4. FACS

FACS analysis was performed to evaluate the quantity and quality of cell suspension from two different patients.

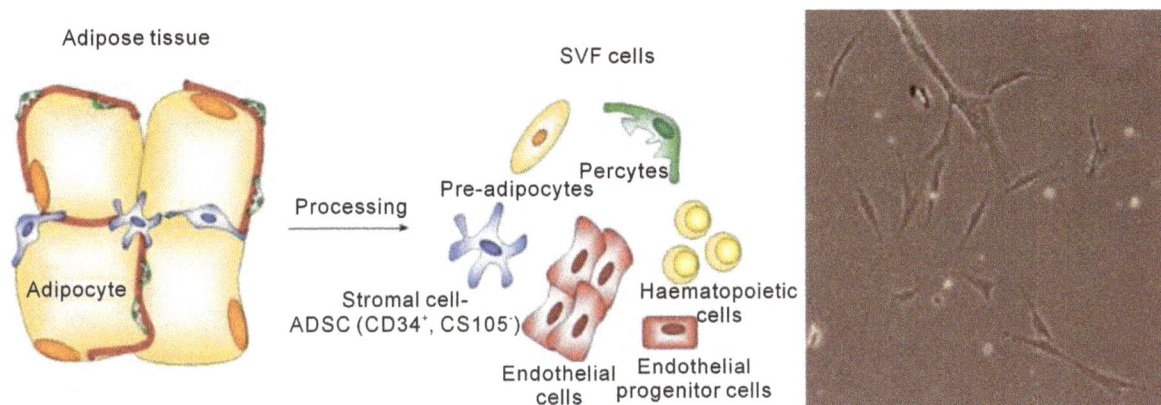

**Figure 1.** Adipose tissue and photo of ADCS by optical microscope.

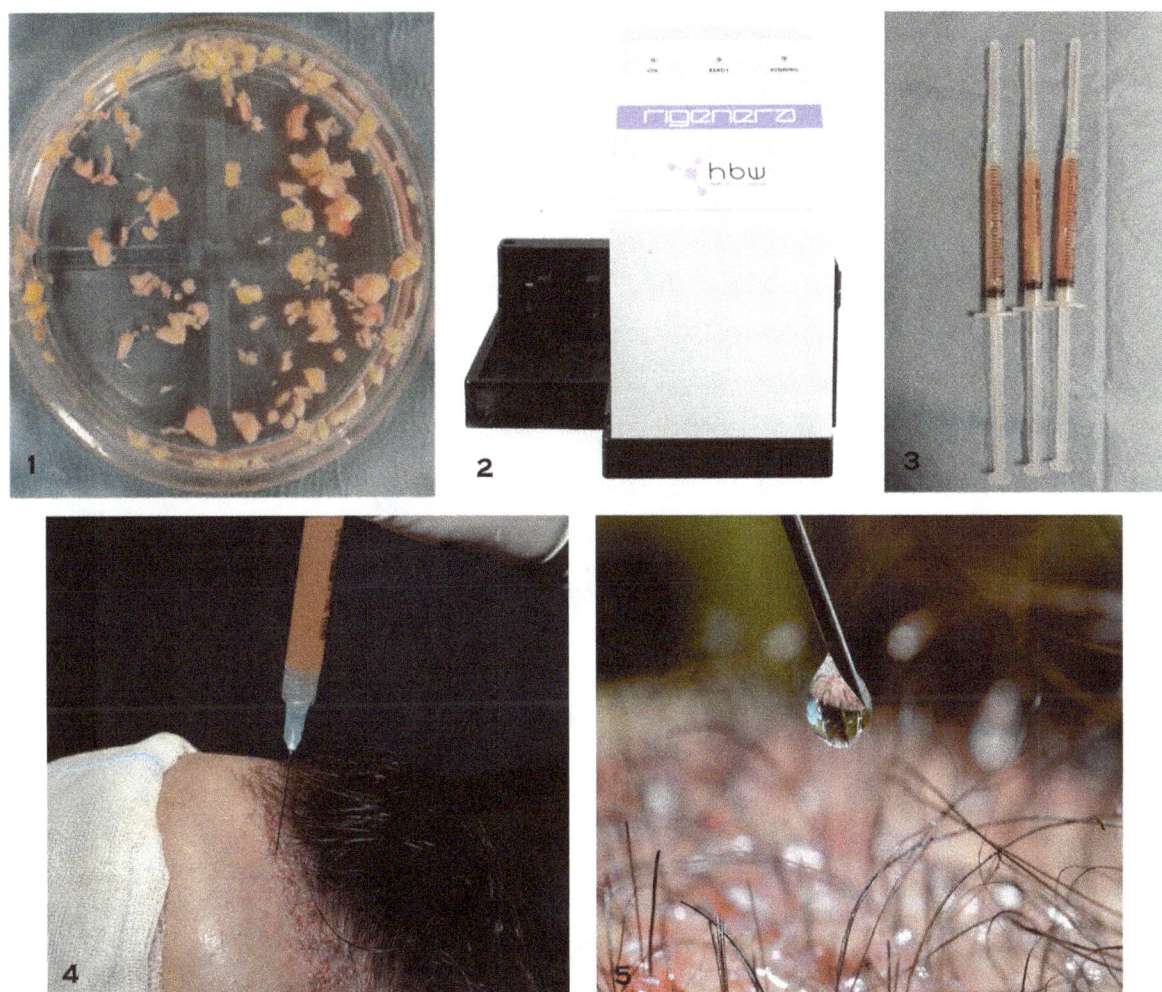

**Figure 2.** Rigenera System: 1) Hypo-derma and adipose tissue from the occipital region; 2) Rigenera system: a piece of tissue +1 ml of saline solution was inserted in Rigeneracons (CE/EC disposable medical devices containing a stainless steel grid with 100 hexagonal holes of 50 μ each surrounded by six micro blades) and mechanically fragmented with Rigenera for 3 min. The cells passed through the grid into the liquid suspension; 3) Cell suspension was collected with a syringe. The disaggregation and filtration results in a physiological saline solution consisting of heterogeneous pool of cells and growth factors; 4) Cell suspension was injected subcutaneously; and 5) Dropped on the micro incisions made for the engraftments of hair. The suspension was applied before and after the hair insertion. (For some patients the suspension was applied also on the donor area wound)

The gating was made for CD146 and CD34, typical of adipose derived mesenchymal stem cells. The cells were also observed at optical microscope.

## 5. Results

### 5.1. Cell Suspension Analysis

The cellular vitality is 93% for the 1st patients and 74% for the 2nd. This represents a good result especially after mechanical fragmentation.

Both gating for CD146 and CD34 shows that the cellular suspension obtained by Rigenera is a heterogeneous pool of cells composed by erythrocytes, epithelial cells, ADSC and 90% of living cells, which correspond to immature adipocytes and ADSC at the first differentiation stage (**Figure 3**).

The cells are in the active phase of the cell cycle; lots of them are doubling and splitting, showing that Rigenera sorting allows the collection of young and active cells, discarding the quiescent and old cells at the end of their functional utility (**Figure 4**).

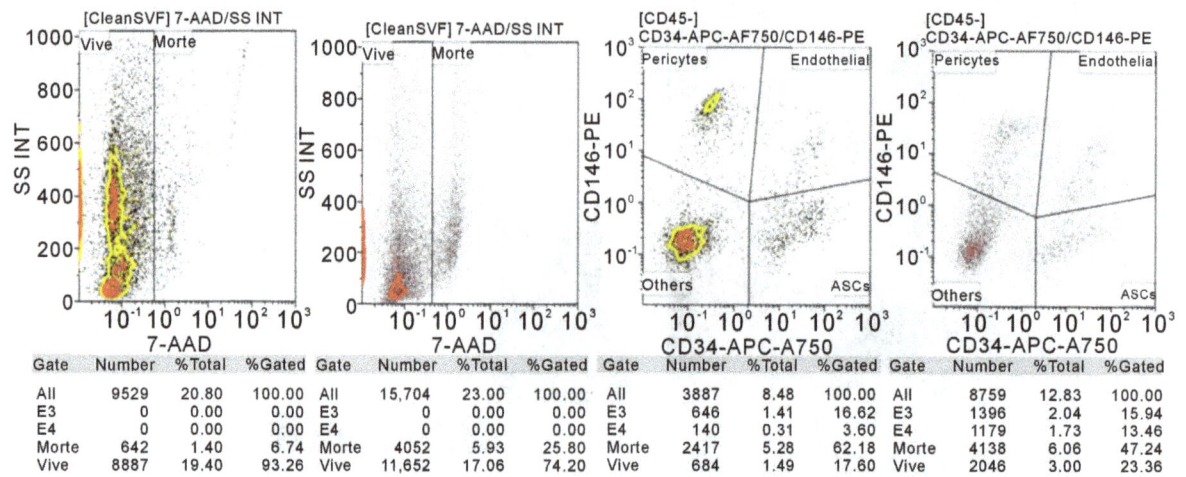

| Gate | Number | %Total | %Gated | Gate | Number | %Total | %Gated | Gate | Number | %Total | %Gated | Gate | Number | %Total | %Gated |
|---|---|---|---|---|---|---|---|---|---|---|---|---|---|---|---|
| All | 9529 | 20.80 | 100.00 | All | 15,704 | 23.00 | 100.00 | All | 3887 | 8.48 | 100.00 | All | 8759 | 12.83 | 100.00 |
| E3 | 0 | 0.00 | 0.00 | E3 | 0 | 0.00 | 0.00 | E3 | 646 | 1.41 | 16.62 | E3 | 1396 | 2.04 | 15.94 |
| E4 | 0 | 0.00 | 0.00 | E4 | 0 | 0.00 | 0.00 | E4 | 140 | 0.31 | 3.60 | E4 | 1179 | 1.73 | 13.46 |
| Morte | 642 | 1.40 | 6.74 | Morte | 4052 | 5.93 | 25.80 | Morte | 2417 | 5.28 | 62.18 | Morte | 4138 | 6.06 | 47.24 |
| Vive | 8887 | 19.40 | 93.26 | Vive | 11,652 | 17.06 | 74.20 | Vive | 684 | 1.49 | 17.60 | Vive | 2046 | 3.00 | 23.36 |

**Figure 3.** FACS made on a pool of cells obtained from the mechanical fragmentation of the hypodermic and adipose tissue from the occipital region of two patients. 1) Vitality of cells; 2) Gating for CD146 and CD34 in order to underline the presence of Adipose Derived mesenchymal Stem Cells (ADSC).

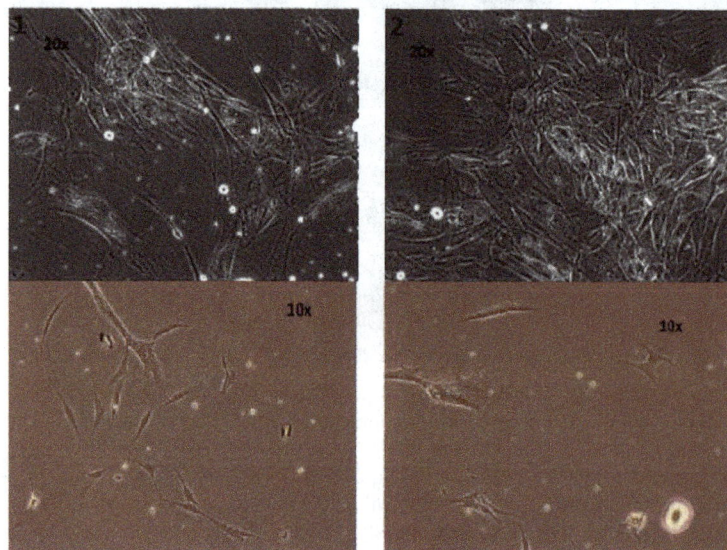

**Figure 4.** Photos of cellular suspension of the two patients by optical microscope.

## 5.2. Patient's Follow-Up

Only two weeks after transplantation the healing of micro wounds was complete. Hair continued growing, greatly improving the patient's mood and self-confidence. Also the wound on the donor area was perfectly healed (**Figure 5**).

Five days after hair restoration surgery, the patient reported a perfect recovery, without any swelling and edema. The small scabs were clean and dry, ready to fall (**Figure 6**).

One month after surgery, a maintenance of transplanted hair and a perfect healing of micro wounds are visible (**Figure 7**).

## 5.3. Patient's Impressions

For all the patients the pain was very mild and for one of them was completely absent.

They also reported a reduction of post operatory edema and swelling. The perception of pain was established by VAS (Visual Analogic Scale) (**Figure 8**).

## 6. Discussion

Rigenera system gives the possibility to extract from tissue only the smallest cells that represent the progenitors responsible for the tissue formation. It allows to cut, without crash, the single extracellular matrix constituents, which are important in reducing the inflammatory process and so to help the healing of tissue. Furthermore, it crashes mature adipocytes freeing up many growth factors. In this way it is possible to maintain a sort of "cellular-niche" in which every cell and growth factor plays its role in tissue regeneration.

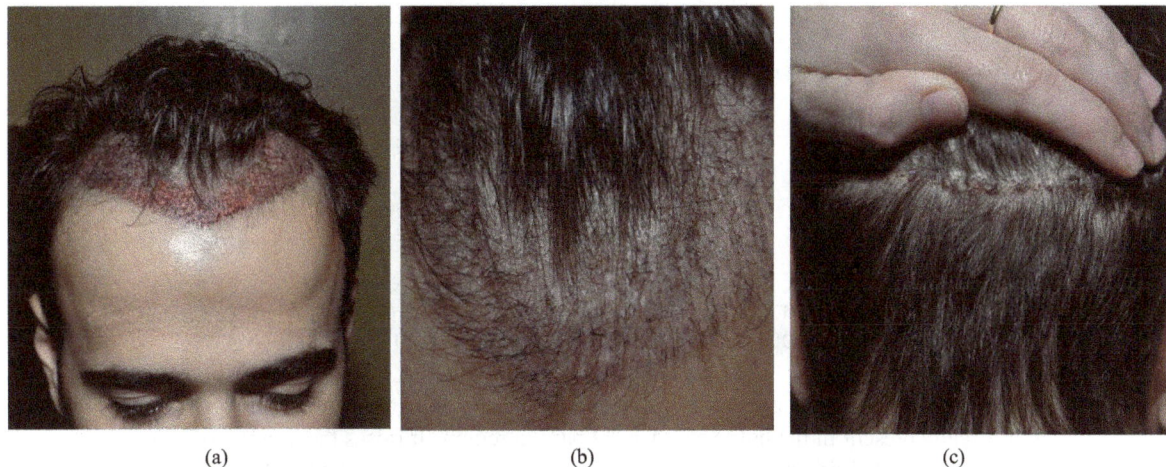

(a)　　　　　　　　　　(b)　　　　　　　　　　(c)

**Figure 5.** Patient 1. (a) Immediately after the hair restoration surgery; (b) and (c) two weeks after.

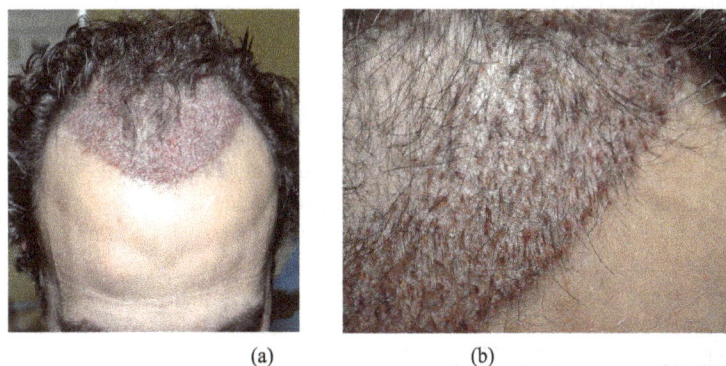

(a)　　　　　　　　(b)

**Figure 6.** Patient 2. (a) Immediately after the hair restoration surgery; (b) Five days after.

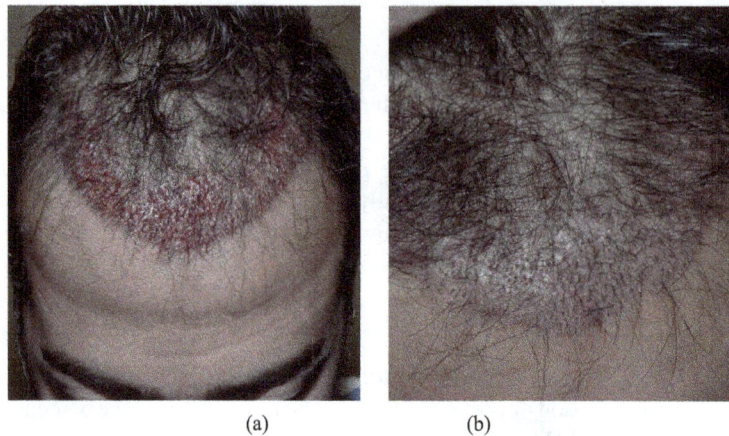

(a)                                              (b)

**Figure 7.** Patient 3. (a) Immediately after the hair restoration surgery; (b) one month after.

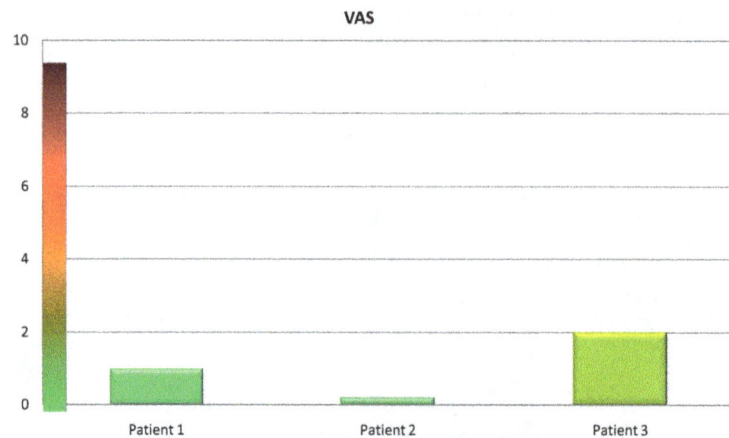

**Figure 8.** Visual analogic scale. The VAS shows the pain suffered by the patients: From 0 to 2 the pain was VERY MILD, from 2 to 4 MILD, from 4 to 6 MEDIUM, from 6 to 8 STRONG, from 8 to 10 VERY STRONG.

Applying these cells in the area of hair transplantation increases the natural background of adipocyte lineage, which is already present in the bulge and dermal papilla region. It raises the amount of growth factors easing the healing process and helping hair growth and engraftment of transplanted hair. It would be wonderful to continue this research to elaborate on the molecular cause behind these satisfying clinical results and to carry out a bigger and more complete clinical trial.

## References

[1]  Park, B.S., Kim, W.S., Choi, J.S., Kim, H.K., Won, J.H., Ohkubo, F. and Fukuoka, H. (2010) Hair Growth Stimulated by Conditioned Medium of Adipose-Derived Stem Cells Is Enhanced by Hypoxia: Evidence of Increased Growth Factor Secretion. *Biomedical Research*, **31**, 27-34. http://dx.doi.org/10.2220/biomedres.31.27

[2]  Lendeckel, S., Jödicke, A., Christophis, P., *et al.* (2004) Autologous Stem Cells (Adipose) and Fibrin Glue Used to Treat Widespread Traumaticcalvarial Defects: Case Report. *Journal of Cranio-Maxillo-Facial Surgery*, **32**, 370-373. http://dx.doi.org/10.1016/j.jcms.2004.06.002

[3]  Yoshimura, K., Sato, K., Aoi, N., *et al.* (2008) Cell-Assisted Lipotransfer for Cosmetic Breast Augmentation: Supportive Use of Adiposederivedstem/Stromal Cells. *Aesthetic Plastic Surgery*, **32**, 48-55. http://dx.doi.org/10.1007/s00266-007-9019-4

[4]  Rosen, E.D. (2002) The Molecular Control of Adipogenesis, with Special Reference to Lymphatic Pathology. *Annals of the New York Academy of Sciences*, **979**, 143-158. http://dx.doi.org/10.1111/j.1749-6632.2002.tb04875.x

[5]   Festa, E., Fretz, J., Berry, R., Schmidt, B., Rodeheffer, M., Horowitz, M. and Horsley, V. (2011) Adipocyte Lineage Cells Contribute to the Skin Stemcell Niche to Drive Hair Cycling. *Cell*, **146**, 761-771. http://dx.doi.org/10.1016/j.cell.2011.07.019

[6]   Sumikawa, Y., Inui, S., Nakajima, T. and Itami, S. (2014) Hair Cycle Control by Leptin as a New Anagen Inducer. *Experimental Dermatology*, **23**, 27-32. http://dx.doi.org/10.1111/exd.12286

[7]   Yano, K., Brown, L.F. and Detmar, M. (2001) Control of Hair Growth and Follicle Size by VEGF-Mediated Angiogenesis. *Journal of Clinical Investigation*, **107**, 409-417. http://dx.doi.org/10.1172/JCI11317

[8]   Tomita, Y., Akiyama, M. and Shimizu, H. (2006) PDGF Induce and Maintain Anagen Phase of Murine Hair Follicles. *Journal of Dermatological Science*, **125**, 873-882.

# 6

# Efficacy Evaluation of Unique Skincare Product Containing Pseudo-Ceramide for Fine Wrinkles in Japanese Female Atopic Dermatitis Patients

**Akihiko Takahashi\*, Katsura Mori, Takahiro Nishizaka, Hisateru Tanabe**

Kao Corporation, R&D, Skincare Product Research, Tokyo, Japan
Email: \*takahashi.akihiko@kao.co.jp

## Abstract

**Background/Objective: Dryness is considered to be an early developmental mechanism of wrinkles, and fine line formation is marked in atopic dermatitis (AD) accompanied by dry skin. To evaluate the efficacy of a skincare product with a moisturizing effect increased by lamellar formulation of pseudo-ceramide for fine lines and wrinkles, a use test was performed applying the product to non-lesional dry skin in patients with atopic dermatitis. Method: The test product was an essence containing pseudo-ceramide formulated in a lamellar structure. The study design was a nine-week single-center non-comparative study, and the evaluation items were the grade of wrinkles at the corners of the eyes judged by a dermatologist, replica analysis, and instrumental measurement (skin surface moisture and transepidermal water loss). Results: Nine-week continuous use of the test product significantly improved the score of wrinkles at the corners of the eyes judged by a dermatologist and wrinkle area ratio on replica analysis of the corners of the eyes and cheeks, compared with those at study initiation. With this improvement, the losses of skin surface moisture and transepidermal water were also significantly improved. Conclusion: It was clarified that the tested pseudo-ceramide-formulated skincare product not only improved the barrier function for atopic dermatitis, but also exhibited an effect on fine lines and wrinkles of dry skin.**

## Keywords

**Pseudo-Ceramide, Fine Lines, Wrinkles, Atopic Dermatitis, Clinical Trial**

---

\*Corresponding author.

# 1. Introduction

Reduced barrier function and dryness of skin are observed in atopic dermatitis (AD), and a lack of intercellular lipids in the stratum corneum, particularly ceramide, is considered to be a cause of this, as it reduces skin surface moisture and increases transepidermal water loss in not only regions with eruptions but also non-lesional regions [1] [2]. Since skin elasticity reduction and wrinkle formation are likely to occur in dry skin, fine lines are readily formed due to reduced skin elasticity in AD, in addition to dryness-induced rough skin surface and scales, and the skin appearance negatively influences the quality of life (QOL) of patients [3] [4]. However, no evaluation of the anti-wrinkle efficacy of ceramide-formulated preparations for non-lesional dry skin of AD patients has been reported.

Improvement of dryness and barrier function by external use of ceramide and ceramide analogues in AD patients have been investigated, and a superior moisturizing effect and improvement of the barrier function have been clarified [5]. In addition, a technique to disperse pseudo-ceramide in a lamellar structure in water has recently been developed, for which a high and persistent moisturizing effect can be expected because the lamellar structure formed by pseudo-ceramide continuously retains water between the lamellar layers [6]. In this study, we performed a use test of a skincare product with a moisturizing effect increased by a lamellar formulation of pseudo-ceramide to confirm its efficacy for fine lines and wrinkles in AD patients.

# 2. Materials and Methods

## 2.1. Test Product

The test product was serum, in which pseudo-ceramide is formulated into a lamellar structure to increase the moisturizing effect (**Table 1**). The chemical structure of the pseudo-ceramide (cetyl PG hydroxyethyl palmitamide) is shown in **Figure 1** [7].

## 2.2. Study Design

The study design was a single-center non-comparative study. After a one-week dry-out period, the test product was applied after face washing twice a day (morning and night) for nine weeks, instead of facial skincare products usually used, and the use of facial moisturizing products (emulsion, cream, and serum) other than the test product was prohibited.

## 2.3. Evaluation

Photography, instrumental measurement, and replica preparation were performed after acclimation to conditions of 22°C (±2°C) temperature and 50% (±5%) humidity for 20 minutes or longer. Skin surface moisture was measured in the cheek using Corneometer® MPA580 (Courage + Khazaka Electronic GmbH, Germany). Transepidermal water loss was measured in the cheek using Tewameter® TM210 (Courage + Khazaka Electronic GmbH, Germany). Photographs were taken using Nikon D3X (Nikon, Japan), and the grade of wrinkles at the corners of the eyes was evaluated based on photographs by a dermatologist. The criteria of the wrinkle level are shown in **Table 2** [8].

Replicas were prepared from the corners of the eyes and cheek. Replica analysis was performed using ASA-03RXD (Asahi Bio-Rad, Japan), and the wrinkle area ratio was calculated by 2-dimensional parameter analysis [8].

## 2.4. Statistical Analysis

In statistical analysis of the grades of wrinkles evaluated by a dermatologist, the p-value was determined employing the Wilcoxon signed-rank test, followed by Bonferroni correction. For instrumental measurement and replica analysis, the p-value was determined employing the paired t-test, followed by Bonferroni correction. The significance level was set at 5% in both tests.

## 2.5. Ethics

An independent ethics committee was established, and the study was approved by this committee (Shinkoukai, Medical Corporation, Tokyo, Japan). The study was performed following the study protocol and ethical guide-

**Table 1.** Ingredients of the test product.

| INCI Name |
| --- |
| Water (Aqua) |
| Glycerin |
| PEG-32 |
| Cetyl-PG Hydroxyethyl Palmitamide |
| Dimethicone |
| Cetyl Alcohol |
| Glyceryl Behenate |
| Butylene Glycol |
| Allantoin |
| Phytosphingosine |
| Glutamic Acid |
| Polyquaternium-52 |
| *Zingiber officinale* (Ginger) Root Extract |
| *Eucalyptus globulus* Leaf Extract |
| Methylparaben |

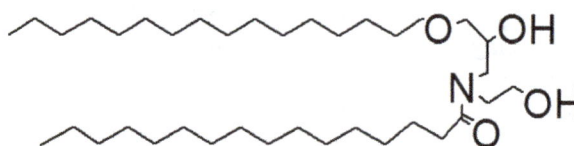

**Figure 1.** Chemical structure of pseudo-ceramide (Cetyl-PG Hydroxyethyl Palmitamide).

lines for clinical studies in conformity with ethical principles based on the Declaration of Helsinki.

# 3. Results

## 3.1. Subjects

Of Japanese female patients diagnosed by a dermatologist with very mild to mild AD based on the atopic dermatitis severity index, 22 patients aged 26 - 51 years (mean: 41 years old) with a specified wrinkle score (1 - 3) of the corners of the eyes who gave informed consent participated in the study (**Table 2**). **Table 3** shows the patients' background. Treatment was discontinued in one patient during the study period due to the development of erythema, scales, and lichenization at sites inconsistent with the region to which the test product had been applied, and this was assumed to be aggravation of AD. Accordingly, the final evaluation was made in 21 patients.

## 3.2. Grade of Wrinkles at the Corners of the Eyes

The grade of wrinkles was significantly improved compared with that at baseline at Weeks 4 and 9 after initiation of test product application (**Table 4**). Digital photographs of a markedly effective case are shown in **Figure 2**.

## 3.3. Analysis of Replicas of Wrinkles at the Corners of the Eyes

The wrinkle area ratio was significantly decreased from the baseline by the test product at Weeks 4 and 9 (**Table 5**).

**Table 2.** Criteria of wrinkle score.

| Grade | State of wrinkles |
|---|---|
| 0 | Wrinkles are absent |
| 1 | Only a few unclear shallow wrinkles are observed |
| 2 | A few clear shallow wrinkles are observed |
| 3 | Clear shallow wrinkles are observed |
| 4 | A few slightly deep wrinkles are observed among clear shallow wrinkles |
| 5 | Slightly deep wrinkles are observed |
| 6 | Clear deep wrinkles are observed |
| 7 | Markedly deep wrinkles are observed |

**Table 3.** Subjects' background.

| Number | Age | Gender | Severity of AD | Onset of AD | Treatment history for AD | Treatment for AD (current) | Complications |
|---|---|---|---|---|---|---|---|
| 001 | 29 | F | Very Mild | 3 yo | Outpatient treatment (external application) | No treatment | |
| 002 | 28 | F | Mild | 0 yo | Outpatient treatment (external application) | No treatment | Pollinosis |
| 003 | 41 | F | Very Mild | 3 yo | Outpatient treatment (external application) | No treatment | Allergic coryza |
| 004 | 43 | F | Mild | 10 yo | Outpatient treatment (external application) | No treatment | Pollinosis |
| 005 | 43 | F | Very Mild | 39 yo | Outpatient treatment (external application) | No treatment | |
| 006 | 40 | F | Mild | 5 yo | Outpatient treatment (external application) | No treatment | Pollinosis, allergic coryza |
| 007 | 43 | F | Very Mild | 10 yo | Outpatient treatment (external application) | No treatment | |
| 008 | 26 | F | Very Mild | 3 yo | Outpatient treatment (external and oral application) | Heparinoid lotion (except face) | |
| 009 | 39 | F | Very Mild | 5 yo | Outpatient treatment (external application) | No treatment | |
| 010 | 41 | F | Very Mild | 5 yo | Outpatient treatment (external application) | Tacrolims ointment (except face) | Pollinosis, contact dermatitis (metal) |
| 011 | 27 | F | Very Mild | 5 yo | Outpatient treatment (external application) | No treatment | Pollinosis |
| 012 | 38 | F | Very Mild | 33 yo | Outpatient treatment (external and orally application) | No treatment | |
| 013 | 48 | F | Very Mild | 35 yo | Outpatient treatment (external application) | No treatment | Allergic coryza |
| 014 | 34 | F | Very Mild | 7 yo | Outpatient treatment (external application) | No treatment | Pollinosis, allergic coryza |
| 015 | 51 | F | Very Mild | 25 yo | No treatment | No treatment | |
| 016 | 31 | F | Very Mild | 8 yo | Outpatient treatment (external application) | No treatment | Pollinosis, allergic coryza |
| 017 | 49 | F | Very Mild | 22 yo | Outpatient treatment (external application) | No treatment | Pollinosis |
| 018 | 41 | F | Mild | 9 yo | Outpatient treatment (external application) | No treatment | |
| 019 | 38 | F | Very Mild | 25 yo | No treatment | No treatment | Pollinosis, allergic coryza |
| 020 | 51 | F | Very Mild | 30 yo | Outpatient treatment (external and oral application) | No treatment | Pollinosis |
| 021 | 45 | F | Mild | 7 yo | Outpatient treatment (external and oral application) | No treatment | |
| 022 | 30 | F | Very Mild | 6 yo | Treatment history for AD | No treatment | |

**Table 4.** Changes in wrinkle score (crow's feet).

| | Mean of wrinkle score | Standard error | Statistical analysis |
|---|---|---|---|
| Baseline | 2.51 | 0.12 | |
| Week 4 | 2.39 | 0.12 | p < 0.05 (vs. baseline) |
| Week 9 | 2.38 | 0.12 | p < 0.05 (vs. baseline) |

The test product improved wrinkles at the corners of the eyes, and the wrinkle scores at Weeks 4 and 9 were significantly lower than at baseline (Wilcoxon signed-lank test followed by Bonferroni correction).

**Table 5.** Changes in wrinkle parameters on replica analysis (crow's feet).

|  | Mean of wrinkle area ratio | Standard error | Statistical analysis |
| --- | --- | --- | --- |
| Baseline | 4.18 | 0.53 |  |
| Week 4 | 3.36 | 0.44 | p < 0.05 (vs. baseline) |
| Week 9 | 3.16 | 0.42 | p < 0.05 (vs. baseline) |

Baseline         Week9

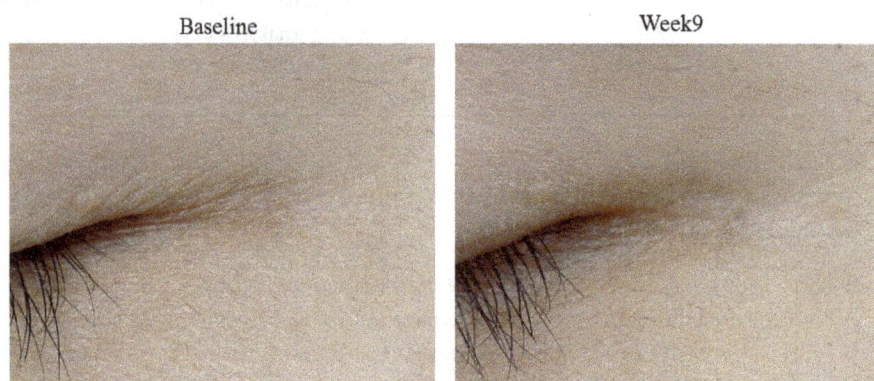

**Figure 2.** An improved case (crow's feet). Digital photographs of a case in which the 9-week use of the test product markedly improved wrinkles at the corners of the eyes.

Photographs of replicas of a markedly improved case are shown in **Figure 3**.

### 3.4. Analysis of Replicas of Wrinkles in the Cheek

The wrinkle area ratio was significantly decreased compared with that before test product application (**Table 6**). Photographs of replicas and digital photographs of the cheek of a markedly effective case are shown in **Figure 4** and **Figure 5**, respectively.

### 3.5. Skin Measurement

Changes in the skin surface moisture from that on the first day of application were analyzed over time. The mean values at Weeks 4 and 9 were significantly higher than at baseline (**Figure 6**). Changes in transepidermal water loss from that on the first day of application were also analyzed over time. The mean value at Week 9 was significantly decreased from the baseline (**Figure 7**).

## 4. Discussion

It has been clarified that wrinkles, a symptom of aging, are formed due to age-related changes in skin elasticity and the degeneration of dermal collagen and elastin, and ultraviolet light and cigarette smoking are involved factors [9] [10]. In photoaging induced by chronic exposure to ultraviolet light, induction of matrix metalloproteinases (MMPs) is enhanced, and accompanying degradation of extracellular matrix, such as collagen Types I and III and elastin, promotes wrinkle formation [11].

In aging, reduction of skin thickness and changes in tissue structure result in fine wrinkles and sagging of skin tissue. In addition, deformity with changes in elasticity induced by reduction of the water content in the stratum corneum is involved in the formation and aggravation of fine wrinkles, for which moisturizing products are widely used to improve wrinkles and smooth the skin surface [12] [13]. In skin with reduced barrier function, the IL-1RA/IL-1$\alpha$ level rises and increases IL-8 [14]. These inflammatory markers enhance MMP-1 and -9 production through the production of reactive oxygen species (ROS), and promote wrinkle formation induced by the degeneration of elastin and collagen [15].

Since dryness and reduced barrier function of the skin are among the causes of wrinkle formation, as described above, patients with skin diseases accompanied by dryness, such as AD, look older than their actual age, even though the severity is very mild with no skin eruption, which negatively influences the QOL of patients.

Baseline    Week4    Week9

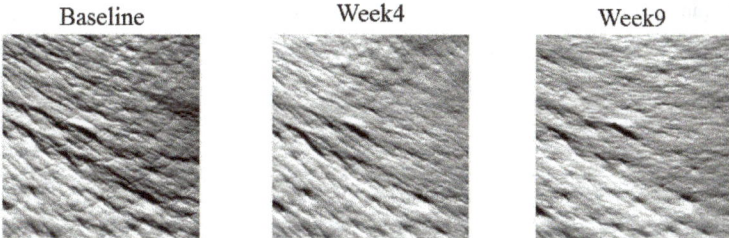

**Figure 3.** An improved case on replica photography (crow's feet). Replica photographs of a case in which the 9-week use of the test product markedly improved wrinkles at the corners of the eyes.

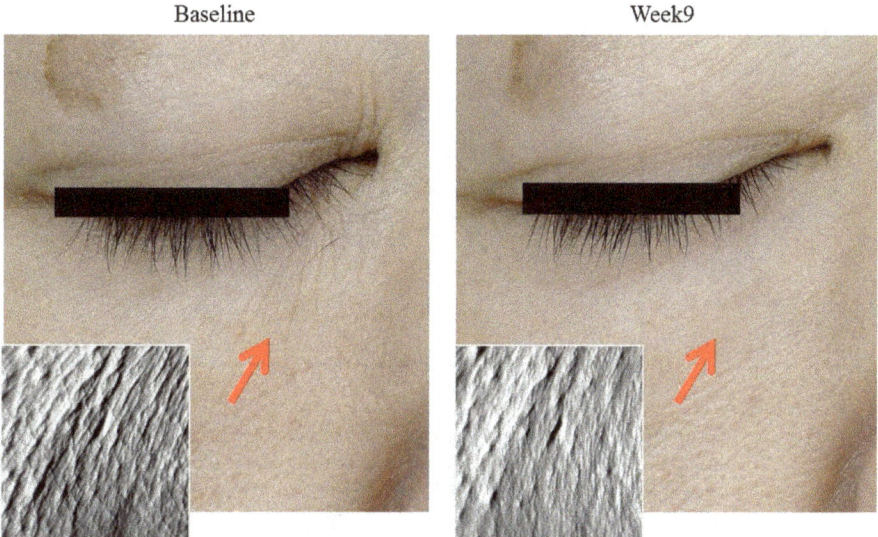

Baseline    Week9

**Figure 4.** An improved case on replica photography (lower eyelid). Replica photographs of wrikles in the lower eyelid markedly improved by the 9-week use of the test product.

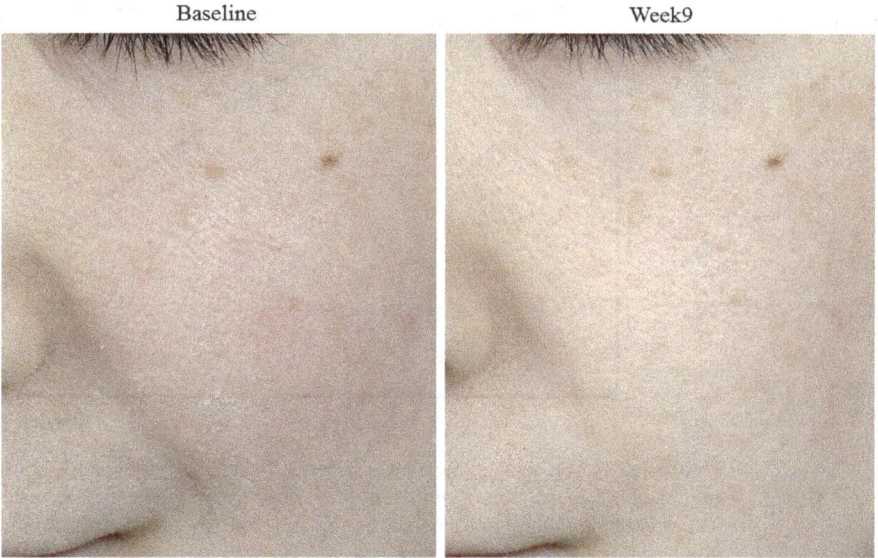

Baseline    Week9

**Figure 5.** Photographs of an improved case. Digital photographs of a case markedly improved by the 9-week use of the test product. Fine wrinkles in the lower eyelid and cheek, nasolabial folds, and scales were improved.

**Table 6.** Changes in wrinkle parameters on replica analysis (lower eyelid).

|  | Mean of wrinkle area ratio | Standard error | Statistical analysis |
|---|---|---|---|
| Baseline | 4.96 | 0.56 |  |
| Week 4 | 3.64 | 0.45 | $p < 0.05$ (vs. baseline) |
| Week 9 | 4.01 | 0.45 | $p < 0.05$ (vs. baseline) |

The wrinkle area ratios in the lower eyelid at Weeks 4 and 9 were significantly lower than at baseline on replica analysis (paired t-test followed by Bonferroni correction).

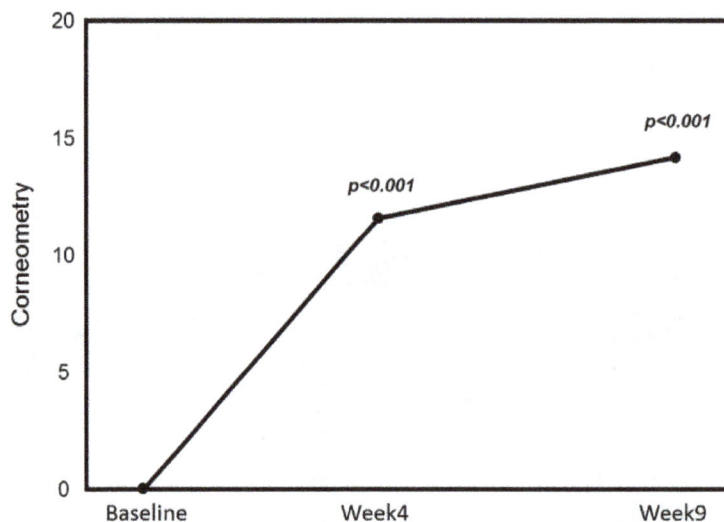

**Figure 6.** Changes in the cheek skin surface moisture. The cheek skin surface moisture was significantly increased at Weeks 4 and 9 compared with that at baseline ($^*$p < 0.05, $^{**}$p < 0.01, paired t-test followed by Bonferroni correction).

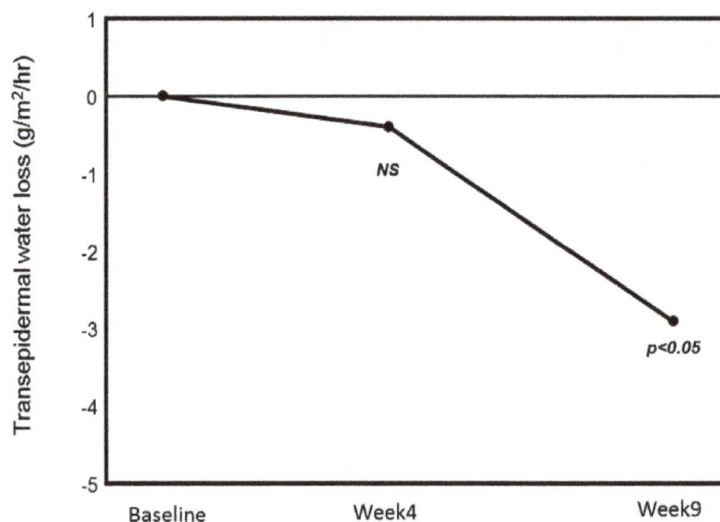

**Figure 7.** Changes in the cheek transepidermal water loss. The cheek transepidermal water loss was significantly decreased at Week 9 compared with that at baseline, improving the skin barrier function ($^*$p < 0.05, paired t-test followed by Bonferroni correction).

The symptom of dryness in AD is considered to be due to insufficient intercellular lipids, particularly ceramide, in the stratum corneum, which reduces the skin barrier function and water retention ability [2]. The efficacy of external use of ceramide preparation for AD has been reported, and improvement of the skin barrier function has been shown, in addition to improvement of the skin appearance, particularly dryness and scales [5]. Kawakita *et al.* discussed that skin elasticity is reduced in AD because the skin barrier function and water retention ability are low [16]. Therefore, dry fine lines may be readily formed even in non-lesional regions in AD patients. However, clinical evaluation of ceramide-formulated skincare products for fine lines and wrinkles in AD has not previously been reported. Thus, we investigated the efficacy of a skincare product containing lamellar-formulated pseudo-ceramide for facial fine lines and wrinkles in patients with very mild to mild AD.

Nine-week application of the product significantly improved the score of wrinkles at the corners of the eyes judged by a dermatologist compared with that at baseline, suggesting that the test product is effective for fine wrinkles in AD patients with reduced barrier function. Various factors are considered to be involved in the improvement of wrinkles. The skin surface moisture was significantly increased and the transepidermal water loss was significantly decreased compared with those at study initiation, suggesting that inhibition of dryness of the stratum corneum through increasing skin surface moisture and inhibiting transepidermal water loss is a cause of improvement of wrinkles. Ceramide plays an important role in the maintenance of barrier function and water retention in the stratum corneum and improvement of the skin barrier function and surface moisture by pseudo-ceramide-formulated preparation has been demonstrated [17] [18]. The pseudo-ceramide formulated in the test product also improved the skin barrier function in AD-induced dry skin measured using the transepidermal water loss and skin surface moisture, which may have smoothed the skin surface. The pseudo-ceramide was formulated in a lamellar structure in the test product, similarly to intercellular lipids in the stratum corneum, and water retention between the layers facilitates persistent high moisture, which may have been effective for fine lines in dry skin. In addition, improved barrier function may have inhibited skin inflammation, which may have reduced MMP production and prevented degeneration of the extracellular matrix, inhibiting wrinkle formation [6]. Kawada *et al.* performed a use test of a niacinamide-formulated skin care product for fine wrinkles in healthy skin, and discussed its efficacy and association with the improvement of skin surface moisture and barrier function [19]. Erol *et al.* reported that positively charged nano-sized emulsion of ceramide lipid improved surface moisture and elasticity of the skin with atopic dermatitis [20]. An increase in the skin surface moisture reduced the wrinkle area ratio in replicas in our study, supporting their discussion.

Adverse events occurred in 2 patients. One was very mild stinging due to the test product. Its remission was achieved by temporarily stopping application of the test product, and application could later be restarted. The other was the development of erythema, lichenization, and scales at sites inconsistent with the region to which the test product had been applied, and these were in remission by 7 days oral treatment (Tauromin®). Since AD exhibits repeated remission and aggravation, this episode may have been due to periodic variation of AD.

Since this was a non-comparative study, the results were limited. However, fine lines were improved on both subjective evaluation (expert grading) and objective measurement (replica analysis), suggesting that the test product exhibits a wrinkle-improving effect. Improvement of fine lines and wrinkles or anti-aging by a ceramide preparation has not previously been reported. This study suggested its potential as a material for novel anti-aging care. Since this test product is very safe, it may be used as an anti-aging product applicable for sensitive skin. To clarify the anti-fine lines effect of ceramide, it is necessary to perform a double-blind study by comparison with a control group.

## Acknowledgements

This study was supported financially by Kao Corporation (Tokyo, Japan). The authors would like to thank Dr. Numano, Dr. Taima, Ms. Kitajima, Mr. Takashima and Ms. Kanazawa for their assistance.

## References

[1] Ishikawa, J., Narita, H., Kondo, N., Hotta, M., Takagi, Y., Masukawa, Y., Kitahara, T., Takema, Y., Koyano, S., Yamazaki, S. and Hatamochi, A. (2010) Change in Ceramide Profile of Atopic Dermatitis Patients. *Journal of Investigative Dermatology*, **130**, 2511-2514. http://dx.doi.org/10.1038/jid.2010.161

[2] Loden, M., Olsson, H., Axell, T. and Linde, Y.M. (1992) Friction, Capacitance and Transepidermal Water Loss (TEWL) in Dry Atopic and Normal Skin. *British Journal of Dermatology*, **126**, 137-141. http://dx.doi.org/10.1111/j.1365-2133.1992.tb07810.x

[3] Jae, W.C., Soon, H.K., Chang, H.H., Kyoung, C.P. and Sang, W.Y. (2013) The Influence of Skin Visco-Elasticity,

Hydration Level and Aging on the Formation of Wrinkles: A Comprehensive and Objective Approach. *Skin Research and Technology*, **19**, e349-e355. http://dx.doi.org/10.1111/j.1600-0846.2012.00650.x

[4]   Juliane, H., Elisabrth, V., Florian, K. and Johannes, R. (2000) Biophysical Characteristics of Healthy Skin and Nonlesional Slin in Atopic Dermatitis: Short-Term Effects of Ultraviolet A and B Irradiation. *Skin Pharmacology and Applied Skin Physiology*, **13**, 174-181. http://dx.doi.org/10.1159/000029923

[5]   Chamlin, S.L., Kao, J., Freiden, I.J., Sheu, M.Y., Fowler, A.J., Fluhr, J.W., Williams, M.L. and Elias, P.M. (2002) Ceramide Dominant Barrier Repair Lipids Alleviate Childhood Atopic Dermatitis: Changes in Barrier Function Provide a Sensitive Indicator of Disease Activity. *Journal of the American Academy of Dermatology*, **47**, 198-208. http://dx.doi.org/10.1067/mjd.2002.124617

[6]   Iwai, H., Fukasawa, J. and Suzuki, T. (1998) A Liquid Crystal Application in Skin Care Cosmetics. *International Journal of Cosmetic Science*, **20**, 87-102. http://dx.doi.org/10.1046/j.1467-2494.1998.171741.x

[7]   Imokawa, G., Akasaki, S., Kawamata, A., Yano, S. and Takaishi, N. (1989) Water-Retaining Function in the Stratum Cornium and Its Recovery Properties by Synthetic Pseudo-Ceramides. *Journal of the Society of Cosmetic Chemists*, **40**, 273-285.

[8]   Task Force Committee for Evaluation of Anti-Aging Function (2007) Guideline for Evaluation of Anti-Wrinkle Products. *J Japanese Cosmet Sci Soc*, **31**, 411-431.

[9]   Leveque, J.L. (1999) EEMCO Guidance for the Assessment of Skin Topography. *Journal of the European Academy of Dermatology and Venereology*, **12**, 103-114.

[10]  Tsuji, N., Moriwaki, S., Suzuki, Y., Takema, Y. and Imokawa, G. (2001) The Role of Elastases Secreted by Fibroblasts in Wrinkle Formation: Implication through Selective Inhibition of Elastase Activity. *Photochemistry and Photobiology*, **74**, 283-290. http://dx.doi.org/10.1562/0031-8655(2001)074<0283:TROESB>2.0.CO;2

[11]  Yin, L., Morita, A. and Tsuji, T. (2001) Skin Ageing Induced by Ultraviolet Exposure and Tabacco Smoking: Evidence from Epidermiological and Molecular Studies. *Photodermatology, Photoimmunology and Photomedicine*, **17**, 178-183. http://dx.doi.org/10.1034/j.1600-0781.2001.170407.x

[12]  Krutmann, J. and Glichrest, B.A. (2006) Photoaging of Skin. In: Glichrest, B.A. and Krutmann, J., Ed., *Skin Aging*, Springer, Heiderberg, 33-43.

[13]  Jae, W.C., Soon, H.K., Chang, H.H., Kyoung, C.P. and Sang, W.Y. (2013) The Influence of Skin Visco-Elasticity, Hydration Level and Aging on the Formation of Wrinkles: A Comprehensive and Objective Approach. *Skin Research and Technology*, **19**, e349-e355. http://dx.doi.org/10.1111/j.1600-0846.2012.00650.x

[14]  Katherine, N. and Ellen, M. (2012) Moisturizers: Reality and the Skin Benefits. *Dermatology and Therapy*, **25**, 229-233. http://dx.doi.org/10.1111/j.1529-8019.2012.01504.x

[15]  Jongh, C.M., Verberk, M.M., Withagen, C.E.T., Jacobs, J.J.L., Rustemeyer, T. and Kezic, S. (2006) Stratum Cornium Cytokines and Skin Irritation Response to Sodium Lauryl Sulfate. *Contact Dermatitis*, **54**, 325-333. http://dx.doi.org/10.1111/j.0105-1873.2006.00848.x

[16]  Shin, M.H., Rhie, G., Kim, Y.K., Park, C.H., Cho, K.H., Kim, K.H., Eun, H.C. and Chung, J.H. (2005) $H_2O_2$ Accumulating by Catalase Reduction Changes MAP Kinase Signaling in Aged Human Skin *in Vivo*. *Journal of Investigative Dermatology*, **125**, 221-229.

[17]  Kawakita, T., Takano, Y., Asano-Kato, N., Tanaka, M., Dogru, M., Goto, E., Tsubota, K., Takahashi, S., Fukagawa, K. and Fujishima, H. (2004) Quantitative Evaluation of Eyelid Elasticity Using the Cutometer SEM575 and Its Clinical Application in Assessing the Efficacy of Tacrolimus Ointment Treatment in eyelid Atopic Dermatitis. *Cornea*, **23**, 468-471. http://dx.doi.org/10.1097/01.ico.0000116521.57227.4c

[18]  Elias, P.M. (1983) Epidermal Lipids, Barrier Function and Desquamation. *Journal of Investigative Dermatology*, **80**, 44s-49s. http://dx.doi.org/10.1038/jid.1983.12

[19]  Leon, K., Firas, H. and Joseph, B. (2013) Atopic Dermatitis, and the Role of Ceramide-Dominant, Physiologic Lipid-Based Barrier Repair Emulsion. *Journal of Drugs in Dermatology*, **12**, 1024-1027.

[20]  Kawada, A., Konishi, N., Oiso, N., Kawara, S. and Date, A. (2008) Evaluation of Anti-Wrinkle Effects of a Novel Cosmetic Containing Niacinamide. *The Journal of Dermatology*, **35**, 637-642. http://dx.doi.org/10.1111/j.1346-8138.2008.00537.x

[21]  Erol, Y. and Hans-Hubert, B. (2006) Effect of Lipid-Containing, Positively Charged Nanoemulsions on Skin Hydration, Elasticity and Erythema—An *in Vivo* Study. *International Journal of Pharmaceutics*, **307**, 232-238. http://dx.doi.org/10.1016/j.ijpharm.2005.10.002

# 7

# Depressed Acne Scars—Effective, Minimal Downtime Treatment with a Novel Smooth Motion Non-Insulated Microneedle Radiofrequency Technology

Yoram Harth[1,2*], Monica Elman[3], Einat Ackerman[2], Ido Frank[2]

[1]Medical OR Center, Herzlya, Israel
[2]EndyMed Medical, Caesarea, Israel
[3]Beit Harofeim, Holon, Israel
Email: [*]skin58@gmail.com

## Abstract

Background: The microneedle fractional RF handpiece used in our study (Intensif Handpiece, EndyMed Medical, Caesarea, Israel) is a novel handpiece that uses a tip with 25 non-insulated, gold plated microneedle electrodes. The needles are inserted into the skin by a specially designed electronically controlled, smooth motion motor minimizing patient discomfort. RF emission delivered over the whole dermal portion of the needle allows effective coagulation resulting in minimal or no bleeding, together with bulk volumetric heating. Study Design/Materials and Methods: The study included 20 patients, treated for depressed acne scars using the Intensif™ Microneedles handpiece (EndyMed PRO Platform System, EndyMed Medical, Caesarea, Israel). The degree of clinical improvement was assessed by the global aesthetic improvement scale (GAIS) and subjects satisfaction by post treatment questionnaires. Results: The number of treatments per patient varied between 1 and 6 (average 3.3 treatments per patient). Eleven patients (55%) reported none to minimal pain, six (30%) moderate discomfort and only three (15%) reported significant pain. Objective evaluation of the improvement by a board certified dermatologist showed improvement in 95% of patients. 25% showed excellent improvement, 50% experienced good improvement, and the 20% showed minimal improvement. One patient showed no improvement. Conclusions: The presented results show that the tested electronically controlled motorized insertion, non-insulated microneedle treatment technology provides a minimal discomfort, minimal downtime, effective and safe treatment for depressed acne scars.

---

[*]Corresponding author.

## Keywords

**Microneedles, Radio-Frequency, Acne Scars, RF, Multisource, Fractional Lasers, Non-Insulated**

## 1. Introduction

Acne scars are one of the most difficult disorders to treat in aesthetic dermatology. Depressed acne scars are divided into 3 categories: boxcar, ice pick and rolling scars. The pathogenesis of the scars relates most probably to thickened bands of collagen under the scars causing a retraction of skin surface. Based on the study of Zheng *et al.* that found that depressed scars may reach a depth of 0.7 mm; an effective treatment will have to reach further into the depth to remodel the retracting collagen fibers under the scar [1]. Based on these findings we may assume that the optimal treatment system for atrophic depressed scars will need to have deep volumetric dermal heating for collagen remodeling in the dermis up to at least 2.5 or 3 mm, and the ability to mechanical disrupt the dystrophic scar tissue. For the patient we will need to allow minimal discomfort, minimal downtime and minimal post treatment side effects.

Fractional ablative or non-ablative lasers are used for minimally invasive treatment of depressed. Ong *et al.* published an extensive review on these lasers found in different studied improvement range of 26 - 83 percent for ablative fractional lasers and lower (26% - 50%) for the non-ablative fractional lasers [2].

Although minimally invasive, the treatment of acne scars with fractional lasers, was accompanied by significant downtime and pain; causing prolonged erythema for up to 11.5 days after ablative fractional laser treatment and up to 7.5 days after fractional non-ablative laser treatment. Pain levels were (5.9 - 8.1) for ablative and (3.9 - 5.6) for non-ablative (on the pain scale of 10). Post inflammatory hyperpigmentation (PIH) incidence was also significant; 0% - 93% (for up to 6 months) after ablative fractional laser treatment and 0% - 13% (for up to 7.5 days) after the non-ablative fractional laser treatment.

Radiofrequency (RF) is non-ionizing electromagnetic radiation used in medicine for nearly 100 years. In contrast to most lasers that target specific chromophores, RF is chromophore-independent and has better penetration to the dermis and hypodermis as compared to light based technologies. Clinical treatment systems using radiofrequency energy (RF) were proven in the last decade to be safe and effective for both non-ablative skin tightening of the face and body, and fractional RF skin resurfacing for skin [3]-[5].

The first generation of microneedle RF delivery technology used insulated needles for skin rejuvenation and acne scars with promising results. These microneedles allowed the heating of small volume of tissue near their needle tip while the rest of the needle was insulated. With these needles the energy flows only through the tip of the needle, resulting in a small coagulated sphere-like shape in the dermis. These devices have several disadvantages, including micro-bleeding during the treatment and the need to perform several passes on the skin at different depths to affect the entire the dermis [5] [6].

Cho *et al.* described treatment of atrophic acne scars with insulated microneedle radiofrequency devices [6]. These authors used needles in which the entire needle electrode is nonconductive expect the tip, (beginning 0.3 mm from the distal end) inserted to a maximum depth of 2 mm. They reported reduction of large pores in 70% of the patients treated. Skin surface roughness, dermal density, and microscopic and composite images also improved, whereas TEWL and sebum measurement did not change. Eight weeks after two sessions of treatment, the grade of acne scars improved in 22 patients (73.3%), did not change in seven (23.3%), and became aggravated in one (3.3%). The mean duration of visible erythema after treatment was 7.8 ± 2.6 days. Pain persisted for longer than 1 day in 10 patients (33.3%) and for longer than 3 days in five (16.7%). Folliculitis was observed in two patients (6.7%).

The microneedle fractional RF handpiece used in our study (Intensif Handpiece, EndyMed Medical, Caesarea, Israel) is a novel FDA cleared handpiece that uses a sterile treatment tip with 25 non-insulated gold plated microneedle electrodes (max diameter of 300 micron at their base gradually tapered to an extra sharp edge) (**Figure 1**). Penetration depth is up to 3.5 millimeter with digitally controlled increments of 0.1 mm. Maximal power is 25 Watts with a maximal pulse duration is 200 milliseconds [7]. The needles are inserted into the skin by a specially designed, electronically controlled, smooth motion motor minimizing patient discomfort. When the needles reach the pre-defined insertion depth the RF is emitted selectively heating the dermis while sparing the epidermis. The difference in electrical impedance between the epidermis (high impedance) and the dermis (low

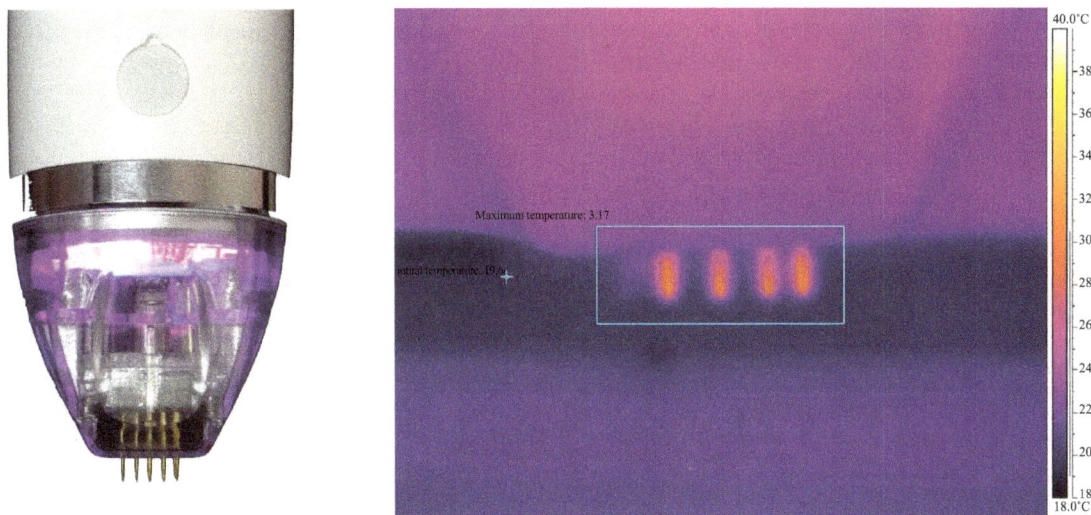

**Figure 1.** Left: EndyMed's Intensif Handpiece. Right: Thermal image of a treatment of laboratory skin model with impedance similar to dermal impedance (Flir Systems, ThermaCAM SC 640).

impedance) further increase selectivity—enhancing RF flow through the dermis. The RF emission delivered over the whole dermal portion of the needle allows effective coagulation resulting in minimal or no bleeding, combined with deep dermal heating.

## 2. Study Design/Materials and Methods

The study included 20 patients treated by two board certified dermatologists for depressed acne scars. We used the EndyMed PRO platform system (EndyMed medical, Caesarea, Israel) equipped with the Intensif™ microneedle RF handpiece. Topical anesthetic cream was applied to the patient skin for 40 minutes before the fractional microneedle RF treatments. The microneedle RF collagen remodeling treatments were performed once a month, (1 to 5 sessions). Patients were photographed by a professional photography assessment system (Fotofinder Systems, Germany and Reveal Imager, Canfield Imaging systems, USA).

The degree of clinical improvement was then given a global aesthetic improvement scale for each patient by the investigator assigning an overall value for reduction in number of scars, reduction in depth of scars and improvement of color uniformity. Excellent improvement (defined as >75% improvement), very good improvement (defined as 51% - 75% improvement), good improvement (defined as 26% - 50% improvement), minimal improvement (defined as 5% - 25% improvement), and no improvement (<5%).

The score was calculated based on blinded comparative analysis of baseline picture and post treatment photographs.

Subjects' satisfaction was assessed by questionnaires that included specific questions about the treatment discomfort and downtime. Subjective assessment of was categorized to excellent, good to very good, moderate to good or none to minimal.

## 3. Results

Twenty patients, fifteen females and five males were included in the study. Treatment was performed by two different board certified dermatologist. Fitzpatrick's skin type was II-2 patients, III-11 patients, IV-5 patients and V-2 patients. Mean age was $32.6 \pm 11.9$ years. Number of treatments varied between one and six, with an average of 3.3 treatments per patient.

Eleven patients (55%) reported none to minimal pain, six (30%) moderate discomfort and only 3 (15%) reported significant pain.

When asked about subjective improvement 19 out of 20 patients (95%) of the treated patients experienced some improvement. 25% experienced very good to excellent improvement (defined as >50% improvement) additional 30% experienced good improvement (defined as 26% - 50% improvement) and the rest reported some improvement (up to 25%). Only one patient did not notice any improvement.

Regarding downtime: 80% of patient reported mild erythema for less than 48 hours (50% percent reported an erythema of a few hours; an additional 30% reported erythema of 1 - 2 days). The rest 20% reported erythema of 72 hours. Edema subsided in less than 24 hours for all patients.

Eighty percent of patients didn't have micro crusts or had a minimal number (up to 5). Twenty percent reported moderate number of visible micro crusts that disappeared in 4 - 5 days. Ninety percent of patients were back to normal activities in less than 48 hours. 65% in less than 24 hours, 25% needed 48 hours and 10 percent needed 72 hours.

No adverse events occurred during the treatments.

Seventy percent of patients said they would recommend the treatment to their friends 25% were not sure and only one patient (5%) said he would not recommend the treatment. Improvement in acne scars was noted starting at 4 weeks after the first treatment improving to a maximum at 3 months follow-up.

Objective evaluation of the improvement by a board certified dermatologist showed improvement in 95% of patients. 25% showed excellent improvement (defined as >75% improvement) additional 50% experienced good improvement (defined as 26% - 50% improvement) and the 20% showed minimal improvement. One patient showed no improvement. None of the patients experienced worsening in their skin condition (**Figures 2-5**).

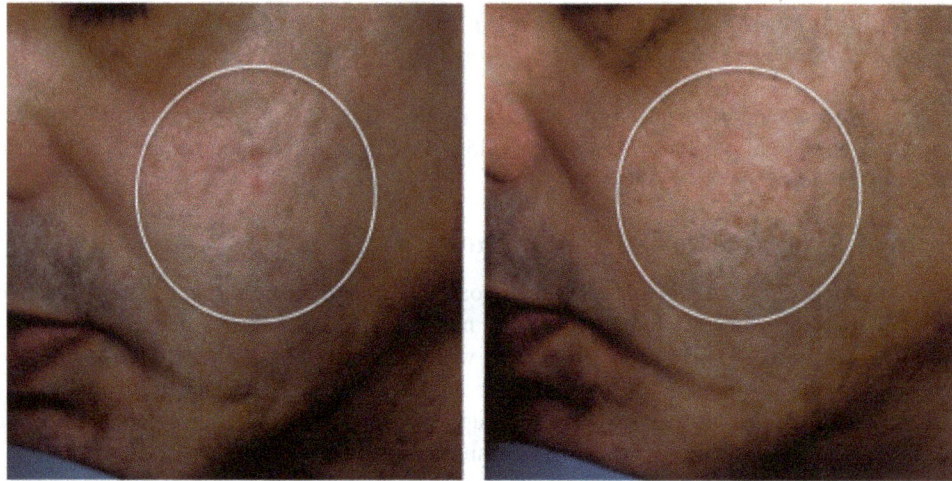

**Figure 2.** Left: Baseline. Right: One month after three microneedle RF treatments sessions. Significant decrease in the depth of the scars and general texture improvement.

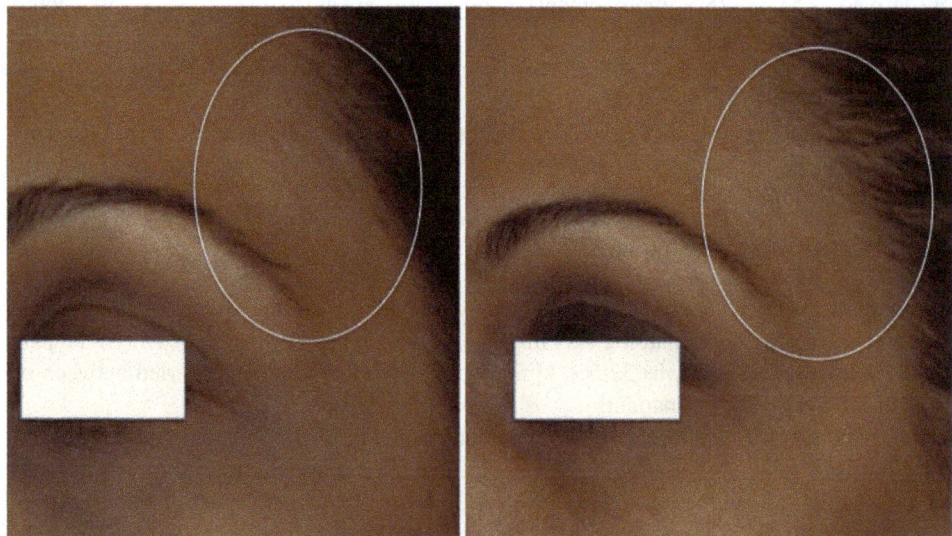

**Figure 3.** Left: Baseline. Right: One month after three microneedle RF treatments sessions. Significant reduction in the number and depth of the scars, with general texture improvement.

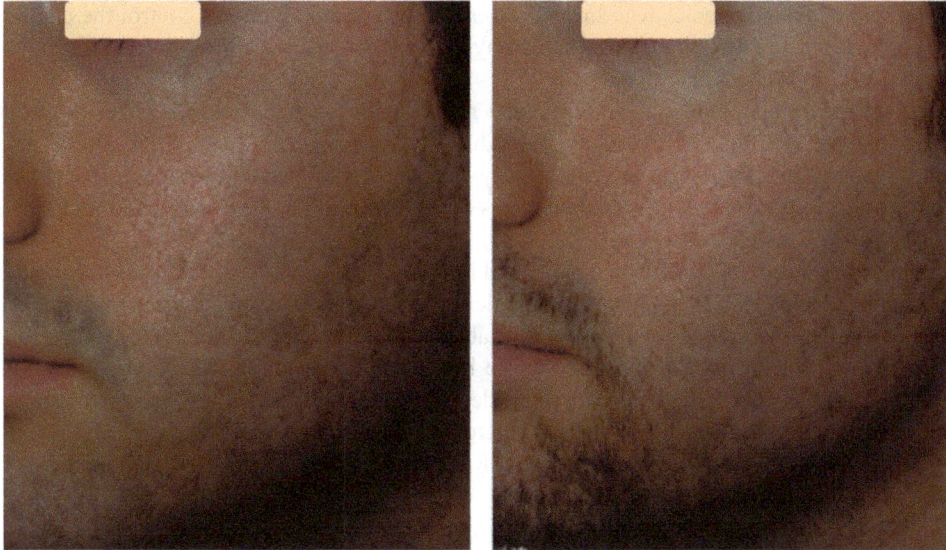

**Figure 4.** Left: Baseline. Right: One month after two microneedle RF treatments sessions. Significant texture improvement with decrease in the depth and number of atrophic and ice pick scars.

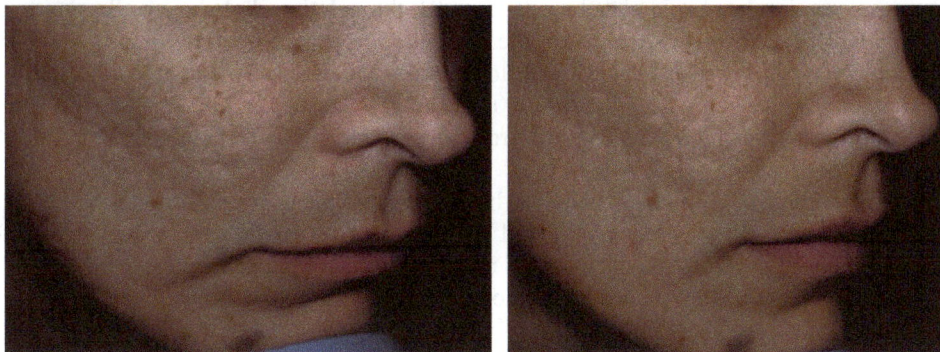

**Figure 5.** Left: Baseline. Right: One month after two microneedle RF treatments sessions. Decrease in the number and depth of the scars.

## 4. Discussion

The current study as a few previous studies proves the efficacy and safety of the microneedles radiofrequency technology in the treatment of depressed acne scars. The efficacy seem to be in the same effectiveness range of ablative fractional lasers and somewhat higher than the non-ablative fractional lasers.

This difference can be explained by considerable higher skin penetration of the microneedles (up to 3.5 mm) vs lower penetration of fractional lasers (up to 0.7 mm) and the additional benefit of the mechanical scar disruption.

Based on recent reviews ablative fractional laser are usually associated with longer post treatment erythema and higher percentage of post inflammatory hyperpigmentation as compared to microneedle RF treatment. Pain is also more significant in ablative and non-ablative fractional lasers than in microneedle RF treatments. This fact may be explained by the ability to use topical anesthesia in microneedles RF treatments. (Not possible for some of the fractional laser procedures.)

Microneedle RF handpieces can be differentiated based on two main features. First is the mode of insertion into the skin (Fixed needles inserted manually, needles inserted mechanically using a "spring" and the latest generation using electronically controlled motorized gradual insertion). Second important differentiating feature involves the needle quality basically the sharpness and coating material.

Our study shows that motorized electronically controlled smooth insertion of the needles allows a minimal pain and downtime procedure with minimal unnecessary trauma to the epidermis and no bleeding. Unlike technologies that use fixed needles with manual insertion, where the user can't control the depth of penetration, the accurate predefined penetration depth enabled by the Intensif system, allows precise treatment for different skin thickness with high safety and efficacy.

Our data show comparable or better clinical results with lower pain level, lower downtime and lower PIH level as compared to fractional ablative or non-ablative lasers [3].

The advantage in efficacy can be explained by considerable higher skin penetration of the microneedles (up to 3.5 mm) vs lower penetration of fractional lasers (up to 0.7 mm) and the mechanical scar disruption effect of the microneedle RF devices.

The lower incidence of PIH may be explained by the difference in physical effects of light and RF. Long term PIH is believed to be caused by damage to the dermo-epidermal junction and dropping of melanin to the dermis. By definition the fractional lasers coagulate or ablate the epidermis with thermal damage to the dermal epidermal junction and upper part of the dermis. We hypothesize that the non-thermal penetration of the epidermis with the smooth motion, extra sharp microneedle is less traumatic to the epidermis and epidermal dermal junction leading to a decreased chance of PIH in microneedle RF treatments.

The reduced pain experience in microneedle RF treatment may be related to sharpness of the needles and the unique smooth needle motorized insertion.

The clinical efficacy of insulated needles is limited by the small volume of heat produced through the small non-insulated part near the tip and significant micro-bleeding through the treatment.

We believe that the use of gold plated non-insulated needles allows multiple clinical advantages over insulated and stainless still needles. In contrast to the insulated needles that emit RF through a small area near their tip the novel non-insulated gold plated needle emit RF through the whole length allowing heating of 3× the volume. While RF is delivered when the needle is inserted to its maximal penetration and dermal impedance is lower than epidermal impedance the RF will flow through the dermis with no epidermal coagulation.

Gold plating allows better RF conductivity than stainless needles and thus better treatment efficacy. In addition, RF emission through the whole needle provides a coagulation effect eliminating micro-bleeding improving the patient experience.

Fixed microneedle RF treatment handpiece have a few disadvantages. Insertion in the skin is manual and thus more uncontrolled and more traumatic. Fixed length of needles would lead to the use of a few tip per patient which will be more costly to the doctor. This may lead to increased pain and risk of PIH. Digitally controlling the penetration depth of the needles with automatic motorized insertion allows better control of patient experience reducing discomfort and side effects.

## 5. Conclusion

This recently introduced FDA cleared non-insulated fractional RF treatment system allows controlled heating to a pre-defined depth of the dermis without epidermal coagulation. This eliminates most of the micro crusting, reduces the risk of post-inflammatory hyperpigmentation associated with epidermal injury, and allows return to normal routine after 24 hours or less. A specially designed smooth motion electronically controlled motor assures minimal trauma to the epidermis and significantly decreases discomfort to the patient. The presented results show that microneedle RF technology with electronically controlled smooth insertion motor and non-insulated gold plated needles is a safe and effective treatment option for atrophic acne scars, providing a minimally invasive, minimal discomfort and minimal downtime for all skin types. This study shows high objective and subjective satisfaction rates with minimal downtime or adverse effects.

## References

[1]   Zheng, Z., Goo, B., et al. (2014) Histometric Analysis of Skin-Radiofrequency Interaction Using a Fractionated Microneedle Delivery System. Dermatologic Surgery, 40, 134-141. http://dx.doi.org/10.1111/dsu.12411

[2]   Elsaie, M.L., Choudhary, S., Leiva, A. and Nouri, K. (2010) Nonablative Radiofrequency for Skin Rejuvenation. Dermatologic Surgery, 36, 577-589. http://dx.doi.org/10.1111/j.1524-4725.2010.01510.x

[3]   Ong, M.W. and Bashir, S.J. (2012) Fractional Laser Resurfacing for Acne Scars: A Review. British Journal of Dermatology, 166, 1160-1169. http://dx.doi.org/10.1111/j.1365-2133.2012.10870.x

[4]   De la Torre, J.R., Moreno-Moraga, J., Muñoz, E. and Navarro, P.C. (2011) Multisource, Phase-Controlled Radiofrequency for Treatment of Skin Laxity: Correlation between Clinical and In-Vivo Confocal Microscopy Results and

Real-Time Thermal Changes Multisource, Phase-Controlled Radiofrequency for Treatment of Skin Laxity: Correlation between Clinical and *In-Vivo* Confocal Microscopy Results and Real-Time Thermal Changes. *Journal of Clinical and Aesthetic Dermatology*, **4**, 28-35.

[5]  Elman, M. and Harth, Y. (2011) Novel Multi-Source Phase-Controlled Radiofrequency Technology for Nonablative and Micro-Ablative Treatment of Wrinkles, Lax Skin and Acne Scars. *Laser Therapy*, **20**, 139-144. http://dx.doi.org/10.5978/islsm.20.139

[6]  Cho, S.I., Chung, B.Y., *et al.* (2012) Evaluation of the Clinical Efficacy of Fractional Radiofrequency Microneedle Treatment in Acne Scars and Large Facial Pores. *Dermatologic Surgery*, **38**, 1017-1024. http://dx.doi.org/10.1111/j.1524-4725.2012.02402.x

[7]  Harth, Y. and Frank, I. (2013) *In Vivo* Histological Evaluation of Non-Insulated Microneedle Radiofrequency Applicator with Novel Fractionated Pulse Mode. *Journal of Drugs in Dermatology*, **12**, 1430-1433.

# 8

# Frictional Melanosis of Rubbing Thighs in Iraqi Patients

Khalifa E. Sharquie*, Adil A. Noaimi, Attaa A. Hajji

Department of Dermatology and Venereology, Baghdad Teaching Hospital, Baghdad, Iraq
Email: *ksharquie@ymail.com, adilnoaimi@yahoo.com, attaa.alhaji2@yahoo.com

## Abstract

Background: Frictional melanosis of rubbing inner thighs is a common problem among Iraqi females causing great psychological and cosmetic impact. It might simulate lifa disease but it is a different entity. It is unfortunately not reported in the medical literatures although commonly encountered in daily clinical practice. Objective: To evaluate the hyperpigmentation of inner aspects of thighs in Iraqi females as an isolated pigmentary problem. Patient and Methods: Sixty patients with frictional melanosis of rubbing thighs were seen in Department of Dermatology, Baghdad Teaching Hospital in this case descriptive, clinical and histopathological study, during the period from April 2011 to March 2012. Any associated skin problems were also noticed like folliculitis and boils at area of friction. Forty individuals were enrolled in the present work as the healthy control group. The pigmentation was assessed by clinical, Wood's light and histopathological examinations (H&E and Fontana stains). Body mass index was obtained for all patients and obesity was graded according to WHO recommendations. Results: The ages of patients ranged between 19 - 52 (32.86 ± 7.65) years, with 59 (98.3%) females and 1 (1.6%) male. By Wood's light examination, accentuation in pigmentation was observed in 39 (58%) patients, while 21 (42%) of lesions showed no change. Body mass index was ranged from 23.3 - 43.6 (34.04 ± 4.13), history of vigorous rubbing of pigmented area with washing tool (lifa) was positive in 46 (76.6%) patients. Skin biopsies in 10 patients showed pure dermal melanophages in 3 of biopsies with slight melanosis of basal layer of epidermis, while the other 7 biopsies showed mainly increase in basal melanin. There was a statistically significant association between obesity and the severity of pigmentation of the inner thighs. Forty control individuals (2 males and 38 females) were assessed, their ages ranged from 19 - 50 (31.72 ± 6.40) years. All females were within normal weight while males were overweight and BMI was ranged from 19.7 - 28.2 (22.49 ± 1.84). All control individuals showed no pigmentation of inner aspects of thighs. Conclusion: Frictional melanosis of rubbing thighs is considered a new entity which had been not reported before in the medical literatures. This is a disease of mostly

---

*Corresponding author.

**young obese females and the effective therapy is weight reduction and possibly liposuction.**

## Keywords

**Frictional Melanosis, Rubbing Thighs, Iraqi Patients**

## 1. Introduction

Melanosis is a major health problem among people with dark complexion and is well demonstrated in a form of facial melanosis, which could be caused by melasma (epidermal and dermal), gazelle eyes like facial melanosis, frictional melanosis, post inflammatory hyperpigmentation especially following lichen planus [1].

Melanosis could be also seen in any part of the body like in lifa disease; described in Iraq by Sharquie, 1993, as a new distinctive condition that followed chronic rubbing and friction with a lifa as washing agent. The distribution of the rash is very characteristic as it is only located over bony prominences [2]. All patients are slim, and using a washing agent (lifa) vigorously during bathing. The lesions are macular, symmetrically distributed with a positive family history of the same problem in 10% of patients [2].

Sharquie, speculated that the mechanism of pigmentation is due to repeated damage to the basal cell layer as a result of squeezing of the epidermis between the underlying bone and the offending wash brush (lifa), that is why the main histopathological picture shows many melanophages in the papillary dermis [3] [4]. Wood's light examination confirms that the melanosis is mainly dermal [2] [4].

Lifa disease could be considered as a variant of macular amyliodosis, as it was found that amyloid deposits were detected in about 10% of the biopsied cases [2] plus the following features:

1) Macular amyloidosis is a common condition among Asian and Middle Eastern people, including Iraqis especially females [5]-[11].

2) The features of pigmentation are similar in both macular amyloidosis and lifa disease. Sometimes might be a combination of both of them in the same patient [12].

3) The histopathology of both conditions consists of dermal melanosis [5] [12] [13].

4) Amyloid deposition could be seen in both diseases but more commonly in macular amyloidosis. Even in the latter, the amyloid deposition might be so small that examination of repeated biopsies and multiple sections is necessary for its detection [12].

Similar pigmentation has been described following chronic rubbing or friction in Japan [8] [10] [13]-[19], India [9] [20] [21], Jordan [3], Italy [22] [23], Oman [24], Israel [25], and UK [26].

Friction is also might be suggested as important cause of melanosis in medial aspects of thighs, although acanthosis nigricans (AN) might attribute to pigmentation of thighs which is the only hyperpigmentary state that is connected to clinical or subclinical insulin resistance and obesity, but hyperpigmentation in this condition is attributed to hyperkeratosis rather than to a mild increase in melanin pigmentation [27]. On contrary, two Iraqi studies of acanthosis nigricans demonstrated basilar hypermelanosis and dermal melanophages [28] [29]. There are no studies in the medical literature related pigmentation of rubbing thighs although there is only single report that described frictional hyperpigmentation on the inner aspects of the thighs and under bra straps as cutaneous manifestations of obesity [30].

Also in post inflammatory hyperpigmentation, pigment might follow injuries like burns, friction [31] and also after recurrent bouts of intertrigo which is a common cutaneous manifestation of obesity [32].

Darkly pigmented individuals are particularly prone to developing this form of hypermelanosis and it is of a greater magnitude, and persists longer [31] [33].

All patients with pigmentary disorders of the skin should be completely undressed and examined fully under both visible and Wood's light [34]. The visual assessment remains one of the "gold standard" methods in the diagnosis and assessment of skin color [29]. Histopathological studies with Hematoxylline and Eosien and other special stains like Fontana masson can assess both presence of melanin and precise site of deposition whether epidermal, dermal or mixed [34].

So, the aim of the present study is to do full clinical and histopathological evaluation and to be differentiated from other frictional melanoses.

## 2. Patients and Methods

This case descriptive clinical and histopathological study was carried out in Department of Dermatology and Venereology, Baghdad Teaching Hospital during the period between April 2011 to March 2012. Sixty patients with hypermelanosis of inner aspects of thighs were included in this study.

Patients with the following conditions were excluded from this study: pregnant females, patients with hyperpigmentation of other flexural areas, skin tags, patients with systemic diseases or using of systemic drugs which could be associated with hyperpigmentation (like oral contraceptive pills), and those with history of using topical treatment within the last 6 months before presentation. No patients with underling diabetes, hypertension or other important medical conditions were noted.

History regarding the following points: age, gender, job, types of usually wearied clothes, duration, associated symptoms and aggravating factors, history of dermatitis (intertrigo), history of rubbing of pigmented skin by any tool, parity, familial history of atopic dermatitis and similar problem (hyperpigmentation of inner aspects of thighs). Thorough clinical examination done, weight and BMI was obtained for all the patients and obesity was graded as in **Table 1**, type of skin according to Fitzpatrick's skin typing.

The pigmentation was assessed by clinical examination regarding exact site, pattern of pigmentation (rippled or confluent), extension of pigmentation away from the area of contact between the two thighs, and associated cutaneous problems (like folliculitis) wasn't mentioned by the patient as a complaint.

*The pigmentation was graded as follows*:

Grade I: Light brown.

Grade II: Dark brown.

Grade III: Bluish (nearly black).

Wood's light was used as an important tool to assess the depth of pigment whether epidermal, dermal or mixed.

Formal consent was taken from all patients after full explanation to the patient about the goal of the present work, nature of disease course and possible modality of treatment. Also, ethical approval was performed by the Scientific Council of Dermatology & Venereology-Arab Board for Medical Specializations.

Photographs were taken for each patient using Sony Cyper-Shot 6.0 Mega pixels camera in the same place and under good illumination in order to reassess pigmentation.

Laboratory investigations were done for female patients including hormonal assays: follicular stimulating hormone (FSH), luteinizing hormone (LH), (LH/FSH ratio) and serum free testosterone, in addition to pelvic sonography as a confirmatory test of PCOS.

The following criteria were used to establish the diagnosis of PCOS: the Rotterdam ESHRE/ASRM-sponsored PCOS consensus workshop group [Revised 2003 criteria (2 out of 3)].

1) Oligo and/or anovulation.

2) Clinical and/or biochemical signs of hyperandrogenism.

3) Polycystic ovaries on U/S examination [presence of ten or more follicular cysts 2 - 8 mm in one plane dis-

**Table 1.** Showing the degree of pigmentation in relation to degree of obesity in patients with frictional melanosis of rubbing thighs.

| BMI | Normal weight (18.5 - 24.9) | Over weight (25 - 29.9) | Obese (over 30) |
|---|---|---|---|
| Grade I (n) | 1 | 7 | 11 |
| % | 100% | 63.6% | 22.9% |
| Grade II (n) | - | 3 | 14 |
| % | - | 27.2% | 29.16% |
| Grade III (n) | - | 1 | 23 |
| % | - | 9.09% | 47.9% |

P value = 0.03.

tributed evenly around the ovarian periphery in a chain like manner (pearl/necklace) with an echo dense ovarian stroma, the ovaries are either normal or enlarged in size].

Incisional skin biopsies were carried out for 10 patients for H&E and Fontana Masson staining (special staining for melanin) was done in order to determine all histopathological features of this disease.

Cosmetic impact assessment was also done according to the patients' awareness of their thighs pigmentation, as some patients feel it as an important cosmetic component causing disabling feature, while others were not interested. Forty apparently healthy individuals were enrolled in the present work as a control group (as patients complaining of other diseases mostly skin infections or companions of patients).

## 3. Results

Sixty patients with hypermelanosis of inner aspects of thighs, 59 (98.3%) females and 1 (1.6%) male, were included in this study. The age of the patients ranged between 19 - 52 years with a mean ± SD of 32.86 ± 7.65 years, 59 female patients with a mean ± SD of 32.91 ± 7.75 years; the duration of hypermelanosis ranged between 2 - 20 years with mean ± SD of 6.4 ± 3.58 years.

Three (5%) patients were unmarried, 19 (31%) patients of females have one child, and all other females have more than one child. Fifty four females were housewives, one student, one driver, and 3 of them are office workers.

Twenty-four (40%) patients using topical whitening commercial mixtures, while history of rubbing of pigmented skin by lifa (washing agent) was positive in 46 (76.7%) patients.

History of bouts of intertrigo was positive in 52 (86.6%) patients, especially during hot humid season. Four (6.6%) patients were atopic, 3 of them had family history of atopy, in addition to 17 (28%) patients had positive family history of atopy. Family history of hypermelanosis of inner aspects of thighs was positive in 46 (77%) of cases.

According to Fitzpatrick's skin typing: 38 (63.3%) patients were skin type IV, 17 (28.3%) patients were skin type III, 3 (5%) patients were skin type V, and 2 patients (3.3%) were skin type II.

Hypermelanotic areas have ill-defined borders confined to areas of maximum contact during walking in the medial sides of upper thighs; in 17 (28.3%) patients, the pattern was rippled in 17(28.3%) patients and confluent homogenous pigmentation was seen in the rest of patients (**Figure 1**).

BMI measurement show that all patients with frictional melanosis of inner thighs were obese except one and the patients were divided according to BMI into three groups: normal weight 1 (1.7%), overweight 11 (18.7%) and obese were 48 (18.4%) patients, BMI was ranged from 23.3 to 43.6 with a mean ± SD of 34.04 ± 4.13 (**Table 1**).

According to grading of pigmentation 19 (31.6%) patients had Grade I pigmentation, 17 (28.3%) had Grade II pigmentation and 24 (40%) had Grade III pigmentation. Statistical analysis showed significant association between degree of obesity and severity of pigmentation P value ≤ 0.03 (**Table 1**, **Figure 2**).

No patient complained of itching of the rash but pseudofolliculitis confined to pigmented area was seen in 16 (26.6%) patients, no itching was reported in all patients as a complaint. Bad odor from pigmented area noticed in

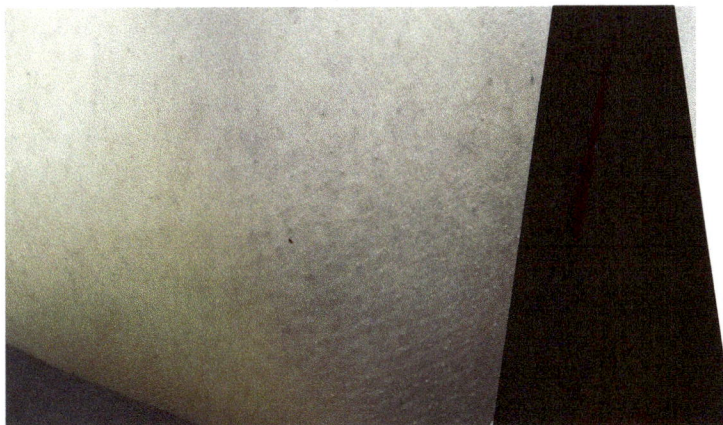

**Figure 1.** A twenty five years old married fertile female with dark brown (Grade 2) pigmentation on upper inner thighs BMI = 42.9.

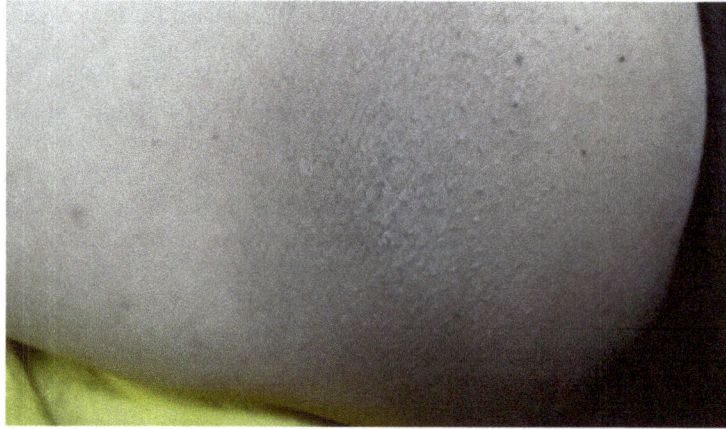

**Figure 2.** A thirty four years old married fertile female with bluish nearly black (Grade 3) pigmentation on upper inner thighs BMI = 36.4.

37 (61.6%) patients.

Wood's light examination revealed accentuation in 39 (58%) lesions which explained as epidermal or mixed (dermal and epidermal) pigmentation, while 21 (42%) of lesions showed no accentuation which represented as dermal pigmentation. Pigmented skin was mildly thickened in comparison with normal non pigmented skin in 27 (45%) of patients.

The cosmetic impact assessment had shown that 44 (73.3%) patients were completely aware of this abnormal pigmentation, as two patients had been divorced because of this problem. At the same time some patients consider it normal familial condition as it is common in their sisters and mothers.

All 10 skin biopsies were obtained from patients with skin type IV. Histopathological examination revealed heterogeneous patterns of pigmentation as 3 of biopsies showed pure dermal melanophages spindle in shape (looks like fibroblast), while the other 7 biopsies showed mainly increase in basal melanin one of these revealed distribution of melanin all over the layers of epidermis although dermal melanophages had been observed in the last group but they were small and scattered (**Figure 3**, **Figure 4**).

Slight perivascular inflammatory infiltrate was observed in 3 (30%) biopsies, no amyloid was seen observed in any of these biopsies (**Table 2**).

Two of female (3.4%) patients fulfilled the criteria of PCOS, another 2 had history of PCOS, 3 (5%) patients were postmenopausal.

Forty control individuals 2 males and 38 females were assessed, their age range from 19 to 50 years old with a mean ± SD of 31.72 ± 6.40 years among 38 females same range with a mean ± SD of 31.52 ± 6.50 years. Five (12.5%) of them were atopic, while 10 (25%) had family history of atopy.

All females were within normal weight, while males were overweight as BMI of them (28.2 and 26.9). BMI was ranged from 19.7 to 28.2 with a mean ± SD of 22.49 ± 1.84, while among 38 females BMI was a mean ± SD of 22.23 ± 1.45. No pigmentation of the inner thighs was noticed.

## 4. Discussion

Hypermelanosis is an important racial feature of black and dark skin individuals and has great psychological and emotional impacts on patients with such problems like melasma, Addison's disease, amyloidosis and its most common type macular amyloidosis, or could be seen as a part of frictional melanosis [4].

Lifa disease which is common among slim bony females with its predilection areas over bony prominences, is a common problem among Asians and Middle East countries especially in Iraq as Sharquie 1993 [2] [4] [29] [35] had reported and named this disease. Since then many other studies had been published in literatures [29].

Frictional melanosis is either induced by rubbing with washing tools like lifa, or by rubbing with hands, scratching [13], or as a result of abnormal counter of the body, like rubbing thighs in obese females.

Pathogenesis of lifa disease is thought to be as a result of squeezing of melanocytes in basal layer by washing agents like lifa against the underlying bony structures. This will cause damage of melanocytes and releasing of their melanosomes to the dermis, which will be seen as melanophages after engulfment by macrophages [4].

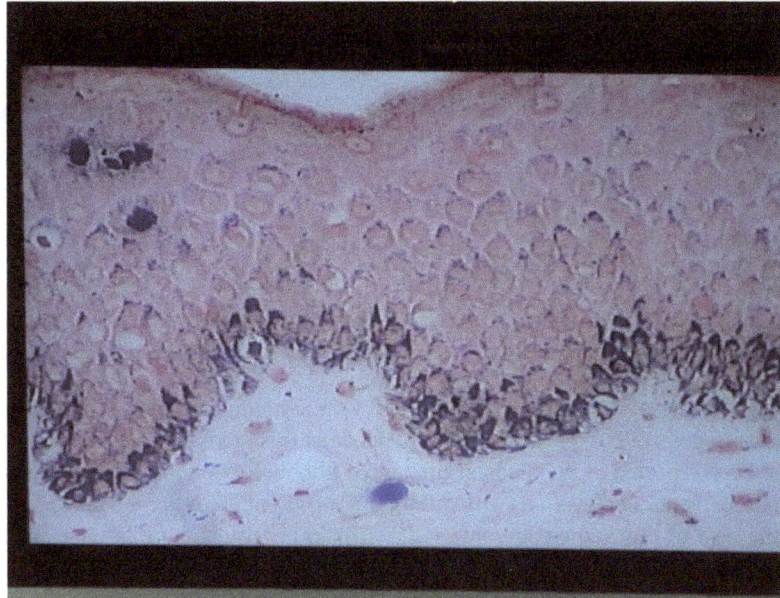

**Figure 3.** Fontana-Masson stained section showing basal hyperpigmentation and scattered melanophages in the dermis.

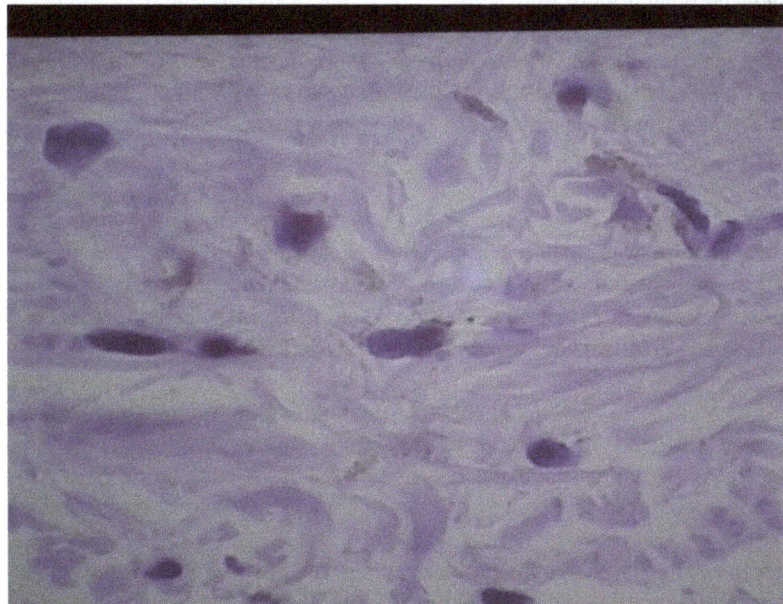

**Figure 4.** Hematoxylin-Eosin stained sections showing dermal melanophages.

**Table 2.** Showing the histopathological features of frictional melanosis of rubbing thighs.

| Feature | No. of patients | % |
|---|---|---|
| Mild hyperkeratosis | 10 | 100% |
| Mild acanthosis | 10 | 100% |
| Perivascular inflammatory infiltrate | 3 | 30% |
| Amyloid | 0 | 0% |
| By Fontana basilar hypermelanosis | 7 | 70% |
| By Fontana dermal melanophages | 3 | 3% |

**Table 3.** Showing the comparison between FM of rubbing thighs and lifa disease.

| FM of rubbing thighs | Lifa disease |
|---|---|
| Benign pigmentary problem resulted from frictional injury. | Benign pigmentary problem resulted from frictional injury. |
| Disease of young adult mostly females. | Disease of young adult mostly females. |
| Disease of obese. | Disease of slim. |
| Friction between two folds of own skin. | Friction between skin and external agent (lifa). |
| Pigmentation over fleshy parts. | Pigmentation over bony prominences. |
| Histopathologicaly Fontana stain showed that pigmentation could be basilar or dermal without amyloid deposition. | Histopathologicaly Fontana stain showed that pigmentation is dermal with possible amyloid deposition. |

Frictional melanosis of rubbing inner thighs is very common problem among Iraqi females causing great psychological and cosmetic impacts on many patients as this study shows (73%), but unfortunately, this melanosis had not been reported in the medical literatures although commonly encountered in daily clinical practice (Sharquie 1990 personal observation). Accordingly the present study was arranged to report this new variety of FM and to the best of our knowledge, this is the first study to clarify this type of pigmentation clinically and histologically.

The present work showed that this variety of melanosis is mostly seen among obese females and the degree of pigmentation went parallel with the degree of obesity (**Table 1**).

Rarity of this condition among males may be related simply to the fact that it is totally cosmetic problem. Although it might be related more to anatomical differences in pelvis and gait between males and females [36], making rubbing of inner aspects of thighs nearly absent in males and even obese one as we reported 2 over weight males in the control group had no pigmentation of inner aspects of thighs (**Table 3**).

This type of hypermelanosis had the positive association with parity. After pregnancy the pigmentation in dark skinned females usually doesn't return to their normal skin color, especially when added to other factors like humidity, friction, using of commercial mixtures with unknown ingredients, and friction by other external agents in hope to decrease pigmentation.

According to this study it is not possible to regard this type of pigmentation as a type of atopic reaction as personal history of atopy was positive only in (6%) of patients.

The pattern of pigmentation was dermal, epidermal or mixed as assessed by clinical, Wood's light and histological examination. This abnormal pigmentation is the main reason behind patients seeking medical therapy.

As this disease has great psychological and cosmetic impacts on these patients (73.3%), accordingly therapy is mandatory needed.

History of vigorous use of washing agent (lifa) in an attempt to remove pigmentation was obtained in (76.7%) of patients, which added to friction produced by rubbing inner thighs.

It is not surprising that only (3.4%) patients had PCOS as we exclude cases of AN and skin tags at same area of friction (inner thighs) the most common cutaneous manifestations of insulin resistance which is the hallmark of PCOS [8] [37].

There are many options to clear this problem either weight reduction with or without giving topical emulsifying cream to minimize friction between rubbing thighs. If these therapeutic measures fail, we can suggest peeling using lactic acid [38] or liposuction as possibly mode of therapy.

## Disclosure

This study was an independent study and not funded by any drug companies.

## References

[1]   Ruiz-Maldonado, R. and Orozco-Covarrubias, L. (2008) Metabolic and Systemic Diseases. In: Bolognia, J., Jorizzo, J. and Rapini, R.P., Eds., *Dermatology*, 2nd Edition, Elsevier, Spain, 672.

[2]   Sharquie, K.E. (1993) Frictional Dermal Melanosis (Lifa Disease) over Bony Prominences. *Journal of the Faculty Medicine (Baghdad)*, **35**, 83-87.

[3]   Al-Aboosi, M., Abalkhail, A., Kasim, O., Al-Khatib, A., Qarqaz, F. and Todd, D. (2004) Frictional Melanosis: A Clin-

ical, Histologic, and Ultrastructural Study in Jordanian Patients. *International Society of Dermatology*, **43**, 261-264. http://dx.doi.org/10.1111/j.1365-4632.2004.01606.x

[4] Sharquie, K.E. and Al-Dorky, M.K. (2001) Frictional Dermal Melanosis (Lifa Disease) over Bony Prominences. *Journal of Dermatology*, **28**, 12-15.

[5] Wong, C.K. (1987) Cutaneous Amyloidosis. *International Journal of Dermatology*, **26**, 273-277. http://dx.doi.org/10.1111/j.1365-4362.1987.tb00187.x

[6] Looi, L.M. (1991) Primary Localized Cutaneous Amyloidosis in Malaysians. *Australasian Journal of Dermatology*, **32**, 39-44. http://dx.doi.org/10.1111/j.1440-0960.1991.tb00681.x

[7] Sharquie, K.E. and Hasson, S.M. (1991) Primary Cutaneous Amyloidosis in Iraqi Patients: Epidemiological, Clinical and Histopathological Study. Diploma Dissertation, University of Baghdad, Baghdad.

[8] Hidano, A., Mizuguchi, M. and Higaki, Y. (1984) Friction Melanosis. *Annales de Dermatologie et de Vénéréologie*, **111**, 1063-1071.

[9] Sumitra, S. and Yesudian, P. (1993) Friction Amyloidosis: A Variant or an Etiological Factor in Amyloidosis Cutis. *International Journal of Dermatology*, **32**, 422-423. http://dx.doi.org/10.1111/j.1365-4362.1993.tb02812.x

[10] Hashimato, K., Ito, K., Kumakiri, M. and Headington, J. (1987) Nylon Brush Macular Amyloidosis. *Archives of Dermatology*, **123**, 633-637. http://dx.doi.org/10.1001/archderm.1987.01660290101025

[11] Tan, T. (1990) Epidemiology of Primary Cutaneous Amyloidosis in Southeast Asia. *Clinics in Dermatology*, **22**, 1082-1087.

[12] Black, M.M. and Jones, E.W. (1971) Macular Amyloidosis: A Study of 21 Cases with Special Reference to the Role of the Epidermis in Its Histogenesis. *British Journal of Dermatology*, **84**, 199-209. http://dx.doi.org/10.1111/j.1365-2133.1971.tb14208.x

[13] Wong, C.K. and Lin, C.S. (1988) Friction Amyloidosis. *International Journal of Dermatology*, **27**, 302-307. http://dx.doi.org/10.1111/j.1365-4362.1988.tb02357.x

[14] Anekohji, K., Maeda, K. and Shigemoto, K. (1983) A Peculiar Pigmentation of the Skin over Bony Regions. *Rinsho Dermatol (Japanese Journal of Clinical Dermatology)*, **25**, 1259-1262.

[15] Asai, Y., Hamada, T., Suzuki, N., Nakano, K., Tanii, T. and Izutani, K. (1983) Acquired Hyperpigmentation Distributed on the Skin over Bones. *Japanese Journal of Dermatology*, **93**, 405-414.

[16] Tanigaki, T., Hata, S., Kitano, Y., Nomura, M., Sano, S. and Endo, H. (1985) Unusual Pigmentation on the Skin over Trunk Bones and Extremities. *Dermatologica*, **170**, 235-239. http://dx.doi.org/10.1159/000249539

[17] Tanigaki, T., Hata, S., Kitano, Y., Sano, S., Nomura, M. and Satoh, K. (1985) Epidemiological Survey of Nylon Clothes Friction Dermatosis. *Nihon Hifuka Gakkai Zasshi*, **95**, 1159-1164.

[18] Iwasaki, K., Mihara, M., Nishiura, S. and Shimao, S. (1991) Biphasic Amyloidosis Arising from Friction Melanosis. *The Journal of Dermatology*, **18**, 86-91.

[19] Hata, S., Tanigaki, T. and Misaki, K. (1987) Incidence of Frictional Melanosis in Young Japanese Women Induced by Using Nylon Towels and Brushes. *The Journal of Dermatology*, **14**, 437-439.

[20] Somani, V.K., Shailaja, H., Sita, V. and Fatima, R. (1995) Nylon Friction Dermatitis: A Distinct Subset of Macular Amyloidosis. *Indian Journal of Dermatology, Venereology and Leprology*, **61**, 145-147.

[21] Probhakara, V.G., Chandra, S. and Krupa, D.S. (1997) Frictional Pigmentary Dermatoses: A Clinical and Histopathological Study of 27 Cases. *Indian Journal of Dermatology, Venereology and Leprology*, **63**, 99-100.

[22] Siragusa, M., Cavallari, V. and Schepis, C. (2000) Macular Amyloidosis Due to Friction by a Horsehair Glove. *Dermatology*, **200**, 82-83. http://dx.doi.org/10.1159/000018327

[23] Siragusa, M., Ferri, R., Cavallari, V. and Schepis, C. (2001) Friction Melanosis, Friction Amyloidosis, Macular Amyloidosis, Towel Melanosis: Many Names for the Same Clinical Entity. *European Journal of Dermatology*, **11**, 545-548.

[24] Venkataram, M.N., Bhushnurmath, S.R., Muirhead, D.E. and Al-Suwaid, A.R. (2001) Frictional Amyloidosis: A Study of 10 Cases. *Australasian Journal of Dermatology*, **42**, 176-179. http://dx.doi.org/10.1046/j.1440-0960.2001.00514.x

[25] Naimer, S.A., Trattner, A., Biton, A., Avinoach, I. and Vardy, D. (2000) Davener's Dermatosis: A Variant of Friction Hypermelanosis. *Journal of the American Academy of Dermatology*, **42**, 442-445. http://dx.doi.org/10.1016/S0190-9622(00)90216-0

[26] Macsween, R.M. and Salhan, E.M. (1997) Nylon Cloth Macular Amyloidosis. *Clinical and Experimental Dermatology*, **22**, 28-31. http://dx.doi.org/10.1046/j.1365-2230.1997.1770598.x

[27] Higgins, S.P., Freemark, M. and Prose, N.S. (2008) Acanthosis Nigricans: A Practical Approach to Evaluation and Management. *Dermatology Online Journal*, **14**, 2.

[28] Sharquie, K.E., Al-Bayatti, A.A., Al-Zaidi, Q.M. and Al-Bahar, A.J. (2004) Acanthosis Nigricans as Skin Manifesta-

tion of Polycystic Ovarian Syndrome in Primary Infertile Female. *Middle East Fertility Society Journal*, **9**, 136-139.

[29] Sharquie, K.E., Noaimi, A.A. and Muhammad Ali, A.H. (2008) Acanthosis Nigricans in Iraqi Patients Clinical, Histopathological and Theraputic Study. Thesis for Fellowship of Iraqi Board for Medical Specializations in Dermatology and Venereology.

[30] García-Hidalgo, L., Orozco-Topete, R., Gonzalez-Barranco, J., Villa, A.R., Dalman, J.J. and Ortiz-Pedroza, G. (1999) Dermatoses in 165 Obese Adults. *Obesity Research*, **7**, 299-302.

[31] Chang, M.W. (2008) Disorders of Hyperpigmentation. In: Bolognia, J., Jorizzo, J. and Rapini, R.P., Eds., *Dermatology*, 2nd Edition, Elsevier, Spain, 946-948.

[32] Bunker, C.B. and Neill, S.M. (2010) The Genital, Perianal and Umbilical Regions. In: Burns, T., Breathnach, S., Cox, N. and Griffiths, C., Eds., *Chap. 71. Rook's Text Book of Dermatology*, 8th Edition, Blackwell Scientific Publication, Singapore City, 4-6.

[33] Costin, G.-E. and Hearing, V.J. (2007) Human Skin Pigmentation: Melanocytes Modulate Skin Color in Response to Stress. *The FASEB Journal*, **21**, 976-994. http://dx.doi.org/10.1096/fj.06-6649rev

[34] Ortonne, J.P. and Nordlund, J.J. (2006) Mechanisms That Cause Abnormal Skin Color. In: Nordlund, J.J., Boissy, R.E., Hearing, V.J., King, R.A., Oetting, W.S. and Ortonne, J.P., Eds., *Chap. 28. The Pigmentary System: Physiology and Pathophysiology*, 2nd Edition, Blackwell Scientific Publication, New York, 521-535.

[35] Sharquie, K.E., Al-Rawi, J.R. and Al-Tamimi, F.F. (2005) The Frequency of Skin Disease in Obese Children and Adult Iraqi Population. *Saudi Medical Journal*, **26**, 1835-1836.

[36] Cho, S.H., Park, J.M. and Kwon, O.Y. (2004) Gender Differences in Three Dimensional Gait Analysis Data from 98 Healthy Korean Adults. *Clinical Biomechanics*, **19**, 145-152. http://dx.doi.org/10.1016/j.clinbiomech.2003.10.003

[37] Sharquie, K.E., Bayatti, A.A., Ajeel, A.I., Bahar, A.J. and Noaimi, A.A. (2007) Free Testosterone, Luteinizing Hormone/Follicle Stimulating Hormone Ratio and Pelvic Sonography in Relation to Skin Manifestations in Patients with Poly Cystic Ovary Syndrome. *Saudi Medical Journal*, **28**, 1039-1043.

[38] Sharquie, K.E., Al-Dhalimi, M.A., Noaimi, A.A. and Al-Sultany, H.A. (2012) Lactic Acid as a New Therapeutic Peeling Agent in the Treatment of Lifa Disease (Frictional Dermal Melanosis). *Indian Journal of Dermatology*, **57**, 444-448.

# 9

# Preparation of Microcapsules Containing Triple Core Materials with Interfacial Condensation Reaction

**Yoshinari Taguchi, Mikihiko Aoki, Masato Tanaka***

Graduate School of Science and Technology, Niigata University, Niigata, Japan
Email: *tanaka@eng.niigata-u.ac.jp

## Abstract

In this manuscript, we describe the novel method for preparing the microcapsules containing $\alpha$-tocopherol oil droplets as the first core material, calcium chloride powder as the second core material and the fine water droplets as the third core material by the interfacial condensation reaction between hydroxyl propyl methyl cellulose and tannic acid. The interfacial condensation reaction was performed between hydroxyl propyl methyl cellulose dissolved in the continuous water phase and tannic acid dissolved in the inner fine water droplets as the third core material. The calcium chloride powder as the second core material was dispersed in the $\alpha$-tocopherol oil droplet as the first core material beforehand. The $\alpha$-tocopherol oil containing the second and the third core materials was dispersed in the continuous water phase to form the [(S + W)/O/W] emulsion. The $\alpha$-tocopherol oil as the first core material was microencapsulated satisfactorily and the contents of the second core material were increased with the concentration of stearic acid as the oil soluble stabilizer. The mechanical strength of microcapsules increased with the concentration of hydroxyl propyl methyl cellulose. Thermal energy could be released by breaking the microcapsules in water and by dissolving calcium chloride in the continuous water phase.

## Keywords

Triple Core Materials-Containing-Microcapsule, Multiple Emulsions, $\alpha$-Tocopherol, Calcium Chloride, Dissolution Heat, Hydroxy Propyl Methyl Cellulose, Tannic Acid

## 1. Introduction

Many kinds of microcapsules have been developed and utilized in the various fields such as cosmetics, food in-

---

*Corresponding author.

dustry, drugs, paintings, adhesives and so on [1]-[4]. Selection of the shell materials of microcapsules depends on the desired functions such as thermal and pH-responsibility, hydrophilicity, hydrophobicity, biodegradability and anti-solubility. It is necessary to develop the new preparation method suitable to these demands. Especially, when the microcapsules are used/utilized in the fields such as food, cosmetics and drug, the microcapsules must be prepared by using the nontoxic shell materials. Also, during microencapsulation of both hydrophobic and the hydrophilic core materials at the same time, it is necessary to develop the effective method for preparing microcapsules with the higher content of core materials. $\alpha$-tocopherol being an antioxidant, reduces risk of diseases such as cardiovascular diseases, and also $\alpha$-tocopherol has been used as supplement. So, if $\alpha$-tocopherol could be kept safely and released at occasion demands, it will be expected that $\alpha$-tocopherolcan be utilized in more fields.

W. Somchue, *et al.* have microencapsulated $\alpha$-tocopherol with protein in order to use the microcapsules as the delivery particles [5]. Song, Y.B., *et al.* have tried to prepare the microcapsules containing $\alpha$-tocopherol with the gellatedpectin and established the optimum preparation conditions [6].

Furthermore, it is well known that calcium chloride is hygroscopic and has heat of dissolution of 285 kJ/kg. If heat of dissolution of calcium chloride is released gradually, its utilization can be expected. For an example, if this heat of dissolution of calcium chloride is gradually released on the face and body skin, it may be expected to keep the face and the body warm. Also, as water can dissolve different kinds of chemicals, various aqueous solutions could be microencapsulated well and the fine droplets containing the aqueous solution can be utilized as the reservoir of water and chemicals. The above stated aims may be accomplished by microencapsulating $\alpha$-tocopherol, the aqueous solution and the calcium chloride powder at the same time.

Authors have developed the preparation method for microencapsulating the eucalyptus oil with the interfacial condensation reaction between hydroxyl propyl methyl cellulose and tannic acid and established the optimum preparation conditions [7]. In the microencapsulation mechanism, authors describe the importance of tannic acid to transfer from the inner water droplets to the interface through the eucalyptus oil phase and subsequent reaction with hydroxyl propyl methyl cellulose. In this study, $\alpha$-tocopherol was used instead of eucalyptus oil and it was tried to microencapsulate the triple core materials and at the same time the microencapsulation mechanism is presented.

The purpose of this study is to investigate whether the $\alpha$-tocopherol oil, the aqueous solution and the calcium chloride powder can be microencapsulated at the same time, and to characterize the microcapsules and to discuss the possible microencapsulation mechanism based on the result obtained.

## 2. Experimental

### 2.1. Materials

Materials used to prepare the microcapsules containing $\alpha$-tocopherol, the fine water droplets and the solid powder of $CaCl_2$ were as follows.

#### 2.1.1. Shell Material
Hydroxyl propyl methyl cellulose (HPMC) (Shinetsu Kagaku Kogyo, Co. Ltd.)
    Tannic acid (TA) (Tokyo Kasei, Co. Ltd.)

#### 2.1.2. Core Materials
$\alpha$-tocopherol ($\alpha$-oil) (Kanto Chemical, Co. Ltd.)
    Calcium Chloride ($CaCl_2$, Kanto Chemical, Co. Ltd.)
    Aqueous solution of tannic acid.

#### 2.1.3. Oil Soluble Stabilizer and Surfactant
Stearic acid (ST) (Kanto Chemical, Co. Ltd.)
    Soybean Lecithin (LC) (Junsei Chemical, Co. Ltd.)

### 2.2. Preparation of Microcapsules

The microcapsules were prepared by modification of the reported methods [7]. **Figure 1** shows the flow sheet for preparing the microcapsules containing the triple core materials together with the schematic diagrams of mi-

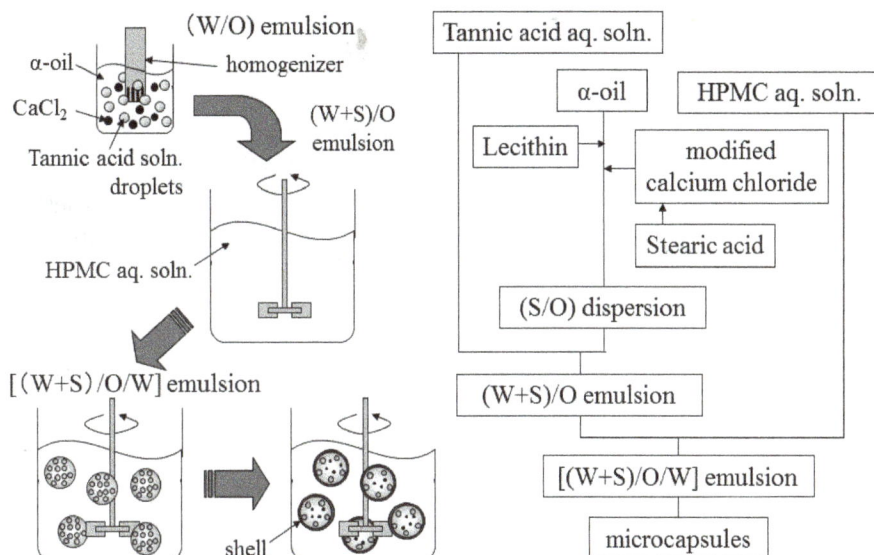

**Figure 1.** Flow chart for preparing microcapsules.

croencapsulation process. $\alpha$-tocopherol ($\alpha$-oil) dissolving soybean lecithin (LC) as an oil soluble surfactant was prepared as the first core material. Tannic acid (TA) aqueous solution was dispersed in $\alpha$-tocopherol ($\alpha$-oil) to form the fine aqueous droplets as the second core material. Here, it is necessary for tannic acid (TA) dissolved in the inner aqueous droplets to transfer through $\alpha$-tocopherol ($\alpha$-oil), to react with HPMC and to form the microcapsule shell. The calcium chloride powder as the third core material was prepared by the following two methods.

First, the calcium chloride powder was modified by mixing with stearic acid as an oil soluble stabilizer to provide hydrophobicity and added to $\alpha$-tocopherol ($\alpha$-oil) to form the (S/O) dispersion. Hereafter, this preparation method will be called the modification method. Second, the calcium chloride powder was dissolved in distilled water. This aqueous solution was added into $\alpha$-tocopherol ($\alpha$-oil) and stirred to form the (W/O) emulsion. Then, the (W/O) emulsion was dried under reduced pressure and 70°C to remove the water and to form the (S/O) dispersion where finer calcium chloride powder was dispersed in $\alpha$-tocopherol ($\alpha$-oil) dissolving stearic acid. Hereafter, this preparation method will be called the breakdown method. The (S/O) dispersion thus prepared was added into the (W/O) emulsion to form [(W + S)/O] emulsion. The [(W + S)/O] emulsion was poured into the HPMC aqueous solution and stirred to form the [(W + S)/O/W] emulsion. Then, temperature of the [(W + S)/O/W] emulsion was raised to 40°C to perform the interfacial condensation reaction between HPMC and tannic acid (TA). It may be expected that tannic acid (TA) may transfer through $\alpha$-tocopherol ($\alpha$-oil) from the inner water droplets to the interface between $\alpha$-tocopherol ($\alpha$-oil) and the continuous water phase and react with HPMC. In this fundamental experiment, the concentrations of HPMC and stearic acid (ST) were changed. The experimental conditions are shown in **Table 1**.

## 2.3. Characterization

### 2.3.1. Observation of Microcapsules
It was observed whether the microcapsules could be prepared or not as follows. Namely, after preparing the microcapsules, the (S + W)/O/W emulsion was set and observed by visual confirmation. If the microcapsules are not be prepared well, the multiple emulsion can be broken rapidly.

Then, the microcapsules were observed by optical microscope and scanning electron microscope (SEM). The shape and inner structure of microcapsule were observed from these photographs and the effects of experimental conditions on them were discussed.

### 2.3.2. Diameter Distribution
The diameter distributions and mean diameters of microcapsules were obtained directly from the photographs taken by the optical microscope. Here, the mean diameters of microcapsules are the mean Sauter diameters.

**Table 1.** Experimental conditions.

| | |
|---|---|
| Distilled water | 270 ml |
| HPMC conc. | 0.05 ~ 0.2 wt% |
| $\alpha$-oil | 27 ml |
| Calcium chloride | 1 g |
| Stearic acid conc. | 0.1 ~ 1.0 wt% oil |
| Lecithin conc. | 3 ml (0.1wt% oil) |
| Tannic acid soln. | 3 ml (0.2 mol) |
| Revolution speed to form (W/O) emulsion | 3000 rpm |
| Revolution time | 10 min |
| Reaction temperature | 40°C |
| Reaction time | 1 h |
| Revolution speed to form [(S + W)/O/W] Emulsion and to prepare microcapsules | 300 rpm |

### 2.3.3. Mechanical Strength of Microcapsules

The mechanical strength of microcapsules was measured by the hardening measurement instrument (Shimazu Seisakusho, Japan, MCT-W500).

### 2.3.4. Microencapsulation Efficiency of Calcium Chloride Powder

The microcapsules of given weight were added in distilled water of 5cc and broken by mechanical pressure to measure temperature of water in the adiabatic vessel. The temperature rise degree was compared with the calibration curve between the calcium chloride concentration and the temperature rise degree. The weight of calcium chloride microencapsulated was obtained from this result. The microencapsulation efficiency (Y) was estimated from the following Equation (1).

$$Y = \frac{\text{weight of calcium chloride microencapsulated}}{\text{weight of calcium chloride in feed}} \tag{1}$$

## 3. Results & Discussion

### 3.1. Confirmation of Microcapsule Formation

In order to confirm whether the microcapsules could be prepared or not according to the microencapsulation mechanism presented in the previous study [7], first, the stability of (W/O)/W emulsion before and after the microencapsulation process without addition of calcium chloride powder was investigated by visual confirmation.

**Figure 2** shows the photographs of the (W/O)/W emulsion without and with the microencapsulation process. These photographs were taken at just after formation of the (W/O)/W emulsion, after 30 s and after 7 days, respectively. In the case of the (W/O)/W emulsion without the microencapsulation process, the (W/O)/W emulsion was formed just after emulsification, however, the (W/O)/W emulsion was broken and the phase separation occurred after 30 s as shown in **Figure 2(a)**. However, in the case of the (W/O)/W emulsion with the microencapsulation process, the (W/O)/W emulsion was formed just after emulsification and kept after 30 s and 7 days as shown in **Figure 2(b)**. Furthermore, the formation of microcapsules could be confirmed by the photograph inserted in **Figure 2(b)**.

Also, the optical microscopic photographs of microcapsules prepared at $C_{HPMC}$ = 0.05 wt% and $C_{HPMC}$ = 0.2 wt% were shown in **Figure 3**. The microcapsules could be prepared at both the highest and the lowest concentrations of HPMC in this experiment.

From **Figure 2** and **Figure 3**, it was found that tannic acid (TA) transferred from the inner water droplets to the interface through $\alpha$-tocopherol ($\alpha$-oil) and reacted with hydroxyl propyl methyl cellulose (HPMC) and the inner aqueous droplets could be microencapsulated well as well as the eucalyptus oil [7].

**Figure 4** shows the dependences of mechanical strength ($S_t$) and mean diameters ($d_p$) of microcapsules on the HPMC concentration ($C_{HPMC}$). The mechanical strength increased with the HPMC concentration and become almost constant at the HPMC concentration larger than $C_{HPMC}$ = 0.15 wt%. The mean diameters increased from

(a) without microencapsulation process

30s    7days

phase separation

oil phase

water phase

(b) with microencapsulation process

30s    7days

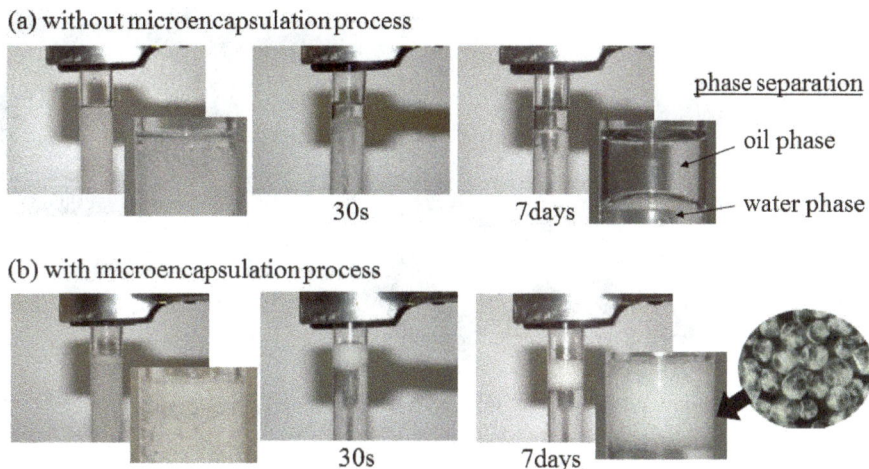

**Figure 2.** Transient features of [(W/O)/W] emulsion.

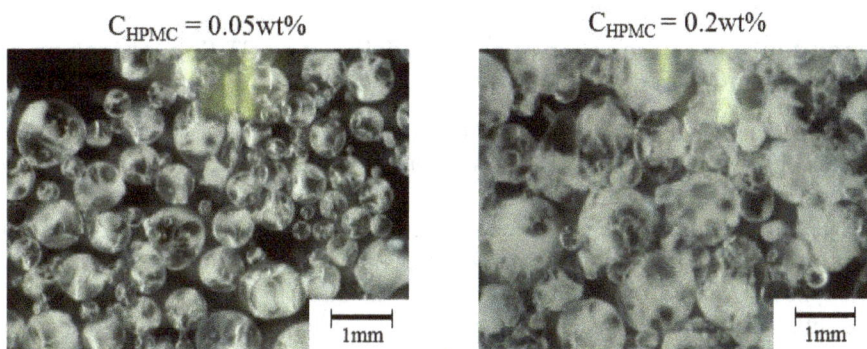

$C_{HPMC} = 0.05wt\%$    $C_{HPMC} = 0.2wt\%$

1mm    1mm

**Figure 3.** Optical microscopic photographs of microcapsules.

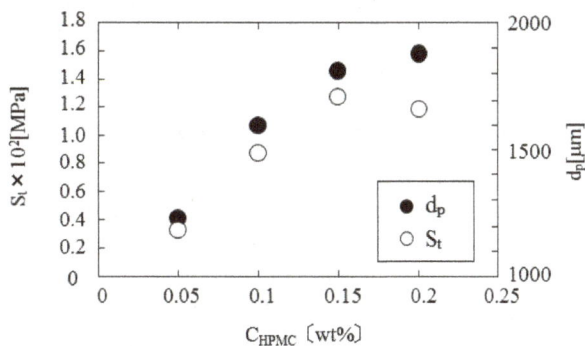

**Figure 4.** Mechanical strength of microcapsules.

1200 μm at $C_{HPMC}$ = 0.05 wt% to 1900 μm at $C_{HPMC}$ = 0.2 wt%. Hereafter, the microcapsules were prepared at $C_{HPMC}$ = 0.2 wt% in order to microencapsulate the calcium chloride powder.

## 3.2. Confirmation of Formation of Microcapsules Containing Calcium Chloride Powder

In the preparation of desired microcapsules, the (S/O) dispersion was added to the (W/O) emulsion prepared beforehand to form the [(W+S)/O/W] emulsion.

**Figure 5** shows the optical microscopic photographs of microcapsules containing the calcium chloride powder at $C_{HPMC}$ = 0.2 wt% and $C_{ST}$ = 0.4 wt%. It was found that the microcapsules could be prepared well and were filled with the calcium chloride powder. The microcapsules are opaque because of dispersion of calcium chlo-

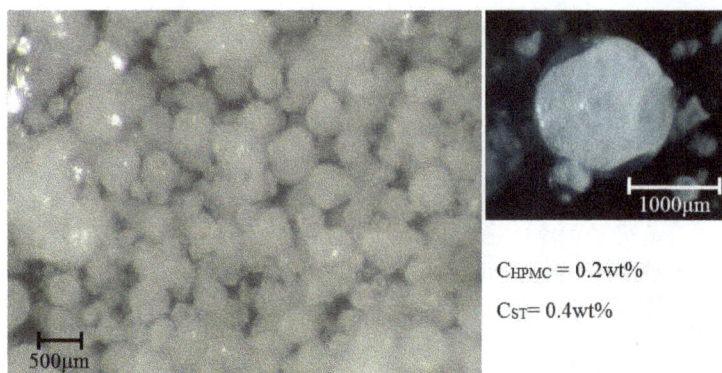

**Figure 5.** Photographs of microcapsules containing triple cores.

ride powder.

From **Figures 2-5**, the microcapsules containing $\alpha$-tocopherol ($\alpha$-oil) as the first core, the calcium chloride powder as the second core and the aqueous droplets as the third core could be prepared well.

### 3.3. Dependence of Microencapsulation Efficiency on ST Concentration and Formation Method of Calcium Chloride Powder

Microencapsulation of solid powder has been mainly performed by selecting the oil soluble surfactant species [8] [9] and by modifying the surface of solid powder due to various coupling agents [10]-[12] in order to obtain the higher content possible.

Here, it was tried to investigate the effect of ST concentration and the (S/O) dispersion preparation method on the content of calcium chloride powder. In this experiment, the calcium chloride powder was modified to become hydrophobic by stearic acid beforehand (modification method) and to finer powder by breaking down the aqueous solution of calcium chloride into finer aqueous droplets and by removing water (break down method).

**Figure 6** shows the dependence of microencapsulation efficiency on the ST concentration for the two preparation methods. It was found that the microencapsulation efficiency for the modification method increased from 8% to 55% with the highest ST concentration. However, the microencapsulation efficiency for the breakdown method increased from 8% to ca. 98%. This result is considered to be due to the fact that calcium chloride powder become more finer and more stable in $\alpha$-tocopherol ($\alpha$-oil).

### 3.4. Rise in Temperature Due to Breakup of Microcapsules

When the calcium chloride powder is released from the microcapsules into the water phase, temperature of aqueous solution may raise due to heat of dissolution of calcium chloride.

**Figure 7** shows the rise in temperature of water phase by dissolving calcium chloride. In **Figure 7**, temperature of the water phase where the microcapsules of a given weight were broken by the finger pressure was plotted, too. It was found that the plots of temperature of the water phase coincided with the correlation plots between temperature of the water phase and the calcium chloride concentration.

From these results, it was confirmed that temperature of the water phase could be raised by breaking the microcapsules of amount designed beforehand.

**Figure 8** shows the microcapsules dried under the room temperature. It was confirmed that the dried microcapsules could be safety kept within twenty days. The microcapsules can be used as the powder material containing the triple core materials.

### 3.5. Microencapsulation Mechanism

The microcapsules containing the triple core materials could be prepared well by the same preparation method as in the previous study. The microencapsulation mechanism may be discussed on the basis of the results obtained above.

**Figure 9** shows the microencapsulation mechanism. The calcium chloride powder as the second core and the

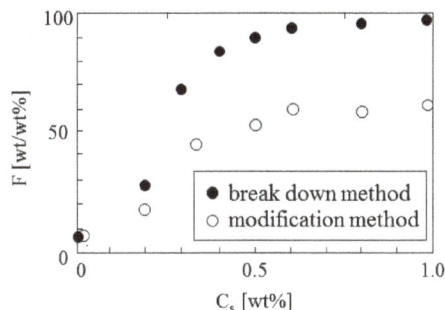

**Figure 6.** Dependence of microencapsulation efficiency of solid powder on ST concentration and preparation method.

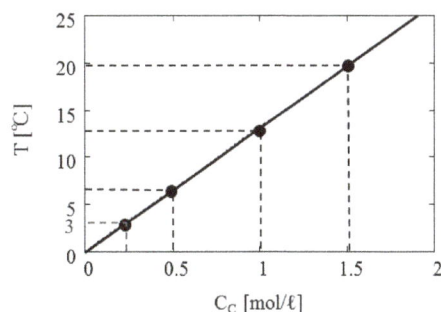

**Figure 7.** Dependence of temperature on calcium chloride concentration.

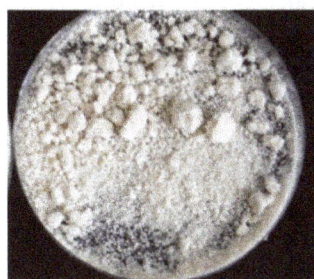

$C_{HPMC} = 0.2wt\%$

$C_{ST} = 0.5wt\%$

Break down method

**Figure 8.** Optical photographs of dried microcapsules.

fine tannic acid (TA) aqueous droplets as the third core were stabilized and dispersed well in the $\alpha$-tocopherol ($\alpha$-oil) droplets as the first core with the help of stearic acid (ST) and lecithin (LC), respectively as shown in **Figure 9(b)**. Tannic acid (TA) dissolved in the inner water droplets should transfer to the interface between $\alpha$-tocopherol ($\alpha$-oil) and the continuous water phase dissolving HPMC through the $\alpha$-tocopherol ($\alpha$-oil) phase and then, reacted with HPMC to form the gelled HPMC shell. The contents of the second and the third core can be considerably increased by decreasing the diameters of inner water droplets and calcium chloride powder and by the stabilizing effect due to the adsorption of lecithin (LC) and stearic acid (ST) on the surface of the aqueous droplets and calcium chloride powder as shown in **Figure 9(b)**. Accordingly, the break down method of calcium chloride powder was very useful to increase the content. Three core materials having the different physical property could be microencapsulated at the same time.

## 4. Conclusions

It was tried to prepare the microcapsules containing the triple core materials with the interfacial condensation reaction between hydroxyl propyl methyl cellulose and tannic acid. The following results were obtained.

1) The $\alpha$-tocopherol oil as the first core, the aqueous droplets as the second core and calcium chloride as the third core could be microencapsulated well at the same time by the microencapsulation mechanism presented in

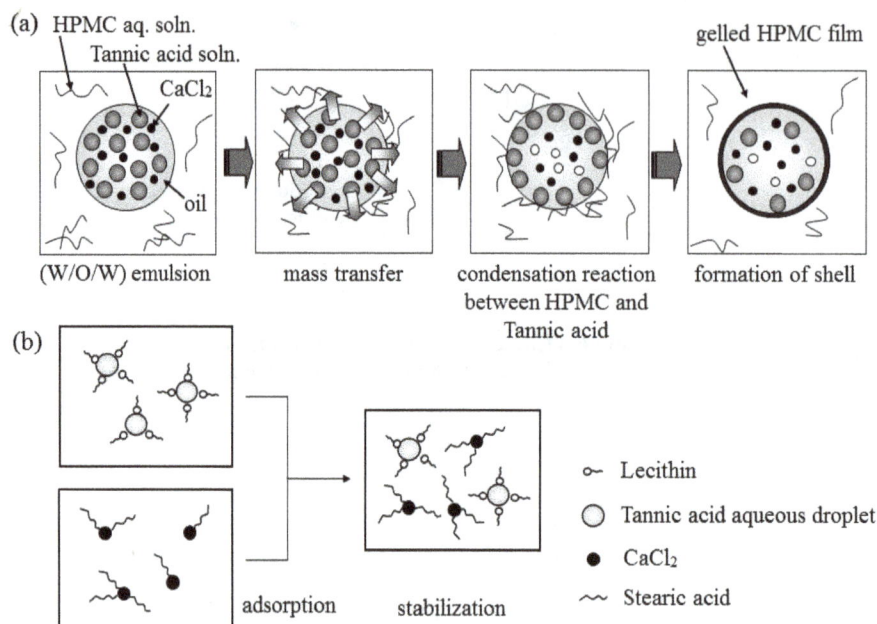

**Figure 9.** Microencapsulation mechanism.

the previous study;

2) The mechanical strength of microcapsules increased with the HPMC concentration;

3) Microencapsulation efficiency of calcium chloride powder could be increased to ca. 98% with the breakdown method as the preparation method of calcium chloride powder;

4) The microcapsules were easily broken by the finger pressure and the calcium chloride powder could be released;

5) Temperature in the water phase was raised to temperature corresponding to the amount of calcium chloride microencapsulated;

6) It may be expected that the microcapsules can be utilized as the face and body cream.

# References

[1]   Kondo, T. and Tanaka, M. (1975) Microcapsules (Preparation, Properties, Application). Sankyo Shuppan, Tokyo.

[2]   Kondo, T. (1967) Saishin Maikurokapseruka Gijutsu (Microencapsulation Technique). TES, Tokyo.

[3]   Tanaka, M. (2008) Key Point of Preparation of Nano/Microcapsules. Techno System Publishing Co. Ltd., Tokyo.

[4]   Koishi, M., Eto, K. and Higure, H. (2005) (Preparation + Utilization) Microcapsules. Kogyo Chosakai, Tokyo.

[5]   Somchue, W., Sermsri, W., Shiowatana, J. and Siripinyanond, A. (2009) Encapsulation of α-Tocopherol in Protein-Based Delivery Particles. *Food Research International*, **42**, 909-914. http://dx.doi.org/10.1016/j.foodres.2009.04.021

[6]   Song, Y.B., Lee, J.S. and Lee, H.G. (2009) α-Tocopherol-Loaded Ca-Pectinate Microcapsules: Optimization, *in Vitro* Release, and Bioavailability. *Colloids and Surfaces B: Biointerfaces*, **73**, 394-398. http://dx.doi.org/10.1016/j.colsurfb.2009.06.014

[7]   Sato, H., Taguchi, Y. and Tanaka, M. (2014) Development of Preparation Method for Microencapsulating Uycalyptus Oil Containing Fine Aqueous Droplets by Use of Interfacial Condensation Reaction between Hydroxy Propyl Methyl Cellulose and Tannic Acid. *Journal of Cosmetics, Dermatological Sciences and Applications*, **4**, 219-227. http://dx.doi.org/10.4236/jcdsa.2014.44030

[8]   Costoyas, Á., Ramos, J. and Forcada, J. (2009) Encapsulation of Silica Nanoparticles by Miniemulsion Polymerization. *Journal of Polymer Science: Part A: Polymer Chemistry*, **47**, 935-948. http://dx.doi.org/10.1002/pola.23212

[9]   Slobodian, P., Pavlínek, V., Lengálová, A. and Sáha, P. (2009) Polystyrene/Multi-Wall Carbon Nanotube Composites Prepared by Suspension Polymerization and Their Electrorheological Behavior. *Current Applied Physics*, **9**, 184-188. http://dx.doi.org/10.1016/j.cap.2008.01.008

[10]  Takahashi, M., Taguchi, Y. and Tanaka, M. (2009) Microencapsulation of Hydrophilic Solid Powder as a Fire Retar-

dant by the Method of *in Situ* Gelation in Droplets Using a Non-Aqueous Solvent as the Continuous Phase. *Polymers & Polymer Composites*, **17**, 83-90.

[11] Takahashi, M., Taguchi, Y. and Tanaka, M. (2010) Microencapsulation of Hydrophilic Solidpowder as a Flame Retardant with Epoxyresin by Using Interfacial Reaction Method. *Polymers for Advanced Technologies*, **21**, 224-228.

[12] Sawatari, N., Fukuda, M., Taguchi, Y. and Tanaka, M. (2004) The Effect of Surface Treatment of Magnetite Powder on a Structure of Composite Particles Prepared by Suspension Polymerization. *Journal of Chemical Engineering of Japan*, **37**, 731-736. http://dx.doi.org/10.1252/jcej.37.731

# Genital Warts in Infants and Children

## —Re-Evaluation of Podophylline 15% as an Effective Topical Therapy

Khalifa E. Sharquie[1,2]*, Adil A. Noaimi[1,2], Mohammed N. Almallah[3]

[1]Department of Dermatology, College of Medicine, University of Baghdad, Baghdad, Iraq
[2]Iraqi and Arab Board for Dermatology and Venereology, Baghdad Teaching Hospital, Medical City, Baghdad, Iraq
[3]Department of Dermatology and Venereology, Baghdad Teaching Hospital, Baghdad, Iraq
Email: *ksharquie@ymail.com, adilnoaimi@yahoo.com, vetmed83@hotmail.com

## Abstract

Background: Condylomataacuminata is an infection caused by Human Papilloma Virus, rarely reported in infants and children. Podophylline as a treatment for this condition has been used cautiously in this age group. Objective: To report the cases of anogenital warts including condy lomataacuminata in infants and children and to evaluate the effectiveness and side effects of 15% podophyllin in treatment of genital warts. Patient and Methods: Thirty infants and young children were seen in Department of Dermatology and Venereology—Baghdad Teaching Hospital in this case descriptive and therapeutic trial, in the period from January 2011 to August 2012. Their ages ranged from 8 - 72 (30.43 ± 15.85) months, 20 females and 10 males with a female:male ratio of 2:1. The duration of the disease ranged from 1 - 12 (5.26 ± 4.00) months. All demographics data were recorded in this study. History and examination were carried out to all patients. Family members including mothers were assessed about the presence of any type of viral warts in other location of body. Podophyllin (15%) in tincture benzoin was applied once weekly to all viral warts and the parents advised to wash out after 2 hours of application. The number of applications was repeated until full recovery. Follow-up after recovery was carried out for 6 months to watch for any relapse and to record local or systemic side effects. Results: The clinical pictures were mostly acondylomata acuminata in a form of cauliflower like warts in 20 (73.33%) patients, while in 10 (26.77%) patients there were ordinary verruca vulgaris like warts. The location of warts was perianal in 23 (76.66%) patients, genital only in 2 (6.66%) patients, and mixed in 5 (16.66%) patients. Topical applications of podophyllin 15% gave a full recovery in 27 (90%) patients, while in 3 (10%) patients there was partial response. The number of applications ranged from 1 - 4 (2.7 ± 1.42) applications. Follow up for 6 months after recovery showed relapse in only one patient, and no side effects were reported in any patients. Conclusion: There is upsurge of cases of anogenital warts among infants and children. Podophyllin (15%) in tincture benzoin is an effective therapy and no local or systemic side effects were recorded in any case.

*Corresponding author.

## Keywords

**Genital Warts in Infants and Children, Podophylline, Topical Therapy**

## 1. Introduction

Anogenital warts (AGWs) are caused by HPV. It is an old disease but the incidence of AGWs in children has increased dramatically all over the world since 1990 [1]-[3]. This increase in incidence of AGWs in children is thought to parallel the increase in incidence of AGWs in the adult population [3].

There are over 200 genotypes of Human Papilloma Viruses (HPV), 30 - 40 of which specifically affect the genital tract [4]. Genital types of HPV are divided into high or low risk according to the association with genital tract cancers.

Low-risk HPV types include Types 6, 11, 42-44, and usually cause benign anogenital warts, while high-risk HPV types include Types 16, 18, 31, 33-35, 39, 45, 51, 52, 56, 58, 59, 66, 68 and 70, and cause mostly anogenital cancers, primarily cervical cancer. Low risk HPV 6 and 11 genotypes are the primary causes of condy lomataacuminata, otherwise known as external genital warts [4].

HPV 16, 18, 31, 45 account for more than 90% of cervical carcinomas [5]. Of these types, HPV-16 is the most often found, accounting for about half of the cervical cancer cases in the United States and Europe [5].

Regarding mode of transmission, sexual abuse has been regarded as a possible cause of childhood genital warts associated with mucosal HPV types. The forms of sexual abuse are oral-genital contact, genital-genital contact, genital-anal contact, fondling and digital penetration of the vagina or anus [6] [7].

Reported frequency of sexual abuse varies considerably depending on the series studied [6] [7]. If sexual abuse is suspected in children, examination should always be performed including behavioral indications of abuse, medical examination to identify the physical indications of abuse, microbiological assessment of other STDs, and age-appropriate interviews of the child and caretakers by skilled personnel [8]-[12].

Most data suggest that AGWs among preadolescent children result from non-sexual transmission acquired either perinatally or postnatally [7]. Vertical transmission of HPVs has been reported to be responsible for at least 20% of AGWs in children [3] and occurs by contamination of the newborn descending through the birth canal, or viralascent through the membranes. In utreo, hematogenus transplacental transmission has been debated but has been supported by the fact that HPV16 DNA was detected in cord blood specimens of seven neonates born to mothers with HPV16 DNA in the peripheral blood mononuclear cells [13].

Horizontal transmission by caregivers in the first days of life is another mode of HPVs contamination in newborns. The concordance of HPVs types detected in the newborns and their mothers, reported to be only 57%, further supports this hypothesis [14], as well as the absence of correlation between HPVs on neonatal fore-skin and maternal abnormal Pap smear [15]. The frequency of transmission through inoculation varies with the child population studied [16].

Autoinoculation of HPVs, e.g. by scratching from one site of the body to another, is also possible [6] [7]. HPV type 2 is frequently detected in lesions of the oral mucosa or lips, and it might be acquired by chewing of common warts present on hands [6] [7].

It has also been shown that infants and children can acquire HPV infections by exposure to contaminated fomites such as underwear [17].

Disagreement exists regarding the incubation period of HPVs. Studies have indicated that HPVs can remain dormant for up to 5 years without causing lesions if transmitted vertically. However, other professionals have concluded that 2 years is the longest period that the HPVs lays dormant following vertical transmission [18].

HPV typing alone cannot determine the mode of transmission, because the virus does not display 100% tropism [19].

AGWs in children are associated with both mucosotropic types HPV6 and 11 and cutaneotropic types 1 and 2. [20].

Other HPV types like 3, 27, and 57 can be detected in both cutaneous and mucosal lesions [21].

In Iraq, the AGWs, has been reported as not uncommon problem but its frequency is increasing over the last 10 years.

Seventy-five percent of AGWs resolves spontaneously within months to a few years in children who have healthy immune systems [22]. Those persisting for more than 2 years are less likely to resolve spontaneously or with treatment [23]. But still therapy is strongly recommended in many cases as the disease bothers the parents.

There are no FDA approved treatments for AGWs in children 12 years of age and younger. Treatments can be divided into nonsurgical and surgical. No approach has been shown to be universally successful, and recurrence is common after any form of treatment. Some children may require combination of therapies. Because recurrence is common. Once a child has had AGWs, the appearance of new lesions after spontaneous resolution or treatment does not necessarily indicate a new exposure [24]. One can choose between cryotherapy, electrodessication, podophyllotoxin, or imiquimod [25].

Imiquimod has been effective even for extensive pediatric AGWs, without causing any significant side effects [26]. Podophyllotoxin has also been reported to be effective and safe in children with genital warts [26].

Podophyllin (15%) has been reported in Iraq to be a safe alternative without any side effect or complications [27].

Therefore the aim of present study was to report the upsurge of cases of AGWs among infants and children, and to confirm that podophyllin (15%) could be a safe weapon against HPVs infections of anogenital area.

## 2. Patients and Methods

This is a case, descriptive, therapeutic trial that was conducted in Department of Dermatology and Venereology—Baghdad Teaching Hospital in the period from January 2011 to August 2012.

A total of 30 infants and children with AGWs were enrolled in this study.

Ages, gender, duration of the disease, clinical type of warts, locations, symptoms, general health, and associated disease were recorded for all children.

AGWs or other types of warts, marital status of the parents, parent's employment status, educational level of the parents were extensively explored.

All patients were examined for any signs of sexual abuse (medical examination, inspection of the genitalia and anus), and the history of the child being placed with relatives and a behavioral history of the child, particularly any unusual behavior, was obtained.

Formal consent was taken from patient's parents following full explanation of the nature of the disease and the procedure of the treatment, and of any possible complications and the need for pre and post treatment photographs. Also, ethical approval was obtained from the Scientific Council of Dermatology and Venereology-Arab Board for Medical Specializations. Fifteen percent podophyllin was prepared by dissolving 15 grams of podophyllum resin (podpphyllin gepulvert, auspodophylumhexandrum, B.P.1973. paul Muggenburg, 2000 HAMBURG1. Ernste Vergiftungsgefahrbeim Verschlucken. Reizt Haut, Augen und Atemwege) in 100 ml benzoinco (COMPOUNlD BENZOIN TINCTURE BP, Friar's Balsam, EVANS, Evans Medical Limited Laughurst Horsham England).

Podophyllin (15%) in benzoin tincture was used in all patients once a week, to applied by a cotton applicator and left on the affected area to dry for a period of time not exceeding 2 hours and after 2 hours it should be washed out. The amount of podophyllin solution did not exceed 1ml/session. The patients were seen once weekly and photographs were taken at each visit.

Follow up was carried out after recovery at month 6 to record any relapse or side effects.

## 3. Results

Thirty patients with AGWs were included in the study, age ranging from 8 - 72 months with a mean ±SD of 30.43 ± 15.85 months, 20 females and 10 males with a female: male ratio of 2:1 (**Table 1**). The duration of the disease ranged from 1 - 12 months with a mean ± SD of 5.26 ± 4.00 months (**Table 2**). Acuminate lesions (**Figure 1**) were seen in 20 cases whereas in 10 patients ordinary verruca vulgaris like were noted. The location of the lesions was primarily perianal (23/30); 1 boy had lesions on the scrotum; 1 girl had lesions on the vulva; 3 girls had lesions simultaneously on the vulva and perianal area; and 2 boys had simultaneously lesions on the scrotum, penis, and perianal (**Table 3**).

Sexual abuse was not confirmed in any case, both on history and clinical examination. Family history of genital warts was denied among all family members apart from one girl and one boy that their mothers had genital warts. In 6 children, a history of common warts could be elicited by the caregivers, and in 1 girl, common warts

**Table 1.** Age of patients in months.

| Age | No. of patients | Percentage |
| --- | --- | --- |
| 1st 6 months | 0 | 0 |
| 7 - 12 | 6 | 20 |
| 13 - 18 | 4 | 13.33 |
| 19 - 24 | 6 | 20 |
| 25 - 36 | 6 | 20 |
| 37 - 72 | 8 | 26.67 |
| Total | 30 | 100 |

**Table 2.** Duration of disease in months.

| Duration | No. of patients | Percentage |
| --- | --- | --- |
| 0 - 3 | 14 | 46.66 |
| 4 - 6 | 9 | 30 |
| 7 - 9 | 2 | 6.67 |
| 10 - 12 | 3 | 10 |
| 13 - 16 | 2 | 6.67 |
| Total | 30 | 100 |

**Table 3.** Location of the warts.

| Location | No. of patients | Percentage |
| --- | --- | --- |
| Perianal | 23 | 76.67 |
| Genital | 2 | 6.67 |
| Both | 5 | 16.66 |
| Total | 30 | 100 |

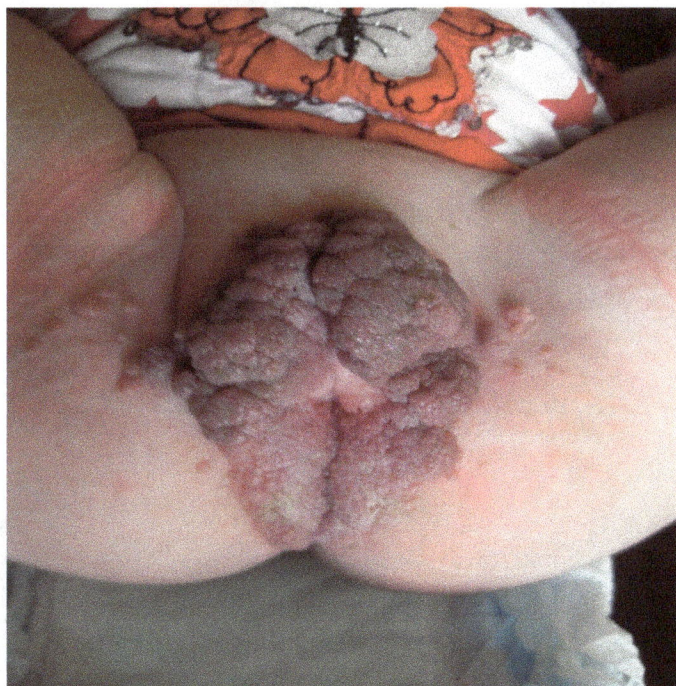

**Figure 1.** Condylomataacuminate in 1-year-old female infant of anogenital area.

affecting her hand were detected. No urethral or vaginal discharge was noticed in any patient.

Podophyllin 15% in tincture benzoin was used once weekly and the number of applications ranged from 1 - 4 applications with a mean ± SD of 2.7 ± 1.42 applications (**Table 4**). The response to therapy was obvious after one week and full recovery was achieved after 4 weeks, apart from 3 cases with partial response (**Figure 2**, **Figure 3**). The cure rate was 90%.

Acuminate lesions had more rapid response to therapy, necessitated less number of applications, and full recovery was seen in all cases, while ordinary viral warts had slow response to therapy, need more applications, and full recovery was seen in 7 out of 10 cases.

In all patients, a slight irritation and swelling of the lesion was noticed after the first application, which did not occur after subsequent applications. No child had any signs of toxicity during the course of therapy and follow up period.

No recurrences were noted apart from one case at 6-month follow-up period.

**Table 4.** Number of treatment sessions.

| No. of sessions | No. of patients | Percentage |
|---|---|---|
| 1 | 3 | 10 |
| 2 | 6 | 20 |
| 3 | 13 | 43.33 |
| 4 | 8 | 26.67 |
| Total | 30 | 100 |

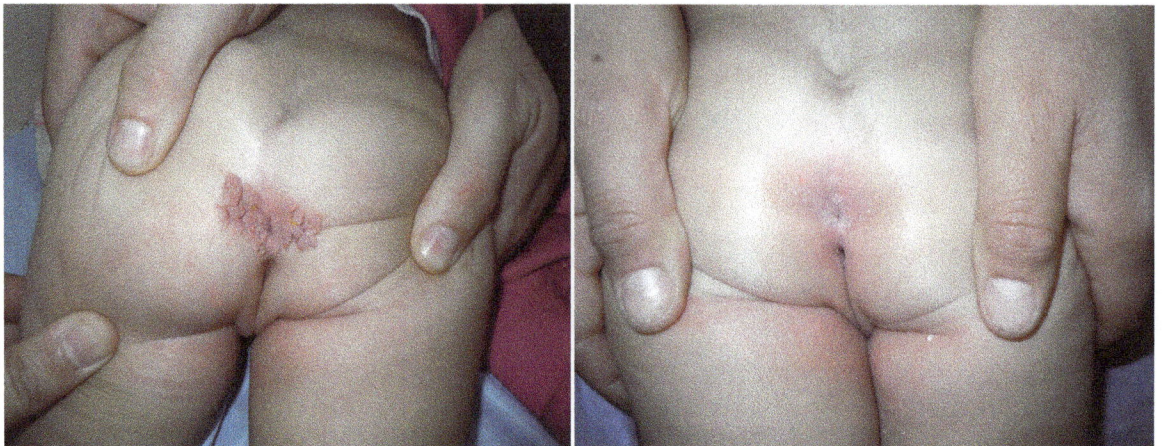

**Figure 2.** (a) One and a half-year-old female before podophyllin treatment; (b) After 3 sessions of podophyllin treatment.

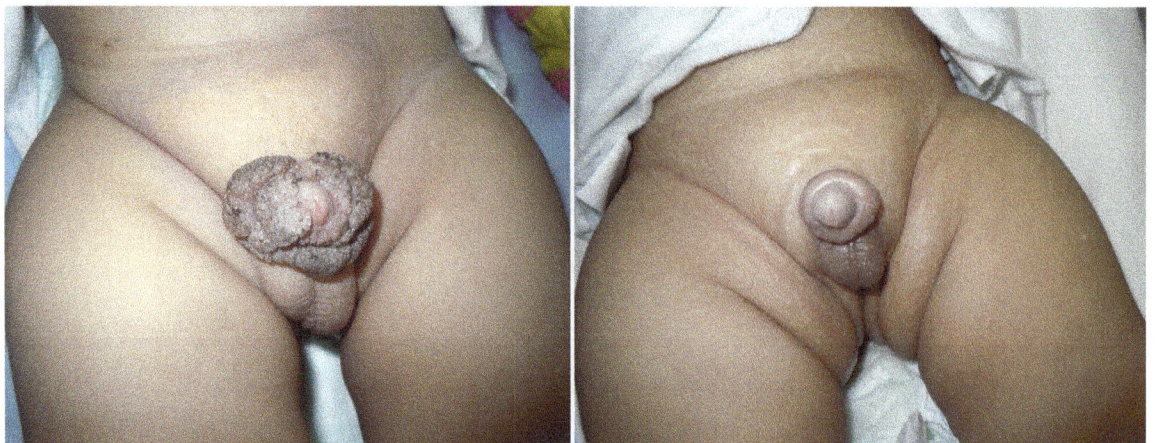

**Figure 3.** (a) One and a half-year-old male before podophyllin treatment; (b) After 3 sessions of podophyllin treatment.

## 4. Discussion

The incidence of anogenital warts in infants and children has increased dramatically all over the world since 1990 [1]-[3]. This is thought to parallel the increase in incidence of AGWs in the adult population [3].

These reasons might explain the increase in the frequency of AGWs in Iraqi infants and children or there might be other contributory.

In children with AGWs, reports of sexual abuse have varied from 0% to 80% [19] [28]. In our study, we did not document any case of sexual abuse by history or physical examination.

However, evaluation is complex, because most children who have been sexually abused will not show carriage of the virus, nor will have evidence of physical trauma [29] [30].

The presence of warts or HPVs DNA alone without supporting social and clinical information is not diagnostic of sexual abuse. An epidemiological study of 124 children with clinical HPVs infection concluded that many children over 2 years of age acquired HPVs from non-sexual contact. The positive predictive value of the presence of AGWs for sexual abuse was 37% for children aged 2 - 12 years, and increased with age (70% for children over 8 years of age) [22]. But still sexual abuse needs to be considered in every case of AGWs, particularly in those over 2 - 3 years of age.

Vertical transmission of HPVs has been reported, HPVs transmission can occur inutero through semen, ascending infection from the mother's genital tract, or transplacentally [3]. Vertical transmission of the HPVs does not mean that warts must be present at birth or shortly after birth. HPVs is a latent virus and can reside in the skin and mucous membranes without causing warts. The warts may not appear until months or even years after birth [18].

Horizontal transmission by caregivers and autoinoculation of HPVs, e.g. by scratching from one site of the body to another, is another possibility of infection [3].

It has also been shown that infants and children can acquire HPVs infections by contaminated fomites such as underwear [17].

HPVs typing does not offer any help to determine whether genital warts in children are sexually transmitted or not [19].

Most of AGWs disappear spontaneously within months to a few years in children who have good immune system [23]. Those persisting for more than 2 years are less likely to resolve spontaneously or with treatment [24].

The decision to treat or not AGWs in children lies on the physician. However, the overwhelming parent's anxiety and the problems that AGWs may cause, such as bleeding or infection, usually lead to a form of treatment.

Many treatments have been used in infants and children, one can choose cryotherapy, electrodessication, podophyllotoxin, or imiquimod [26].

After the discovery of podophyllum resin in 1835 by John King [31], it was put to numerous innovative therapeutic uses over the next century ranging from a laxative to treatment of cancers. However, in the 1940s, it has been used topically for treatment of various skin lesions, especially for venereal warts, and also has antineoplastic effect, as it has been shown in a very recent study

Podophyllin resin is an antimitotic and caustic agent with antiviral activity [32] [33]. The possible mechanism of action is that it arrests cellular mitosis in metaphase, accomplished by reverse binding to tubuline which is the protein subunit of the spindle microtubules at a site that is the same of overlaps with the colchicines binding site thereby preventing polymerization of tubuline into microtubules. So it will disturbs the cellular cytoskeleton; it blocks oxidation enzymes in tricaboxylic acid cycle, and interferes with nutrition of cells; it inhibits axonal transport, protein, RNA, and DNA synthesis and also inhibits mitochondrial activity and reduction of cytochrome oxidase activity [34] [35].

Side effects include local erythema, tenderness, burning, erosions, and edema [36]. If podophyllin is used in an extensive area or injected or ingested, central nervous system toxicity and respiratory depression may result [35].

Experimental studies in animals have clearly demonstrated that podophyllin is embryotoxic and has a strong growth retarding effect on pregnancy [36] [37]. Fetal anomalies suspected to have been induced by podophyllin include preauricular skin tags, limb malformations, simian crease, septal heart defects and polyneuritis [38] [39]. Intrauterine death has also followed the application of podophyllin on vulvarwarts [40].

Bargman [41] has reviewed the whole subject of systemic toxicity to podophyllin including its reported teratogenicity. He noted that in almost all cases there were factors (such as alcohol or drug abuse, recent surgical procedures, general anaesthesia) which may have potentiated the toxicity of podophyllin. Since nearly all reported cases have been blacks, he also considered the possibility of an unsuspected racial susceptibility. He concluded that the dangers of podophyllin toxicity have been overplayed, and that it is an extremely safe drug when used properly.

Accordingly, podophyllin has been widely used in Iraq in the treatment of genital warts among infants and children, and proved to be a safe drug when applied cautiously and wisely. Its safety has been well documented by an Iraqi study in 2006 among infants and children with AGWs, where in 18 patients with conylomata acuminate were treated with podophyllin 15% during the period from January 1996 to January 2000, effectively with a cure rate 100%, and no side effects were reported during therapy and follow up [28].

In this study, a greater number of patients were included for a shorter study duration indicating a possible increase in incidence.

We had also proved that podophyllin application is an effective therapy for genital warts in infants and children and no case showed any symptoms and signs of toxicity. The cure rate was 90% and was more effective in acuminate lesions.

Sundharam in 2011 put precautions based on the recommendations of Fisher [42], Miller [43] and others [38]-[40], so the following precautions are considered obligatory in this table:

| Precautions No. | Precautions |
|---|---|
| 1 | Podophyllin should be applied only by the physician. |
| 2 | The drug should be applied only to small areas of intact skin. Biopsies if taken, should be allowed to heal completely before the application of podophyllin. |
| 3 | Alcohol should be avoided before and for several hours after the application. General anaesthesia and central nervous system depressant drugs should be avoided. |
| 4 | The drug should be avoided in the oral cavity. |
| 5 | It should not be used in pregnant women. |
| 6 | Initially, a test application should be left on for a period of one hour. If there is no irritation, subsequent applications should be allowed to remain for 4 - 6 hours. |
| 7 | The volume of liquid applied should be kept to the minimum (von Krogh [44] recommends a volume not exceeding 0.4 - 0.5 ml for *P. emodi* based podophyllin and 0.9 -1.2 nil for *P. peltatum* based podophyllin). |
| 8 | The drug should be stored in narrow-mouthed bottles, otherwise undue evaporation might lead to an increased concentration of podophyllin. Preparations containing a sludge or precipitate and old, dried, gritty preparations should be discarded. |

But our practice doesn't agree with many of these precautions, and we recommend the following guidelines of therapy:

1) The drug should be applied by physician or by very careful parents.

2) Podophyllin should be used in low concentrations not above 15% and kept for not more than 2 hours, possibly half an hour is enough, and then washed away.

3) The drug used once a week and could be repeated according to the response.

4) Infants and children should be kept under clinical supervision to watch any side effect, and laboratory test like liver function test, renal function test, complete blood picture might be needed.

These recommendations agrees with bargman who concluded that the danger of podophyllin toxicity have been overplayed and could be used safely when used in correct way.

After the use of podophyllotoxin, which is much safer and less irritating than podophyllin, podophyllin has been largely replaced. However, it is a useful alternative and its use should not be completely abandoned.

## 5. Conclusion

Podophyllin (15%) in tincture benzoin is an effective therapy for AGWs in infants and children and no adverse effects were noted in any case.

# References

[1] Cohen, B.A. (1997) Warts and Children: Can They Be Separated? *Contemporary Pediatrics*, **14**, 128-149.

[2] Siegfried, E., Conley, R., Cook, J., Leonardi, C. and Monteleone, J. (1998) Human Papillomavirus Screening in Pediatric Victims of Sexual Abuse. *Pediatrics*, **101**, 43-47. http://dx.doi.org/10.1542/peds.101.1.43

[3] Syrjänen, S. and Puranen, M. (2000) HPV Infections in Children: The Potential Role of Maternal Transmission. *Critical Reviews in Oral Biology Medicine*, **11**, 259-274. http://dx.doi.org/10.1177/10454411000110020801

[4] Garland, S. (2002) Human Papillomavirus Update with a Particular Focus on Cervical Disease. *Pathology*, **34**, 213-224. http://dx.doi.org/10.1080/00313020212469

[5] Muñoz, N., Bosch, F.X., de Sanjosé, S., Herrero, R., Castellsagué, X., Shah, K.V., *et al.* (2003) Epidemiologic Classification of Human Papilloma Virus Types Associated with Cervical Cancer. *New England Journal of Medicine*, **348**, 518-527.

[6] Syrjänen, K. and Syrjänen, S. (2000) Papillomavirus Infections in Human Disease. Wiley & Sons, New York, 1-615.

[7] Syrjänen, S. (2003) HPV Infections in Children. Invited Review. *Papillomavirus Report*, **14**, 93-110. http://dx.doi.org/10.1179/095741903235001425

[8] Hornor, G. (2004) Ano-Genital Warts in Children: Sexual Abuse or Not? *Journal of Pediatric Health Care*, **18**, 165-170. http://dx.doi.org/10.1016/j.pedhc.2003.01.001

[9] Gutman, L.T., Claire, K., Herman-Giddens, M.E., Johnston, W.W. and Phelps, W.C. (1992) Evaluation of Sexually Abused and Non-Abused Young Girls for Intravaginal Human Papillomavirus Infection. *American Journal of Diseases of Children*, **146**, 694-699.

[10] Gutman, L.T., Claire, K.K., Everett, V.D., Ingram, D.L., Soper, J. and Johnston, W.W. (1994) Cervical-Vaginal and Intra Anal Human Papillomavirus Infection of Young Girls with External Genital Warts. *The Journal of Infectious Diseases*, **170**, 339-344. http://dx.doi.org/10.1093/infdis/170.2.339

[11] Gutman, L.T. (1990) Sexual Abuse and Human Papillomavirus Infection. *Journal of Pediatrics*, **116**, 495-496. http://dx.doi.org/10.1016/S0022-3476(05)82863-X

[12] Muram, D. (1989) Anal and Perianal Abnormalities in Prepubertal Victims of Sexual Abuse. *American Journal of Obstetrics & Gynecology*, **161**, 278-281. http://dx.doi.org/10.1016/0002-9378(89)90498-5

[13] Tseng, C.J., Lin, C.Y., Wang, R.L., Chen, L.J., Chang, Y.L., Hsieh, T.T. and Pao, C.C. (1992) Possible Transplacental Transmission of Human Papillomaviruses. *American Journal of Obstetrics & Gynecology*, **166**, 35-40. http://dx.doi.org/10.1016/0002-9378(92)91825-U

[14] Alberico, S., Pinzano, R., Comar, M., Toffoletti, F., Maso, G., Ricci, G. and Guaschino, S. (1996) Maternal-Fetal Transmission of Human Papillomavirus. *Minerva Ginecologica*, **48**, 199-204.

[15] Roman, A. and Fife, K. (1986) Human Papillomavirus DNA Associated with Foreskins of Normal Newborns. *Journal of Infectious Diseases*, **153**, 855-861. http://dx.doi.org/10.1093/infdis/153.5.855

[16] Handley, J., Hanks, E., Armstrong, K., Bingham, A., Dinsmore, W., Swann, A., Evans, M.F., McGee, J.O.D. and O'Learj, J. (1997) Common Association of HPV 2 with Anogenital Warts in Prepubertal Children. *Pediatric Dermatology*, **14**, 339-343. http://dx.doi.org/10.1111/j.1525-1470.1997.tb00976.x

[17] Bergeron, C., Ferenczy, A. and Richart, R. (1990) Underwear: Contamination by Human Papillomaviruses. *American Journal of Obstetrics & Gynecology*, **162**, 25-29. http://dx.doi.org/10.1016/0002-9378(90)90813-M

[18] Frazier, L. (1998) Genital Warts in Children. *The American Professional Society of the Abuse of Children Advisor*, **11**, 9-12.

[19] Armstrong, D.K. and Handley, J.M. (1997) Anogenital Warts in Prepubertal Children: Pathogenesis, HPV Typing and Management. *International Journal of STD & AIDS*, **8**, 78-81. http://dx.doi.org/10.1258/0956462971919598

[20] Joyasinghe, Y. and Garland, S.M. (2006) Genital Warts in Children: What Do They Mean? *Archives of Disease in Childhood*, **91**, 696-700. http://dx.doi.org/10.1136/adc.2005.092080

[21] Singlair, K., Woods, C., Kirse, D. and Sinal, S.H. (2005) Anogenital and Respiratory Tract Human-Papillomavirus Infections among Children: Age Gender and Potential Transmission through Sexual Abuse. *Pediatrics*, **116**, 815-825. http://dx.doi.org/10.1542/peds.2005-0652

[22] Culton, D.A., Morrell, D.S. and Burkhart, C.N. (2009) The Management of Condyloma Acuminata in the Pediatric Population. *Pediatric Annals*, **38**, 368-372. http://dx.doi.org/10.3928/00904481-20090622-05

[23] Allen, A.L. and Siegfried, E.C. (1998) The Natural History of Condyloma in Children. *Journal of the American Academy of Dermatology*, **39**, 951-955. http://dx.doi.org/10.1016/S0190-9622(98)70268-3

[24] Sinclair, K.A., Woods, C.R. and Sinal, S.H. (2011) Venereal Warts in Children. *Pediatrics in Review*, **32**, 115-121.

http://dx.doi.org/10.1542/pir.32-3-115

[25] Stefanaki, C., Barkas, G., Valari, M., Bethimoutis, G., Nicolaidou, E., Vosynioti, V., Kontochristopoulos, G., Papado-georgaki, H., Verra, P. and Katsarou, A. (2012) Condylomata Acuminata in Children. *The Pediatric Infectious Disease Journal*, **31**, 422-424.

[26] Moresi, J.M., Herbert, C.R. and Cohen, B.A. (2001) Treatment of Anogenial Warts in Children with Topical 0.05% Podophilox Gel and Imiquimod Cream. *Pediatric Dermatology*, **18**, 448-450. http://dx.doi.org/10.1046/j.1525-1470.2001.1980a.x

[27] Sharquie, K.E., Al-Waiz, M.M. and Al-Nuaimy, A.A. (2005) Condylomata Acuminata in Infants and Young Children. Topical Podophyllin an Effective Therapy. *Saudi Medical Journal*, **26**, 502-503.

[28] Moscicki, A. (1998) Genital Infections with Human Papillomavirus (HPV). *Pediatric Infectious Disease Journal*, **17**, 651-652. http://dx.doi.org/10.1097/00006454-199807000-00014

[29] Atabaki, S. and Paradise, J. (1999) The Medical Evaluation of the Sexually Abused Child: Lessons Learned from a Decade of Research. *Pediatrics*, **104**, 178-186.

[30] Berenson, A.B., Chacko, M.R., Wiemann, C.M., Mishaw, C.O., Friedrich, W.N. and Grady, J.J. (2000) A Case-Control Study of Anatomic Changes Resulting from Sexual Abuse. *American Journal of Obstetrics & Gynecology*, **182**, 820-834. http://dx.doi.org/10.1016/S0002-9378(00)70331-0

[31] Zakon, S. (1952) Discovery of Podophyllum Resin. *JAMA Dermatology*, **65**, 620-622. http://dx.doi.org/10.1001/archderm.1952.01530240112022

[32] Sharquie, K.E. and Noaimi, A.A. (2012) Basal Cell Carcinoma: Topical Therapy versus Surgical Treatment. *Journal of the Saudi Society of Dermatology and Dermatologic Surgery*, **16**, 41-51. http://dx.doi.org/10.1016/j.jssdds.2012.06.002

[33] United States Pharmacopeia Committees (2004) Podophyllin. In: *Drug Information for the Health Care Professional*, 24th Edition, Rev. US Convention Inc., Thomason Micromedex, 2341-2348.

[34] Oslen, D.G. and Dart, R.C. (2004) Skin and Mucous Membrane Agents. In: *Medical Toxicology*, 3rd Edition, Vol. 165, Walters Kluwer Company, Philadilphia, 1003-1004.

[35] Moore, M.M. and Strober, B.E. (2008) Topical and Intralesional Cytotoxic Agent. In: Wolff, K., Goldsmith, L.A., Katz, S.I., Gilchrest, B.A., Paller, A.S. and Leffell, D.J., Eds., *Fitzpatrick's Dermatology in General Medicine*, 7th Edition, McGraw-Hill-Company, New York, 220, 224.

[36] Thiersch, J.B. (1963) Effect of Podophyllin and Podophyllotoxin on the Rat Litter in Utero. *Proc. Soc. Exp. Biol. Med.*, **113**, 124.

[37] Joneja, M.G. and Leliever, W.C. (1974) Effects of Vinblastine and Podophyllin on DBA Mouse Fetuses. *Toxicology and Applied Pharmacology*, **27**, 408-414. http://dx.doi.org/10.1016/0041-008X(74)90211-7

[38] Cullis, J.E. (1962) Congenital Deformities and Herbal "Slimming Tablets". *Lancet*, **280**, 511-512. http://dx.doi.org/10.1016/S0140-6736(62)90387-2

[39] Karol, M., Conner, C., Watanabe, A.S. and Murphrey, K. (1980) Podophyllum: Suspected Teratogenicity from Topical Application. *Clinical Toxicology*, **16**, 283-286. http://dx.doi.org/10.3109/15563658008989950

[40] Chamberlein, M.J., Reynolds, A.L. and Yeoman, M.B. (1972) Toxic Effect of Podophyllum Application in Pregnancy. *British Medical Journal*, **3**, 391-392. http://dx.doi.org/10.1136/bmj.3.5823.391

[41] Bargman, H. (1988) Is Podophyllin a Safe Drug to Use and Can It Be Used in Pregnancy? *JAMA Dermatology*, **124**, 1718-1729. http://dx.doi.org/10.1001/archderm.1988.01670110074020

[42] Fisher, A. (1981) Sever Systemic and Local Reaction to Topical Podophyllin Resin. *Cutis*, **28**, 233-236.

[43] Miller, R.A. (1985) Podophyllin. *International Journal of Dermatology*, **24**, 491-498. http://dx.doi.org/10.1111/j.1365-4362.1985.tb05535.x

[44] Von Krogh, G. (1983) Condylomata Acuminate 1983 an Updated Review. *Semin Dermatol*, **2**, 109-129.

# 11

# Usefulness of a Newly-Developed Device, the Power Tree®, for Body Massage: Evidence from a Medical Evaluation

Kentaro Ishii[1], Mayumi Kotani[1], Akihito Fujita[1], Shinichi Moriwaki[2]

[1]Bloom Classic Co., Matsuyama, Japan
[2]Department of Dermatology, Osaka Medical College, Takatsuki, Japan
Email: der002@poh.osaka-med.ac.jp

## Abstract

We investigated the effectiveness and usefulness of a novel tool: the Power Tree®, for body massage in 10 healthy female volunteers (age range, 24 - 55 years; mean age, 40.5 years) by evaluating several dermatological and psychological parameters, such as the amount of dermal collagen, the skin temperature, the level of salivary amylase and the scores on the State-Trait Anxiety Index (STAI). After 60-minute Power Tree®-mediated body massage, both the dermal collagen score determined from the DermaLab® images and skin temperature measured by infrared thermography were found to have increased significantly in several body sites compared to those before the treatment (p < 0.01 and p < 0.001, respectively). Although the level of stress estimated by the amount of amylase in the saliva was not significantly different pre- and post-procedure (p = 0.3), the treatment significantly reduced both the state anxiety (SA) and trait anxiety (TA) scores on the STAI (p < 0.001 for the SA, p < 0.01 for the TA). The treatment with this device was smoothly performed without any burden on the therapists during the present study. These data suggest that the newly-developed device is a powerful and useful tool for reflexology when used for full body massage therapy, and massage therapy using this device may produce beneficial, physiological effects as well as psychosocial improvements.

## Keywords

Dermal Collagen Score, Hand Massage, Power Tree®, Salivary Amylase, Skin Temperature, STAI

## 1. Introduction

There are a number of procedures used in the aesthetic and aesthetic dermatological field, where people can receive non-invasive treatments for the purpose of anti-skin aging or slimming.

Among these procedures, a hand massage can be a good alternative not only to a facial but also to a full body treatment. It can be a relaxing, rejuvenating and sometimes becomes a therapeutic method for flabby skin. However, there have been only a few studies that have evaluated the effectiveness of a hand massage based on medical approaches [1]-[4].

The application of a treatment by hand or a hand massage is one of the commonly used non-invasive cosmetic procedures, and it not only provides the skin with nourishment and improves the circulation, resulting in rejuvenated skin, but also is known be a good way to relieve stress. On the other hand, therapists have to continue to work for long hours and utilize their skin and muscles in every possible type of motion and injuries of the hands and back are common among manual therapists. In addition, therapists sometimes become exhausted after performing the hard work for several days in succession, although certain breathing and stretching exercises may help.

In such situation, the similar massage can be performed with appropriate products, such as stones or sticks. The quality or the effect of the treatment depends on how well therapists have been trained, how skilled they are, and how they feel when they are performing the treatment. Therefore, a treatment with these products may be helpful for practitioners, because it enables them to uniformly and stably add power and to control the intensity of the power applied to the subjects' skin, making them more comfortable. For example, a hot stone massage is a special kind of massage where therapists use and handle smooth, heated stones to massage the subject. By using the stones, the therapists can work more accurately, more quickly and more easily compared with the treatment using just their hands without the stones.

We recently developed a new device for body treatment using a tree instead of a stone. The device is made from Hinoki cypress and has a peculiar shape, which is perfectly configured for full body of humans. In this study, we examined the effectiveness and usefulness of this novel tool (Power Tree®) for body massage by evaluating several dermatological and psychological parameters.

## 2. Materials and Methods

We enrolled 10 healthy female volunteers (age range, 24 - 55 years; mean age, 40.5 years) in the present study. We applied the newly developed novel-shaped tool, the Power Tree®, made from Hanoi cypress, for a full massage body massage (**Figure 1**).

A typical full body massage consists of effleurage, friction, pressure, smoothing and kneading, and these treatments are performed in order on appropriate sites of the body with a mixture of massage oil (**Table 1**), typically for 60 minutes. In all of these steps, the Power Tree® was used instead of the hands and the treatments were performed by three female therapists in the present study.

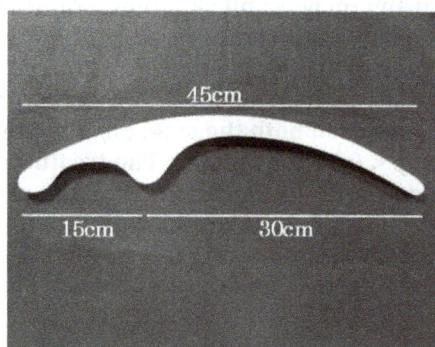

**Figure 1.** The newly-developed device, the Power Tree®, made of Hinoki cypress.

**Table 1.** The major chemical constitutions of the essential oils used in the study.

| | |
|---|---|
| Hydrogenated poly (C6-12 olefin) | 35% |
| Oryza sativa (rice) bran oil | 35% |
| Cetylethylhexanoate | 30% |

We analyzed the changes in the dermal collagen score, skin temperature and release of the salivary enzyme alpha-amylase, before and immediately after the body massage treatment by using a SkinLab Ultrasound system (DermaLab®, Cortex Technology, Denmark), a Thermo Shot F20 (NEC Avio Infrared Technologies Co., Ltd, Japan) and a Cocoro Meter (Nipro Co., Japan), respectively according to the manufacturers' instructions. The cross-sectional skin image obtained by the SkinLab device represents the intensity of collagen signals, where high density (yellow or red) areas contain abundant collagen. Before and after the procedure, ultrasound images were compared with an average density in the range 0 - 100. The higher the density in the dermis, the higher the collagen score is. This dermal collagen score was measured at the lateral site of the left thigh. The skin temperature was measured at three points; the center of the bilateral scapulae and the bilateral posterior site of the thigh before and after the procedure by using infrared thermal imaging camera. The Cocoro Meter is a stress detector and the level of the comprehensive stress can be evaluated by measuring the amount of amylase in the saliva with this meter after putting its spatula on the subject's tongue for 60 seconds. In addition, the Spielberger State-Trait Anxiety Index (STAI) (Chiba Test Center Co., Ltd, Tokyo) was measured as described previously [5] [6] to assess the subject' levels of anxiety. The STAI inventory is used to assess both state and trait anxiety (SA and TA) separately. Each type of anxiety has its own scale of 20 different questions that are scored. Scores range from 20 to 80, with higher scores correlating with greater anxiety. All of the measurements were carried out immediately after the therapy and there was no skin abnormality including edema and erythema.

All of the analyses were performed after obtaining institutional approval and written informed consent from the subject and the study was conducted according to the principles of the Declaration of Helsinki. The results are expressed as the means with SD. The statistical analyses were performed using the two-tailed student's t test for independent samples. Significant differences were recognized at p values $\leq 0.05$.

## 3. Results

The sixty-minute treatment with this device was smoothly performed without any burden on the therapists in the present study.

The dermal collagen score assessed by the SkinLab system increased from $55.5 \pm 13$ to $67.5 \pm 18.5$ by the treatment (**Figure 2(a)**, **Figure 2(b)**) and this change was statistically significant (p = 0.005). In addition, the skin temperature of the back, right thigh and left thigh (mean $\pm$ SD pre-treatment: $34.5 \pm 0.9$, $32 \pm 0.7$ and $32.4$

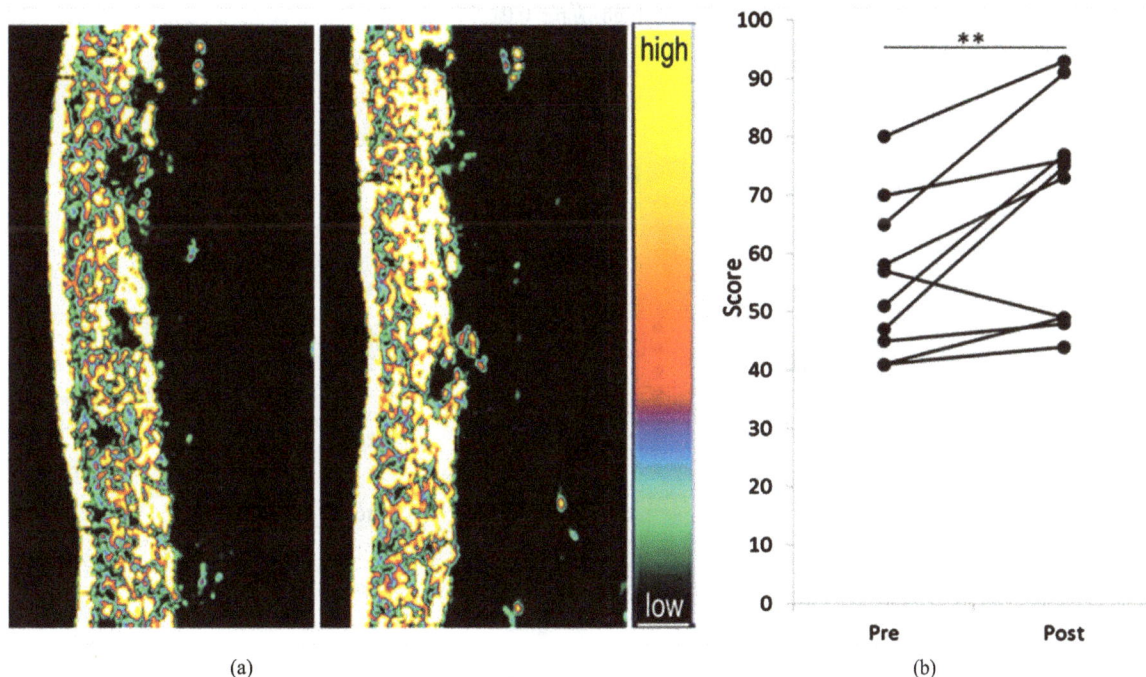

(a)                                                                                    (b)

**Figure 2.** An image showing the changes in dermal collagen score in a representative subject (a) and all of the data regarding the changes in the dermal collagen score (b). **p < 0.01.

± 0.7, respectively) was increased significantly by the treatment (post-treatment 36.1 ± 1, 35.1 ± 1 and 35 ± 0.9, respectively, p < 0.001) (**Figure 3(a)**, **Figure 3(b)**).

Regarding the level of general stress, the concentration (kU/l) of amylase in the saliva was not significantly different pre- and post-procedure (mean + SD: 58 + 40, 64 ± 28, respectively) (p = 0.3) (data not shown). However, the mean ± SD of SA and TA scores before the procedure were 43 ± 8 and 46 ± 10, respectively, and changed to 27 ± 5 and 42 ± 9, respectively, after the treatment. Both of these changes were statistically significant (p = 0.0002 for the SA, p = 0.009 for the TA) (**Figure 4**).

## 4. Discussion

There have been several reports of the psychological and physiological efficacy of hand massage therapy;

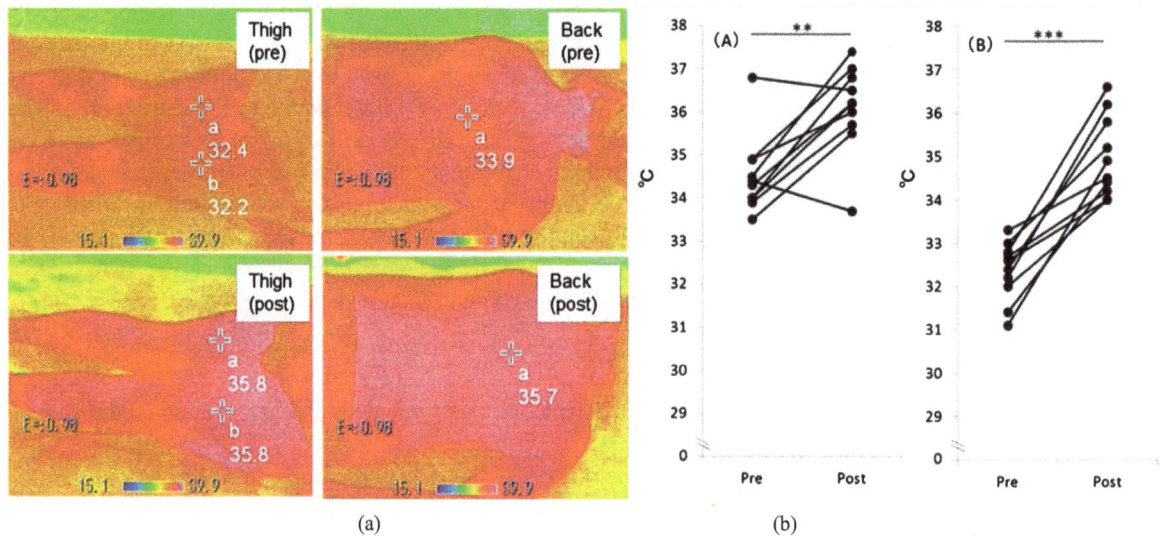

**Figure 3.** A representative image showing the changes in the skin temperature in a subject (a) and all of the data for the changes in skin temperature ((A) back; (B) left thigh). **p < 0.01, ***p < 0.001.

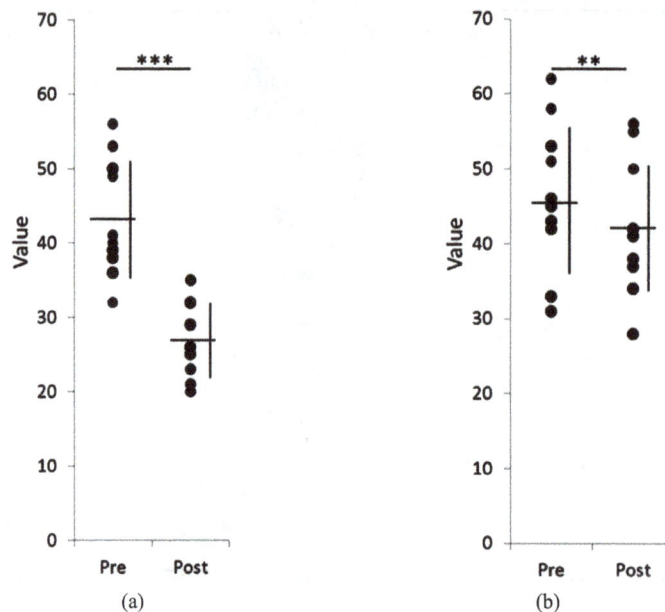

**Figure 4.** The changes in the STAI score. (a) State anxiety; (b) Trait anxiety. Vertical bar = SD, horizontal bar = mean value. **p < 0.01, ***p < 0.001.

relaxation, improvement of the score estimated by the STAI and a decrease in the levels of cortisol and nor epinephrine [1]-[5].

In the present study, we evaluated the usefulness of a special tool; the Power Tree®-mediated massage therapy by assessing various parameters including the dermal collagen score, skin temperature, the level of stress based on the concentration of salivary amylase as well as the STAI score. The collagen stimulating effect of the Power Tree®-mediated treatment in the dermis visualized by the DermaLab® system was confirmed.

We also observed that the Power Tree® increased the skin temperature after the massage. However, there was little or no change in the level of salivary amylase after the procedure. The level of salivary amylase is one of the valuable biological indicators of physiological and psychological stress reactions. The lack of any differences between the salivary amylase levels before and after treatment may have been due to a lack of stress pre-procedure or the discomfort associated with the use of the Power Tree®, even though they were receiving a treatment considered to have a relaxing effect.

In the present study, we examined the psychological effects of the massage by evaluating the STAI scores, and we observed that the post-procedure scores were significantly lower for both the SA and TA compared to those pre-procedure. These results suggest that beneficial effects in terms of anxiety reduction were obtained by the full body massage using the Power Tree®. The improvement of the TA following the procedure implies the possibility that there is a healing effect induced by Power Tree®-mediated message therapy.

## 5. Conclusion

In conclusion, a newly-developed device, the Power Tree®, is a powerful and useful tool for reflexology during full body massage therapy, as evaluated by several medical parameters. By using this device, massage therapy may produce beneficial physiological effects as well as psychosocial improvement.

Because we performed this study in only a small number of subjects, and examined the data over a short period before and immediately after the treatment, it is necessary to validate the effects a longer period of time after the Power Tree®-mediated massage in a future study, and to examine the impact of the treatment in patients experiencing high levels of stress prior to the treatment.

## Conflict of Interests

One of the authors (S.M.) is a research adviser for the Bloom Classic Co.

## References

[1]  Kuriyama, H., Watanabe, S., Nakaya, T., Shigemori, I., Kita, M., Yoshida, N., Masaki, D., Tadai, T., Ozasa, K., Fukui, K. and Imanishi, J. (2005) Immunological and Psychological Benefits of Aromatherapy Massage. *Evidence-Based Complementary and Alternative Medicine*, 2, 179-184. http://dx.doi.org/10.1093/ecam/neh087

[2]  Noto, Y., Kudo, M. and Hirota, K. (2010) Back Massage Therapy Promotes Psychological Relaxation and an Increase in Salivary Chromogranin A Release. *Journal of Anesthesia*, 24, 955-958. http://dx.doi.org/10.1007/s00540-010-1001-7

[3]  Lee, Y.H., Park, B.N.P. and Kim, S.H. (2011) The Effects of Heat and Massage Application on Autonomic Nervous System. *Yonsei Medical Journal*, 52, 982-989. http://dx.doi.org/10.3349/ymj.2011.52.6.982

[4]  Rapaport, M.H., Schettler, P. and Bresee, C. (2012) A Preliminary Study of the Effects of Repeated Massage on Hypothalamic-Pituitary-Adrenal and Immune Function in Healthy Individuals: A Study of Mechanisms of Action and Dosage. *Journal of Alternative and Complementary Medicine*, 18, 789-797. http://dx.doi.org/10.1089/acm.2011.0071

[5]  Hashizume, H., Horibe, T., Ohshima, A., Ito, T., Yagi, H. and Takigawa, M. (2005) Anxiety Accelerates T-Helper 2-Tilted Immune Responses in Patients with Atopic Dermatitis. *British Journal of Dermatology*, 152, 1161-1164. http://dx.doi.org/10.1111/j.1365-2133.2005.06449.x

[6]  McVicar, A.J., Greenwood, C.R., Fewell, F., D'Arcy, V., Chandrasekharan, S. and Alldridge, L.C. (2007) Evaluation of Anxiety, Salivary Cortisol and Melatonin Secretion Following Reflexology Treatment: A Pilot Study in Healthy Individuals. *Complementary Therapies in Clinical Practice*, 13, 137-145. http://dx.doi.org/10.1016/j.ctcp.2006.11.001

# 12

# Documentation and Phytochemical Screening of Traditional Beauty Products Used in Missenyi District of Tanzania

**Sheila M. Maregesi\*, Godeliver A. Kagashe, Fatuma Felix**

Pharmacognosy Department, School of Pharmacy, Muhimbili University College of Health and Allied Sciences, Dar es Salaam, Tanzania
Email: \*smaregesi@hotmail.com

Academic Editor: Pierfrancesco Morganti, Mavicosmetics, Italy

## Abstract

Background Information: The concept of beauty and cosmetics is as old as mankind and civilization. Raw materials for beauty products are dominated by petroleum and synthetic products. In recent years, there has been an increase of natural product-based cosmetics along with creating beauty from the inside by consumption of nutraceuticals. Tanzania traditional beauty products are still in use especially rural areas, but the documentation is lacking. Objectives: This work aimed at documenting traditional beauty products in Kagera region as an effort to avoid loss of useful information and available useful traditional findings for safe utilization in beauty products. Methodology: Information was obtained from knowledgeable people in Missenyi district by focus group discussion. Collected materials were identified in Botany and Zoology Departments at the University of Dar es Salaam followed by literature search and phytochemical screening. Results: This study afforded to record 13 plants, 4 animal products, mineral and other organic products. Most products are used for skin care (57%) followed by hair care (22%). Literature search supported the use of some of the products and plants subjected to qualitative analysis showed presence of phytochemicals relevant to beautification. Discussion: Some of the recorded plant and animal products are incorporated in natural based cosmetic products. Hazardous practice of using skin lightening plant products and dry cell powders was noted. Conclusion: The use of products which are already incorporated in the cosmetic products especially in countries where these products are well regulated should be promoted. Products reported for the first time require scientific studies to establish their effectiveness and safety. Since this study recorded the use of some dangerous materials, people need to be educated through media.

---

\*Corresponding author.

## Keywords

**Tanzania, Traditional Beauty Products, Phytochemicals**

## 1. Introduction

A cosmetic product refers to any substance or preparation intended to be applied on various external parts of the human body (epidermis, hair system, nails, lips and external genital organs) or on the teeth and the mucous membranes of the oral cavity with a view of cleaning them, perfuming them, changing their appearance and/or correcting body odors and/or protecting them or keeping them in good conditions [1]. Since ancient times, raw materials for preparing these products have been derived from plants, animals and minerals [2].

Cosmetic beautification outcomes are also associated with nutritional and/medicinal effects. Hence, emergence of nutracosmetics is a class of health and beauty aid products that combine the benefits of nutracosmetical ingredients with the elegance, skin feel, and delivery systems [3]. Vitamins (A, C and E) obtained from vegetables and fruits protect cells and tissues against damaging effect of free radicals [4]. On the other hand, some ingredients from natural products are incorporated in cosmetic preparations due to their various therapeutic properties, e.g. sunscreen (skin protection effects), antiaging, moisturizing, antioxidant, antiinflammatory and antimicrobial effects, hair repair/growth stimulants, etc. [5].

The skin has a highly differentiated and complex organizational structure that is particularly vulnerable to free radical damage because of its contact with oxygen and other environmental stimuli [6]. When the skin is exposed to sunlight and other atmospheric conditions production of reactive oxygen species is stimulated. The reactive oxygen species then react with cellular DNA, proteins and fatty acids, causing oxidative damage and impairment of antioxidant system in the body. As a result, regulation pathways of skin are altered and lead to photo aging and sometimes skin cancer development [7].

The effects of aging include wrinkles, roughness, loss of skin elasticity and hyper or depigmentation marks. Herbal extracts or cosmetics containing herbal ingredients act on these areas and produce healing, softening, rejuvenating and sunscreen effects due to the antioxidant activity of phenolic compounds (tannins and flavonoids) present in most of the herbal products used for cosmetic purpose. The antioxidant activity is mainly due to their redox properties, which allow them to act as reducing agents, hydrogen donors and quenchers of singlet oxygen. In addition, they may also possess metal chelating properties [8]. Compared with synthetic cosmetic products, herbal products are mild, biodegradable and assumed to have low mammalian toxicity [8] [9].

In Tanzania, traditional beauty products have been overtaken by imported synthetic and herbal cosmetics. To a great extent, this is due to lack of documentation and research and development of these products that lead to unawareness of their existence among the young generation especially in urban areas. This situation prompts us to start recording such information from rural areas where these products are still meaningful for preserving indigenous knowledge with an anticipation of possible production of local products in more acceptable formulations and packaging in the future. Kagera region was chosen based on the fact that people of the Haya tribe are known for maintaining their culture and traditions that include the use of traditional beauty and products.

## 2. Methodology

**Study site**: Traditional beauty natural products were recorded in six different villages of Missenyi district in Kagera region namely; Byeju, Bulembo-Kyaka, Igayanza, Minziro, Mutukula and Ngando.

**Study design:** Focus group discussion with information providers being mainly those who are expert for decorating young girls during wedding ceremonies.

**Data solicitation:** Data was collected using semi-structured questionnaires and interviews in Kiswahili and Haya languages. Various questions about cosmetic products and their methods for preparation and use were asked to women who have traditional knowledge, about traditional beauty products used for cosmetics purposes *i.e.* maintaining/uplifting their appearance. The questionnaire consisted of the four parts:

1. What traditional cosmetic products do use for beatification purposes?
2. How are each of the mentioned product(s) prepared?
3. For what cosmetic/hygiene purposes do the mentioned product(s) used for? (*i.e.* face, hair, skin, nails, the oral tract, decoration of eyes and the maintenance of the skin health.)

4.  What are the outcomes for the mentioned product(s)? E.g. smoothness of the skin and slightly lightening.

Some of the botanical species and the insect mentioned by the participants were collected and identification done in Zoology and Botany Departments at the University of Dar es Salaam, Tanzania.

## 2.1. Collection and Preparation of Plant Materials

Plant materials for both herbaria preparation and phytochemical screening and the insect mentioned were collected from Missenyi district. Identification was done in Botany and Zoology Departments at the University of Dar es Salaam. The drying of plant materials was done in open under shade and took 7 to 10 days.

## 2.2. Extraction

Chemical reagents and solvent were all of the analytical grade solvents and reagents were purchased from Lab Equip Tanzania Ltd. (Dar es Salaam, Tanzania) and Scharlau Company (South Africa).

Dried aerial part of the plant materials were powdered and weighed (29 g of Bidens schimperi and 22 g of Cyphostemma adenocaule and 30 g of Cyphostemma maranguense). Each sample was defatted using petroleum ether followed exhaustive extraction with 80% methanol by maceration (4 × 600 ml) for the seven days. Extracts for each solvent were pooled together, filtered and concentrated to dryness under vacuum at 40°C using a Buchi RE 111 rotary evaporator from Gemini BV, The Netherland.

## 2.3. Phytochemical Analysis

Petroleum ether, methanol, and distilled water extracts of the three plants were used to determine chemical groups using the standard procedures using relevant reagents [10].

**Test for tannins:** About 0.5 g of each methanol extract was boiled in 20 ml of water in their respective test tubes and then filtered. A few drops of 0.1% ferric chloride was added to each test tube. A brownish green or blue-black coloration indicates the presence of tannins.

**Phlobatannins:** An aqueous extract of each plant sample was boiled with 1% aqueous hydrochloric acid. A deposition of a red precipitate indicates the presence of Phlobatannins.

**Saponins:** To 400 ml of distilled water was added 50 g of powdered sample in a conical flask and boiled for 5 min. The mixture was filtered when still hot and 5 ml of sterile distilled water added to a test tube containing equal amounts of cooled filtrate. The test tube was shaken vigorously for 30 seconds and then allowed to stand for 30 min. Formation of honey comb froth indicates the presence of saponins.

**Flavonoids:** 5 ml of dilute ammonia solution was added to a portion of the aqueous filtrate of each plant extract followed by addition of concentrated $H_2SO_4$. Formation of yellow color indicates the presence of flavonoids.

**Steroids:** 2 ml of acetic anhydride was added to 0.5 g of the methanol extract with 2 ml $H_2SO_4$. The change in colour from violet to blue or green indicates the presence of steroids.

**Terpenoids:** 5 ml of the extract was mixed with 2 ml of chloroform, and concentrated $H_2SO_4$ (3 ml) carefully added to form a layer (Salkowski test). A reddish brown coloration on the interface indicates the presence of terpenoids.

**Sterols:** To 5 ml of the extract, equal volume of Salkowski's reagent was added. A bluish-red solution that slowly changes to violet-red, with the fluorescence showed the presence of sterols.

**Essential oils:** To 2 ml of the extract, 0.1 ml of 2 M sodium hydroxide was added, followed by a small quantity of 2 M hydrochloric acid and shaken. A white precipitate indicates the presence of essential oils.

**Phenols:** To 2 ml of the extract, 2 ml of Iron III chloride was added to the solution. A deep bluish-green solution indicates the presence of phenols.

**Alkaloids:** To 1 ml of the extract, concentrated sulphuric acid was added followed by potassium dichromate crystals. An olive-green colour indicates the presence of alkaloids.

## 3. Results

### Ethno-Cosmetic Data

This study recorded 23 products used for beauty purposes in Missenyi district. The major sources of these products were plants, animals, minerals and others. Proportions of these products are shown in **Figure 1** and the applications are given in **Figure 2**. Details of the products are presented in **Tables 1-3**.

**Table 1.** Plant derived cosmetic products used in Missenyi district.

| Botanical Name and Family Name | Vernacular Name | Parts Used and Preparation | Uses |
|---|---|---|---|
| *Abrus precatorius* L. **Fabaceae** | | The bright seeds are strung make jewelry. | Necklaces and hair bands especially by female children. |
| *Bidens schimperi* **Compositae** | Luongwa | Flowers are macerated in water, mixed with papaya latex and applied on the skin. | To lighten the skin. |
| *Carica papaya* L. **Caricaceae** | Omupapari | Latex obtained from the stem and applied directly on the skin three times a day. | To lighten the skin, emollient. |
| *Citrus limon* **Rutaceae** | | Fruit juice mixed with egg albumin, honey and cucumber applied on the skin everyday at night. | To smoothen facial skin, treatment of acne. |
| *Cyphostemma adenocaule* **Vitaceae** | Ibombo | Aerial parts are macerated in water and applied on skin. | To lighten the skin. |
| *Cyphostemma maranguense* **Vitaceae** | | Juice made from leaves is applied on the normal skin or affected areas, every day. Also can be mixed with water and boiled for drinking to increase CD4 count in HIV patients. | Emollient, Skin diseases treatment: eczema, wounds, bacterial and fungal infection. |
| *Diospyros usambarensis* **Ebenaceae** | omudawa | Root barks applied on the teeth. | To whiten the teeth and oral hygiene. |
| *Eucalyptus globulus* **Myrtaceae** | Omukalitusi | Leaves boiled with ghee, and the steam is applied on the skin. | To smoothen the skin. |
| *Ficus thonningii* **Moraceae** | Mtoma | The milky latex often turning pinkish is used alone or mixed with lemon juice and applied to the vagina early in the morning every day. | Create artificial virginity in women. |
| *Lawsonia inermis* L. **Lythraceae** | Ehina | Leaves are grounded and suspended in water and applied on hair or mixed with lemon juice and soot and applied on nails. | To dye hair; To color the nails. |
| *Musa paradisiaca* L. **Musaceae** | Engemu | Stem is cut into small pieces and boiled, the juice is applied on the skin or the warm stem is rubbed on the skin directly once or twice a day for three months. Banana peels are cooked and the steam is directed to skin. This is done once or twice every day for three months. | To smoothen the skin; To lighten the skin. |
| *Persea americana* Mill. **Lauraceae** | | Fruit is mixed with the egg yolk and applied on hair. | Moisturizer, anti-dandruff: to strengthen hair and prevent hair loss. |
| *Phytolacca dodecandra* **Phytolacaceae** | Omuoko | Seeds are mixed with papaya latex and applied on cracked feet. | To smoothen the skin. |
| *Zea mays* **Poaceae** | | Corn silk (stigma) aqueous extract is used to wash the skin while fresh ground corn silk is used as body ointment especially after intense sun exposure. | To rejuvenate the skin. |

**Table 2.** Animal mineral and others sources used for beauty in Missenyi district.

| Ingredients | Preparation | Use |
|---|---|---|
| Bicycle tyre inner tubes | With petroleum jelly, applied on eye blows. | To decorate eyes, similar to eye liner. |
| Cercopid nymph secretion | Secretions are collected and applied on the face. 10mls three times a day with or without lemon juice for treatment of gastric ulcers and cough. | To remove unwanted facial hairs. |
| Snail slime | Slime is collected and rubbed on the cracked feet. | To treat cracked feet. |
| Egg yolk | Mixed with avocado fruit and applied on hair. | To strengthen the hair. |
| Honey | Mixed with cucumber and lemon juice and applied directly on the skin at bedtime. | To smoothen the skin. |
| Kerosene | Applied on the nails three times a day. | To strengthen the nails. |
| Clay (red clay) | With or without water, applied on face at night. | To give a special softness to skin. |

**Continued**

| Mercury oxide from battery (dry cells) powder | With water or petroleum jelly applied on the hair. | Hair dye. |
| Soft charcoal | Applied on teeth. | To whiten the teeth. |
| Soft charcoal e.g. *Zea mays stem* charcoal | Crushed and mixed with petroleum jelly and applied on hair. | Hair dye. |
| Sooty | Fine powder is mixed with petroleum jelly and applied on eyes blows (eye liner). | To decorate the eyes. |

**Table 3.** Detected Phytochemicals and relative amounts of *Cyphostemma adenocaule*, *Cyphostemma maranguense* and *Bidens schimperi*.

| Phytochemical Group | B. schimperi | C. maranguense | C. adenocaule |
|---|---|---|---|
| Alkaloids | - | +++ | +++ |
| Essential oils | + | + | + |
| Flavonoids | +++ | - | ++ |
| Phenols | ++ | - | ++ |
| Phlobatannins | + | - | - |
| Saponins | - | - | - |
| Steroids | - | +++ | +++ |
| Sterols | - | + | ++ |
| Tannins | +++ | + | +++ |
| Terpenoids | +++ | - | - |

Key: + = little; ++ = high; +++ = higher.

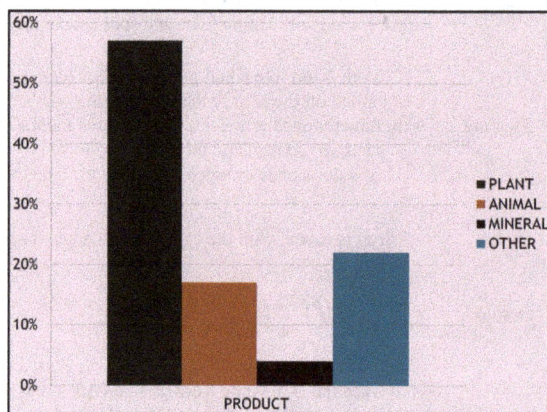

**Figure 1.** Proportions of beauty product sources.

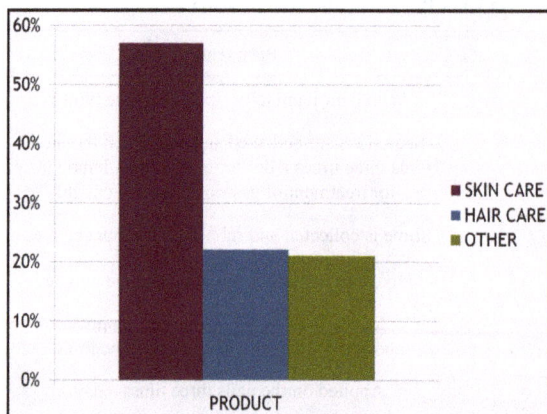

**Figure 2.** Proportions of product applications.

## 4. Discussion

### 4.1. General Observation

Proportions of products for application to the skin were (57%) and hair (22%) this matches with people's concern on skin complexion especially the face and hair look. Regarding the skin, smooth complexion and lightening are main expected beauty outcomes. Information providers were aware of the fact that, besides topical application of cosmetic products, beauty can also result from eating certain foods (concept of nutracosmetics), e.g. banana stems and fruits. Majority of beauty products recorded in this work are supported by scientific results previous studies as described below.

### 4.2. Beauty Products from Plant Sources: Previous Reports on Uses, the Phytohemical Constituents, Pharmacological and Biological Activity

*Abrus precatorius*: Unlike other plant beauty products topically applied or eaten, the bright seeds of *A. precatorius* are strung on a thread to make necklaces and bangels which are worn to enhance good looking. In India the natives value bright coloration of *A. precatorius* seeds and use them for making necklaces and other ornaments worn by both children and adults [11].

*Carica papaya* latex: Latex from unripe fruits, leaves or stem of the papaya tree contains proteolytic enzymes such as papain enzymes which soften and dissolve dead skin layers and simultaneously nourish and support the creation of healthy skin. The enzymes also strengthen collagen tissue due to their ability of protecting and repairing damaged elastic collagen fibers, offering protection to the skin from developing wrinkles [12]. Externally the papaya latex is known to cause contact dermatitis [13]. Cosmetically, papain is used in some dentifrices, shampoos, and face-lifting preparations [14].

*Citrus limon*: Lemon juice contains citric acid and is very rich in vitamin C, which provide many health benefits for all types of the skin. The citric acid is able to exfoliate the skin, which is an important step in treating acne or pimples. It also has astringent properties, thus drying the blemish itself [15]. The juice acts as an antiaging remedy due to its antioxidant activity and can remove wrinkles and blackheads. Lemon juice is also a natural skin lightener, so it can act to reduce a pimple's redness, speeding up the healing process and cause temporary bleaching to improve the look of the skin. However, citric acid may cause skin irritation [16].

*Diospyros usambarensis* root bark: The antibacterial activity of 7-methyljuglone exhibited against oral pathogenic bacteria: S*treptococcus sp.* and *Porphyromonas* [17] and *Diospyros species* possession of naphthaquinones [18] justify the use of root bark for oral hygiene and as a teeth whitener.

*Eucalyptus globulus* oil: Due to its antiseptic and antifungal properties, eucalyptus oil can keep the scalp healthy by preventing microbial growth and getting rid of dandruff. It promotes hair growth, maintains strength and elasticity of hair, improves blood circulation which can help to eliminate the build-up of oil and bacteria in the hair follicles as well as revitalizing dull hair and improve hair texture by increasing the production of ceramide [19].

*Ficus thonningii* latex: Hayas are among those societies from different parts of the world were virginity is highly valued thus forbidden to have sex intercourse before marriage. Some people would attempt to restore virginity by applying some natural products including *Ficus thonningii* latex. Supporting this practice, literature search shows that, there are various herbs that can be used to overcome loose vagina or restore vaginal muscle elasticity, vaginal prolapse, vaginal dryness and discharge, and overall health of the vagina. Examples include *Hamamelis virginiana* and the oak plant which offer fast action in tightening vaginal walls due to its natural phenol content-tannins [20] [21]. Previous study on *Ficus thonningii* stem bark revealed the tannins among other chemicals and antibacterial activity [22].

*Lawsonia inermis*: This is used and well known worldwide as hair and nail dye whose active component, lawsone, binds to keratin. It is therefore considered semi-permanent to permanent, depending on a person's hair type. Most people will achieve a permanent color from henna, especially after the second dye. With repeated use the orange color builds up into red and then auburn [23] [24].

*Musa spp*: Banana fruit is used worldwide for its nutritional values and the different parts of banana plant are used to treat different diseases such as hypertension, diarrhea, peptic ulcer and cardiac diseases in human [25]. Bananas have a variety of skin care benefits. The fruit peels have antimicrobial activity against *Staphylococcus* and *Pseudomonas* [26] and high potassium content which makes them ideal for treating acne prone skin. The spread of bacteria in skin cells is diminished allowing pimples or blemishes to heal at a faster rate. They are known to contain antioxidants such as dopamine, ascorbic acid and flavonoids [27] [28] that provide anti-aging properties. Bananas also contain Vitamin C known to inhibit melanin production, the substance that the skin produces in response to sunlight, which darkens the skin. Banana stem juice contains manganese peroxide enzyme which causes enzymatic degradation of the skin melanin. [29] [30] Thus, skin lightening effect can be associated with anti-melanin formation and/or degradation. The antiinflamatory properties provide soothing effect for dry itchy skin preparation made from banana peels and stem. Ingested stem juice help to detoxify the body, increase skin circulation, boost collagen levels exerts antibacterial and antioxidant activity, as well as providing an overall youthful, fresh looking, smoother and glowing appearance [31].

*Persea americana* (Avocado oil): Supporting the use of avocado is the fact that, avocado oil present in the avocado fruit has essential nutrients like proteins, Vitamins A, D, E and B6, magnesium, copper, iron, amino acids and folic acid, all of which is extremely essential for hair growth and nourishment. Lecithin contained in the oil gives it good penetrative qualities. The avocado oil is also known to have natural sunscreen properties that can protect the hair and scalp from the damage caused by the harmful UVA and UVB rays of the sun. This oil is also effective in getting rid of dandruff [32].

*Phytolacca dodecandra*: It is used as a detergent, common medicinal uses include treatment of skin itching (ringworm), abortion, gonorrhea, leeches, intestinal worms, anthrax and rabies [33].

*Zea mays*: Chemical constituents of corn silk include; protein/amino acids, carbohydrates, flavonoids, phenols, tannins, steroids, alkaloids, terpenoids, saponins, glycosides, fat/oils fibers, vitamins and minerals (calcium, potassium, magnesium and sodium salts) [34] [35]. Corn silk is an ingredient in cosmetic face powder. Skin rejuvenation can be associated with antioxidant activity of flavonoids and tannins.

## 4.3. Current Phytochemical Results

In addition to documentation, phytochemical screening of three plants we performed revealed the presence of chemical classed that could be correlated with their use for beauty purposes as follows.

*Bidens schimperi* flower: Flavonoids and tannins are among other phytochemicals, shown in this study. Skin smoothening effect could be due to antioxidant activity of these compounds.

*Cyphostemma adenocaule* and *Cyphostemma maranguense* leaves: Both species showed same phytochemical profile with the presence of alkaloids, flavonoids, steroids and tannins in the similar proportions based on the colour intensity observation. However, *C. maranguense* contained less amounts of sterols and tannins than *C. adenocaule*. Saponins, triterpanods and phlobatannis could not be detected. Presence of steroids may be associated with their application for skin lightening since steroids have catabolic and antianabolic effect on the skin which results to the thinning of the skin, making the skin appear lighter [36]. The reported itching effect can be associated with the presence of oxalic acid which exist in form of calcium oxalate crystals known to cause dermatitis upon skin contact [37] [38].

## 4.4. Beauty Products from Animal Sources: Chemical Constituents, Pharmacological and Biological Activity

**Chicken egg yolk:** Using egg yolk as a natural hair conditioner or in combination with avocado pulp to nourish and strengthen hair is supported by essential nutrients present in egg yolk. These including; protein, vitamins like A, E and D, high amount of sulfur and fatty sulfur and Vitamin B12 help the hair to grow faster and possession of healthy appearance [39].

**Honey:** The medicinal use of honey and its incorporation in cosmetic products is well known. When applied to wounds or burns, the high sugar content prevents infections, specifically from *Staphylococcus* bacteria strains, as well as *E. coli* and *Candida albicans*. It is thus recommended for skin-care purposes like promoting wound healing and preventing bacterial or fungal skin infections [40].

**Snail secretion (slime):** Its use is well supported; the secretion is rich in proteins of high and low molecular weight hyaluronic acid and antioxidants. It has a double function when applied to human skin: (i) to stimulate the formation of collagen and elastin; (ii) dermal components that repair the damaged skin and to minimize effect of free radicals that are responsible for premature skin aging [41].

**Spittlebug nymphs:** Spittlebug nymphs foam contains anti-repellant chemicals: fatty acid-derived alcohols c-lactones and a single 1-monoacylglycerol, as well as the polyol pinitol and the polyhydroxyalkanoate, poly-3-

hydroxybutyrate [41] [42]. Application in cosmetic products is reported for polyhydroxybutyrate a plastic-like and biodegredable material having skin oil absorbing properties incorporated in skin cleansing products, polyol pinitol having skin moisturizing properties incorporated into skin creams, sunscreens and lotions products and monoacylglycerol used as emulsifying agent [43] [44].

## 4.5. Other Sources for Beauty Products

**Red clay:** Clay is a natural substance with a slightly grainy texture which helps the exfoliation, while the nutrients in the clay tone, firm, and nourish the skin. It is able to draw dirt, oils and toxins, resulting in deeply cleansed and softened skin [45]. Red clay in particular is richer in iron oxide, having absorbent properties and is especially good for oily skin. It tones, stimulates, and cleanses the skin pores resulting in skin smoothening and protection against pimples [46].

**Unusual products:** These include dry cells and inner tube of bicycle tyre. The later contain mercury oxide which has been banned in most countries because of health concerns. Mercury is toxic to the central and peripheral nervous systems. The inhalation, ingestion or dermal exposure of any form of mercury can cause neurological and behavioural disorders, harmful effects to digestive and immune systems, lungs, skin and kidneys, and may be fatal. Symptoms include tremors, insomnia, memory loss, neuromuscular effects, headache cognitive and motor dysfunction [47].

## 5. Conclusion

This type of study was done for the first time in Tanzania. It afforded to record 13 plants, 4 animal products, minerals and organic products. Skin care products were the most reported products followed by hair care products. Some of the mentioned products are known ingredients that are incorporated in cosmetics based on natural products. These include eucalyptus oil, honey, avocado, papaya latex, egg yolk, lemon oil and corn silk. Most of these are incorporated in body creams, lotions and shampoos. Traditional beauty products reported in this study but with no scientific support require further investigation to determine their safety. Also, people should be educated on the hazardous human health effects of products like dry cells and bicycle inner tubes through mass media such as TV news paper and flares.

## Acknowledgements

Our thanks are due to Ms. Rehema Amlan Nyamichwo for the facilitation of the focus group discussion and all information providers in Missenyi district for their willingness to reveal traditional natural products used for beauty purposes.

## References

[1]  Pieroni, A., Quave, C.L., Villanelli, M.L., Mangino, P., Sabbatini, G., Santini, L., Boccetti, T., Profili, M., Ciccioli, T., Rampa, L.G., Antonini, G., Girolamini, C., Cecchi, M. and Tomasi, M. (2004) Ethnopharmacognostic Survey on the Natural Ingredients Used in Folk Cosmetics, Cosmeceuticals and Remedies for Healing Skin Diseases in the Inland Marches, Central-Eastern Italy. *Journal of Ethnopharmacology*, **91**, 331-344. http://dx.doi.org/10.1016/j.jep.2004.01.015

[2]  Schneider, G., Gohla, S., Schreiber, J., Kaden, W., Schönrock, U., Schmidt-Lewerkühne, H., Kuschel, A., Petsitis, X., Pape, W., Ippen, H. and Diembeck, W. (2005) Skin Cosmetics: Ullmann's Encyclopedia of Industrial Chemistry. Wiley-VCH, Weinheim.

[3]  Chanchal, D. and Swarnlata, S. (2008) Novel Approaches in Herbal Cosmetics. *Journal of Cosmetic Dermatology*, **7**, 89-95. http://dx.doi.org/10.1111/j.1473-2165.2008.00369.x

[4]  Mukherjee, S. and Mitra, A. (2009) Health Effects of Palm Oil. *Journal of Human Ecology*, **26**, 197-203.

[5]  Aburjai, T. and Natsheh, F.M. (2003) Plants Used in Cosmetics. *Phytotherapy Research*, **17**, 987-1000. http://dx.doi.org/10.1002/ptr.1363

[6]  Calabrese, V., Scapagnini, G., Randazzo, S.D., Randazzo, G., Catalano, C., Geraci, G. and Morganti, P. (1999) Oxidative Stress and Antioxidants at Skin Biosurface: A Novel Antioxidant from Lemon Oil Capable of Inhibiting Oxidative Damage to the Skin. *Drugs under Experimental and Clinical Research*, **25**, 281-287.

[7]  Rocha, H.M., Galindo, I., Huerta, M., Trujillo-Hernandez, B., Elizalde, A. and Cortes-Franco, R. (2002) UVB Pho-

to-Protection with Antioxidants: Effects of Oral Therapy with d-α-Tocopherol and Ascorbic Acid on the Minimal Ery-thema. *Acta Dermato Venerologica*, **82**, 21-24. http://dx.doi.org/10.1080/000155502753600830

[8]   Gulcin, I., Huyut, Z., Elmastas, M. and Aboul-Enein, H.Y. (2010) Radical Scavenging and Antioxidant Activity of Tannic Acid. *Arabian Journal of Chemistry*, **3**, 43-53. http://dx.doi.org/10.1016/j.arabjc.2009.12.008

[9]   Chanchal, D. and Swarnlata, S. (2008) Novel Approaches in Herbal Cosmetics. *Journal of Cosmetic Dermatology*, **7**, 89-95. http://dx.doi.org/10.1111/j.1473-2165.2008.00369.x

[10]  Ahumuza, T. and Kirimuhuzya, C. (2011) Qualitative (Phytochemical) Analysis and Antifungal Activity of *Pentas decora* (De Wild), a Plant Used Traditionally to Treat Skin Fungal Infections in Western Uganda. *Research in Pharmaceutical Biotechnology*, **3**, 75-84.

[11]  Acharya, D., Shrivastava, A., Pawar, S. and Sancheti, G. (2010) The Medicinal Value of Indian Herb *Abrus precatorius* Used in Herbal Medicines in India.
      http://www.disabled-world.com/medical/alternative/herbal/abrus-precatorius.php

[12]  Silva, L.G., Garcia, O., Lopes, M.T.P. and Salas, C.E. (1997) Changes in Protein Profile during Coagulation of Latex from *Carica papaya*. *Brazilian Journal of Medical and Biological Research*, **30**, 615-619.
      http://dx.doi.org/10.1590/S0100-879X1997000500007

[13]  Aravind, G., Debjit, B., Duraivel, S. and Harish, G. (2013) Traditional and Medicinal Uses of *Carica papaya*. *Journal of Medicinal Plants Studies*, **1**, 7-15.

[14]  Duke, J.A. (1983) Handbook of Energy Crops. Unpublished. http://www.rain-tree.com/papaya.htm

[15]  Stratford, S.J. (2013) Using Lemon Juice to Help Pimples.
      http://skincare.lovetoknow.com/Lemon_Juice_Help_Pimples

[16]  Riggins, K. (2011) Lemon Juice and Health. http://www.livestrong.com/article/422902-lemon-juice-health

[17]  Jeon, J.H., Lee, C.H., Kim, M.K. and Lee, H.S. (2009) Antibacterial Effects of Juglone and Its Derivatives against Oral Pathogens. *Journal of the Korean Society for Applied Biological Chemistry*, **52**, 720-725.
      http://dx.doi.org/10.3839/jksabc.2009.119

[18]  Maridass, M. (2008) Phytochemicals from Genus *Diospyros* (L.) and Their Biological Activities. *Ethnobotanical Leaflets*, **12**, 231-244.

[19]  Chandramita, B. (2013) Eucalyptus Oil for Hair. http://www.buzzle.com/articles/eucalyptus-oil-for-hair.html

[20]  Sarina, D. and Florian, S. (2011) Investigation on the Phenolic Constituents in *Hamamelis virginiana* Leaves by HPLC-DAD and LC-MS/MS. *Analytical and Bioanalytical Chemistry*, **401**, 677-688.
      http://dx.doi.org/10.1007/s00216-011-5111-3

[21]  Jamil, M., Haq, I., Mirza, B. and Qayyum, M. (2012) Isolation of Antibacterial Compounds from *Quercus dilatata* L. through Bioassay Guided Fractionation. *Annals of Clinical Microbiology and Antimicrobials*, **11**, 11 p.
      http://www.ann-clinmicrob.com/content/11/1/11 http://dx.doi.org/10.1186/1476-0711-11-11

[22]  Usman, H., Abdulrahman, F.I. and Usman, A. (2009) Qualitative Phytochemical Screening and *in Vitro* Antimicrobial Effects of Methanol Stem Bark Extract of *Ficus thonningii* (Moraceae). *African Journal of Traditional, Complementary, and Alternative Medicines*, **6**, 289-295.

[23]  Corbett, J.F. (1998) Hair Colorants: Chemistry and Toxicology. Micelle Press, Dorset.

[24]  Thompson, R.H. (1957) Naturally Occuring Quinones. Academic Press, New York.

[25]  Imam, M.Z. and Akter, S. (2011) *Musa paradisiacal* L. and *Musa sapientum* L.: A Phytochemical and Pharmacological Review. *Journal of Applied Pharmaceutical Science*, **1**, 14-20.

[26]  Alisi, C.S., Nwanyanwu, C.E., Akujobi, C.O. and Ibegbulem, C.O. (2008) Inhibition of Dehydrogenase Activity in Pathogenic Bacteria Isolates by Aqueous Extracts of *Musa paradisiaca* (var. Sapientum). *African Journal of Biotechnology*, **7**, 1821-1825.

[27]  Yin, X.Z., Quan, J. S. and Kanazawa, T. (2008) Banana Prevents Plasma Oxidative Stress in Healthy Individuals. *Plant Foods for Human Nutrition*, **63**, 71-76. http://dx.doi.org/10.1007/s11130-008-0072-1

[28]  Vijayakumar, S., Presannakumar, G. and Vijayalakshmi, N.R. (2008) Antioxidant Activity of Banana Flavonoids. *Fitoterapia*, **79**, 279-282. http://dx.doi.org/10.1016/j.fitote.2008.01.007

[29]  Yadav, P., Singh, V.K., Yadav, M., Singh, S.K., Yadava, S. and Yadav, K.D. (2012) Purification and Characterization of Mn-Peroxidase from *Musa paradisiacal* (Banana) Stem Juice. *Indian Journal of Biochemistry & Biophysics*, **49**, 42-48.

[30]  Mohorcic, M., Friedrich, J., Renimel, I., Andre, P., Mandin, D. and Chaumont, J.P. (2007) Production of Melanin Bleaching Enzyme of Fungal Origin and Its Application in Cosmetics. *Biotechnology and Bioprocess Engineering*, **12**, 200-206.

[31] Yakinican (2014) Health Benefits of Bananas Inside and Out. http://skincareonthescars.blog.com/2014/11/01/health-benefits-of-bananas-inside-and-out/#

[32] Mukherjee, B. (2011) Benefits of Egg Yolk on Hair. http://www.buzzle.com/articles/benefits-of-egg-yolk-on-hair.html

[33] Esser, K.B., Semagn, K. and Wolde-Yohannes, L. (2003) Medicinal Use and Social Status of the Soap Berry *Endod* (*Phytolacca dodecandra*) in Ethiopia. *Journal of Ethnopharmacology*, **85**, 269-277. http://dx.doi.org/10.1016/S0378-8741(03)00007-2

[34] Bhaigyabati, T., Kirithika, T., Ramya, J. and Usha, K. (2011) Phytochemical Constituents and Antioxidant Activity of Various Extracts of Corn Silk (*Zea mays*. L). *Research Journal of Pharmaceutical, Biological and Chemical Sciences*, **2**, 986-993.

[35] Hasanudin, K., Hashim, P. and Mustafa, S. (2012) Corn Silk (*Stigma maydis*) in Healthcare: A Phytochemical and Pharmacological Review. *Molecules*, **17**, 9697-9715. http://dx.doi.org/10.3390/molecules17089697

[36] Katzung, B.G., Masters, S.B. and Trevor, A.J. (2009) Basic and Clinical Pharmacology. 11th Edition, McGraw-Hill Medical, New York.

[37] Bosch, C.H. (2004) *Cyphostemma adenocaule* (Steud. ex A.Rich.) Wild and R.B. Drumm. In: Grubben, G.J.H. and Denton, O.A., Eds., *PROTA* 2: *Vegetables/Légumes*, PROTA Foundation, Wageningen, 279-300.

[38] Nakata, P.A. (2012) Plant Calcium Oxalate Crystal Formation, Function, and Its Impact on Human Health. *Frontiers in biology*, **7**, 254-266. http://dx.doi.org/10.1007/s11515-012-1224-0

[39] Mukherjee, B. (2011) Benefits of Egg Yolk on Hair. http://www.buzzle.com/articles/benefits-of-egg-yolk-on-hair.html

[40] Molan, P.C. (2009) Honey: Antimicrobial Actions and Role in Disease Management. In: Ahmad, I. and Aqil, F., Eds., *New Strategies Combating Bacterial Infection*, Wiley VCH, Weinheim, 229-253.

[41] Iglesias, M.C., Sanz-Rodríguez, F., Zamarrón, A., Reyes, E., Carrasco, E., González, S. and Juarranz, A. (2012) A Secretion of the Mollusc *Cryptomphalus aspersa* Promotes Proliferation, Migration and Survival of Keratinocytes and Dermal Fibroblasts *in Vitro*. *International Journal of Cosmetic Science*, **34**, 183-89. http://dx.doi.org/10.1111/j.1468-2494.2011.00699.x

[42] Del Campo, M.L., King, J.T. and Gronquist, M.R. (2011) Defensive and Chemical Characterization of the Froth Produced by the Cercopid *Aphrophora cribrata*. *Chemoecology*, **21**, 1-8.

[43] Maeda, M., Sudesh, K.K. and Iwata, T. (2008) Biodegradable Oil Absorbing Film. USPTO Application. US Patent No. 20080226580A1.

[44] Agati Group (2012) Active for Cosmetics. http://agatigroup.com/actives-for-cosmetics/

[45] Frontier Natural Products Co-Op (2013) Clay Masks. http://www.frontiercoop.com/learn/claymasks.php

[46] Carretero, M.I. and Pozo, M. (2010) Clay and Non-Clay Minerals in the Pharmaceutical and Cosmetic Industries Part II. Active Ingredients. *Applied Clay Science*, **47**, 171-181. http://dx.doi.org/10.1016/j.clay.2009.10.016

[47] World Health Organization (2013) Mercury and Health. Fact Sheet No. 361.

# 13

# Combination (5% Hydroquinone, 0.1% Tretinoin and 1% Hydrocortisone) Cream in Treating Facial Hyperpigmentation: A Retrospective Patient Satisfaction Survey

John Fleming*, Saqib Bashir

Dermatology Department, King's College Hospital, London, UK
Email: *jdfleming@gmail.com

## Abstract

Background: Melasma and post-inflammatory hyperpigmentation provide a significant source of psychosocial morbidity, especially in those with Fitzpatrick skin types III-VI. In Europe, a proprietary product aimed at treating these conditions, similar to Kligman's formula but with a longer expiry date, has become available. Objectives: To assess patient satisfaction with a newly available combination de-pigmenting preparation. Methods: We conducted a small study to see if patients felt that this new product affected their quality of life and skin symptoms from hyperpigmentation. 41 subjects, who had all been prescribed a 15 g tube to use sparingly at night for 90 days within the last 12 months were telephoned to rate the effect the cream had on their quality of life and skin symptom improvement. Each patient also had their Dermatology Life Quality Index (DLQI) score assessed. Results: Out of the 29 patients who responded to the study, 22 had melasma and 7 had post-inflammatory hyperpigmentation from acne. 21 subjects felt that the cream made either a marked or moderate improvement on their quality of life and 23 subjects felt that the cream made either a marked or moderate improvement on their skin symptoms. Conclusion: Patients reported improvement in both hyperpigmentation and quality of life, suggesting a high level of satisfaction with treatment. The long shelf life of the product may also promote compliance and reduce health- care costs.

## Keywords

Melasma, Chloasma, Acne-Scarring, Hydroquinone, Tretinoin, Kligman's Solution

*Corresponding author.

## 1. Introduction

Melasma and post-inflammatory hyperpigmentation provide a significant source of psychosocial morbidity, especially in those with Fitzpatrick skin types III-VI. Kligman's formula was the mainstay of topical depigmenting therapy but occasionally induced skin irritation [1]. Further, it has a short shelf life and high cost, when compounded to order by pharmacists. In Europe, a proprietary product, with a long expiry date, has become available, which may influence treatment effectiveness by reduced cost manufacture from compounding and increased patient use as a result of the longer shelf life. Its ingredients, hydroquinone 5%, tretinoin 0.1% and hydrocortisone 1%, are similar to Kligman's formula.

## 2. Methods

We studied the effect the proprietary cream had in improving a patient's quality of life and the symptoms they experienced from their skin. 41 subjects, who had all been prescribed a 15 g tube to use sparingly at night for 90 days within the last 12 months were telephoned to rate the effect the cream had on their quality of life and skin symptom (subjective hyperpigmentation assessment) improvement. They were each asked to rate this as either a marked, moderate or mild improvement or as no improvement. Each patient also had their Dermatology Life Quality Index (DLQI) score assessed.

## 3. Results

The mean post treatment DLQI was 4.4 (range 1 - 10). Those patients deriving the most benefit from the treatment were those making a 15 g tube last 60 days or more. Of the 7 patients reporting skin irritation and peeling following use, [5] had finished a 15 g tube of cream in less than 30 days (**Figure 1**).

## 4. Discussion

Melasma and post-inflammatory facial acne scarring are notoriously difficult conditions to treat. Topical agents, superficial chemical skin peels or laser treatment, are often required to attempt to reduce the appearances of hyperpigmentation. Laser treatment has significant risks of worsening hyperpigmentation, especially in darker skin types III-VI. Other agents in addition to photo and oestrogen avoidance to managemelasma include topical methimazole [2], oral tranexamic acid [3], kojic acid [4] and mulberry [5] (*Morus alba*). Patients in our study reported improvement in both skin symptoms (92%) and quality of life (88%), suggesting a high level of satis-

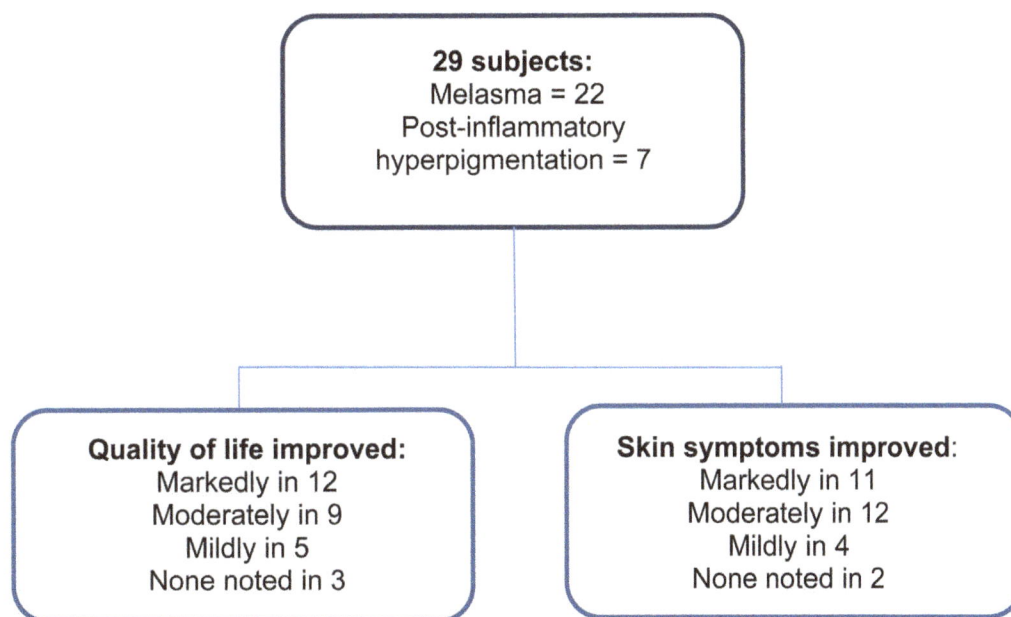

**Figure 1.** Consort diagram results summary.

faction with treatment. The advantages of the long shelf life product may also include decreased cost via decreased physician and pharmacist time. The data collected indicate that treatment with the new product effectively improves self-assessed quality of life and hyperpigmentation.

## References

[1]   Ball Arefiev, K.L. and Hantash, B.M. (2012) Advances in the Treatment of Melasma: A Review of the Recent Literature. *Dermatologic Surgery*, **38**, 971-984. http://dx.doi.org/10.1111/j.1524-4725.2012.02435.x

[2]   Malek, J., Chedraoui, A., Nikolic, D., Barouti, N., Ghosn, S. and Abbas, O. (2013) Successful Treatment of Hydroquinone-Resistant Melasma Using Topical Methimazole. *Dermatologic Therapy*, **26**, 69-72. http://dx.doi.org/10.1111/j.1529-8019.2012.01540.x

[3]   Tse, T.W. and Hui, E. (2013) Tranexamic Acid: An Important Adjuvant in the Treatment of Melasma. *Journal of Cosmetic Dermatology*, **12**, 57-66 http://dx.doi.org/10.1111/jocd.12026

[4]   Sheth, V.M. and Pandya, A.G. (2011) Melasma: A Comprehensive Update: Part II. *Journal of the American Academy of Dermatology*, **65**, 699-714. http://dx.doi.org/10.1016/j.jaad.2011.06.001

[5]   Alvin, G., Catambay, N., Vergara, A. and Jamora, M.J. (2011) A Comparative Study of the Safety and Efficacy of 75% Mulberry (*Morus alba*) Extract Oil versus Placebo as a Topical Treatment for Melasma: A Randomized, Single-Blind, Placebocontrolled Trial. *Journal of Drugs in Dermatology*, **10**, 1025-1031.

# 14

# Kerosene-Induced Panniculitis in Iraqi Patients

**Khalifa E. Sharquie[1]\*, Adil A. Noaimi[1], Maha S. Younis[2], Bashar S. Al-Sultani[3]**

[1]Department of Dermatology, College of Medicine, University of Baghdad, Baghdad, Iraq
[2]Department of Psychiatry, College of Medicine, Baghdad University, Baghdad, Iraq
[3]Department of Dermatology, Baghdad Teaching Hospital, Medical City, Baghdad, Iraq
Email: \*ksharquie@ymail.com, adilnoaimi@yahoo.com, Maha.younis@gmail.com, bashar-sami83@yahoo.com

## Abstract

Background: Kerosene is a common household stuff that has been used as accidental oral poisoning material in children and as suicidal attempt in adults. In the last decade intradermal kerosene injection has been commonly used to induce dermatitis artefecta as a part of emotional upset. Objective: To evaluate the clinical cases of intradermal kerosene injection in Iraqi patients. Patients and Methods: This is a descriptive case study that had been conducted in Department of Dermatology Baghdad Teaching Hospital, Baghdad, Iraq during the period from Jan. 2003 to Dec. 2012. History and full clinical examination were performed including all sociodemographic aspects associated with this condition. Psychiatric evaluation was done for each patient. Results: All eleven patients had single lesion except that two had two lesions. They were distributed on accessible areas on the limbs. The exact diagnosis was not reached for at least few weeks after kerosene injection. The patients denied any kerosene injection, but after a while they all admitted that the cause of their rash, severe emotional tension was observed at the time of kerosene injection as they had sociopsychological disturbances. The initial rash was erythematous indurated tender plaque that was gradually increasing in size simulating the picture of panniculitis and then followed by rupture of lesion and associated pyoderma, forming chronic discharging ulcer. Patients were managed by topical and systemic antibiotics until complete resolution leaving a big ugly scar that was treated by topical steroids to improve its cosmetic appearance. Conclusions: Kerosene intradermal injection is an increasing problem among Iraqi adult females and it should be suspected in any patient with chronic discharging ulcer on accessible areas like limbs.

## Keywords

Kerosene, Panniculitis, Emotional Tension

---

\*Corresponding author.

## 1. Introduction

Kerosene is one of petrolatum products that are commonly used for heating in houses during winter time. Kerosene poisoning is frequently encountered in Iraqi hospitals as children and toddlers accidently ingest it, probably due to its unlabeled containers. In the last few years we have come across cases of kerosene injection as an attempt for suicide. Kerosene is a hydrocarbon compound that is known to cause toxicity which affects many different organs according to the dose and route of exposure, whether through ingestion, inhalation, intravenous injection or dermal injection. The chemical properties of the individual hydrocarbon determine the specific toxicity, while the dose and route of ingestion affect organs which are exposed to the toxicity. If these hydrocarbons come in contact with the skin surface, they can cause dryness, scaling and sometimes severe dermatitis [1]. Skin absorption of kerosene has been demonstrated to be fairly rapid, but it is limited to approximately 10% - 15% after 24 hours of the applied dose [2]. When injected into skin, kerosene causes an intense local inflammatory reaction with necrosis of the skin, fatty tissue and possibly underlying muscle [3] [4]. Chronic exposure can result in renal failure and/or degenerative changes of livers or kidneys. Signs and symptoms of overexposure include giddiness, headache, dizziness, nausea, vomiting, incoordination, narcosis, stupor, coma, unconsciousness, weight loss, anemia, renal failure, and pains in the limbs peripheral numbness, parasthesia, drying and cracking of skin, and rashes or spots on skin.

Intradermal kerosene injection causing fasciitis and necrosis is self mutilation practice that has been reported among adults [5] [6], however only four cases are documented and all of them are in Arab communities.

In Iraq it is not an uncommon problem among children to have accidental oral ingestion or inhalation of kerosene while for adults oral intake or bathing with kerosene is used as a suicidal attempt.

During Iran-Iraqi war 1980-1988 it is a well known practice among soldiers during army attacks to do intradermal injection of kerosene to induce dermatitis in order to have sick leave (Sharquie observations).

In the last ten years and specifically after American occupation of Iraq there is a new trend among young adults to induce self infliction by intradermal kerosene injection under the pressure of their emotional problems.

Although household kerosene is a familiar tool for committing suicide whether an attempt or complete by self burning in Middle East countries [7]. Very few literatures report cases using it for self mutilation [8]. General studies that assess suicidal behavior are rare in the Arab world given the fact that suicide is considered as a disgraceful act prohibited by religion, condemned by society and intrigued by legal consequences [7].

Psychiatric evaluation should be done for the attempters in order to assess the presence of any psychological disorders. In reviewing the clinical picture, time was an important factor [9]. Delay in management would have allowed the noxious agents to cause much irreversible necrosis and possible suppuration. Since the injected material penetrates slowly, immediate and adequate surgical debridement with possible fasciatomy is the best initial treatment, followed by repeated and relentless debridement with dressings [10].

So the aim of the present work is to report cases of intradermal kerosene injection causing panniculitis and fasciitis and to evaluate the different clinical and psychological aspects of this self-induced disease.

## 2. Patients and Methods

This is a descriptive case study that had been carried out in Department of Dermatology and Venereology Baghdad Teaching Hospital, Baghdad, Iraq during the period from Jan. 2003 to Dec. 2012.

Eleven cases—ten females and one male were seen, whose ages range from 17 - 25 year with a mean 21.5 years. Full history and examination was carried out to evaluate the sociopsychological aspects and the emotional tension of the patients and to evaluate the course of the disease from the time of the injection. Digital photographs were taken using SONY Cyber-Shot T300 10.1 MP for each patient in good illumination.

Formal consent was taken from each patient after full explanation about the nature and the goal of the present work. Ethical approval was obtained from the Scientific Council of Dermatology and Venereology-Arab Board for Medical Specializations.

## 3. Results

All eleven patients (**Table 1**) had severe emotional tension as a result of social, economical and psychological problems. All patients denied the self injection of kerosene but when confronted with the injection, they all admitted the cause. Psychiatric assessment revealed absence of psychotic disorders or cognitive impairment

**Table 1.** Showing features of cases with kerosene intradermal injection.

| No. | Age | Gender | Site | Type |
|-----|-----|--------|------|------|
| 1 | 23 | M | Both Forearm | Ulcer & Pyoderma |
| 2 | 19 | F | Forearm | Ulcer & Pyoderma |
| 3 | 21 | F | Forearm | Ulcer & Pyoderma |
| 4 | 20 | F | Thigh | Ulcer & Pyoderma |
| 5 | 17 | F | Buttock | Ulcer & Pyoderma |
| 6 | 25 | F | Arm | Ulcer & Pyoderma |
| 7 | 23 | F | Wrist | Ulcer & Pyoderma |
| 8 | 24 | F | Both Popliteal Fossae | Ulcer & Pyoderma |
| 9 | 20 | F | Forearm | Ulcer & Pyoderma |
| 10 | 23 | F | Forearm | Ulcer & Pyoderma |
| 11 | 19 | F | Forearm | Ulcer & Pyoderma |

for any reason. There was no history of alcohol/drug abuse or serious anti-social behavior. The site of injection was usually on accessible areas and all seen on the limbs. One case study of patient number eleven is reported here. A thorough psychiatric semi-structured interview has been conducted with one of the patients as a detailed example:

A 19-year old Iraqi Muslim single girl, a student in the college of education, living in Baghdad with her parents and younger two brothers, was brought to the emergency Department of Baghdad Teaching Hospital Medical City in March 2010 after three days of outpatient treatment by a private local doctor, where she received cortisone ointment and analgesic tablets for suspected erosive contact dermatitis on her left arm without improvement. The lesion was expanding to involve the whole arm with generalized redness and swelling and in ability to move it freely with intensifying pain and tenderness for which she was referred for consultation. The Patient admitted using a 5 ml disposable syringe filled with household kerosene injecting it into her left arm just below the cubital fossa. This was in response to her total failure in her first term examination four days before consultation. She was taught about this method by a friend in the college. Urgent surgical debridement of the all necrotic and a vascular tissues was done under anesthesia. Minor injury to the flexors of the forearm occurred, but did not affect full movement. She had neither previous medical or psychiatric problems nor family history of mental illness. She was described as a pleasant friendly girl by her mother with no record of impulsivity or anti-social behavior. The patient denied any emotional or family conflict. Both parents were college graduates and government employees living in comfortable accommodation with a reasonable financial status. On assessing her mental state, she was fully conscious and alert with the injured arm wrapped up to the wrist and an intravenous fluid containing anti-biotic running in the healthy arm, but looked pale and gloomy. Speech was coherent and logical, there were no thought or perceptual disorders, her affect were sad and congruent with her mood. She expressed full ignorance of the toxic nature of kerosene and denied any suicidal thoughts justifying her act as a self punishment for school failure. She denied feeling psychological relief by the injection and expressed regret and concerns about future disfigurement or paralysis. The patient was jointly followed up in the skin clinic and psychiatry outpatient clinic in the Medical City Teaching Hospital according to an appointment protocol.

In eight cases the injection was on the upper arms specifically on the forearms while three cases on the lower limbs specifically thigh, buttock, popliteal fossae.

Patients were seen after few days to few weeks following the injection. The course of the disease started as erythematous plaques that were hot and tender simulating a picture of panniculitis, after awhile there was rupture of the lesions leaving discharging deep ulcers. No smell of kerosene was detected in any lesion. These ulcers were managed by antiseptic clearance, topical and oral antibiotics were given, and the healing time took few too many weeks. In all cases there was disfiguring scar at the site of injection and one patient with the wrist injection left severe fibrosis and contracture of the wrist and hand.

The scars were managed by strong topical steroid ointment with oral antihistamine to improve the cosmetic appearance (**Figure 1** and **Figure 2**).

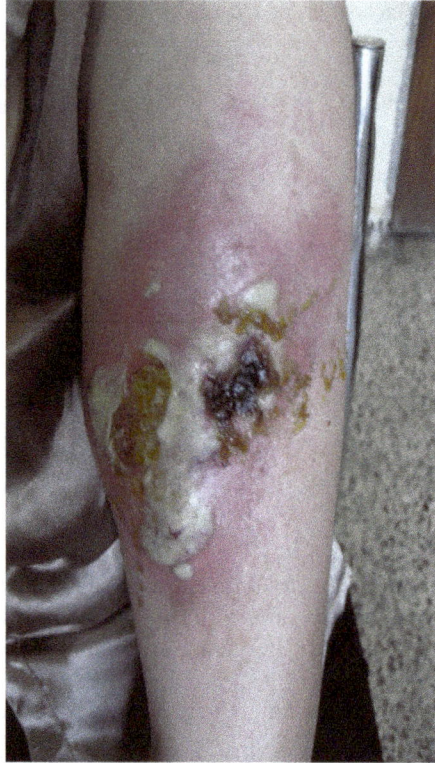

**Figure 1.** Showing female patient with kerosene intradermal injection presented with pyoderma of right upper arm.

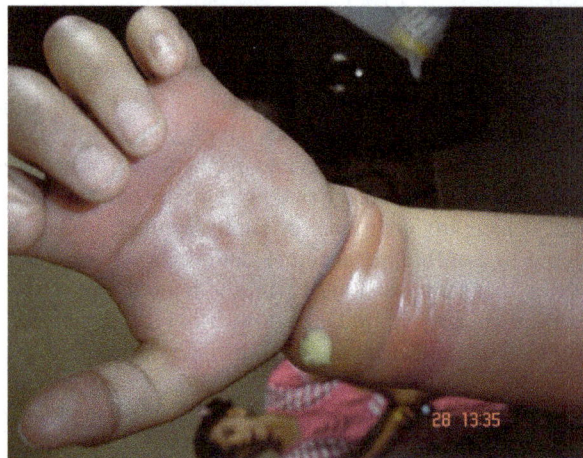

**Figure 2.** Showing panniculitis is and pyoderma in the left wrist in female patient.

## 4. Discussion

US Occupation of Iraq caused severe economic, social and psychological problems among population and one of these medical problems is doing kerosene injection. Kerosene is a mixture of hydrocarbons [11] [12], which can cause severe inflammation and necrosis of all layers of the skin even and can involve the fascia and the underlying muscles. But clinically as seen in the present work all features of panniculitis were observed. So we preferred the term panniculitis rather than fasciitis. As a kind of chronic ulcer it might also simulate the picture of pyoderma gangrenosum. In searching the medical literatures, we came across only four cases of so called fasciitis and panniculitis, which were all in Arab world [8]-[10]. In Iraq, there is an increasing report about this problem within the last ten years [13].

Initial diagnosis is very essential in order to achieve successful management of these cases, so any panniculitis like pictures on accessible area commonly the upper arms of young female, kerosene injection should be highly suspected. Immediate management including hospital admission and urgent surgical debridement should be carried out to evacuate the remaining kerosene in the tissue with full antibiotic cover, while the condition is seen as chronic discharging ulcer and management including cleaning with antiseptic, topical antibiotic and systemic antibiotics cover. In late cases scarring could be managed by topical steroid ointment and cosmetic surgery might be arranged.

Emotional tensions that can lead to skin diseases are those like dermatitis artefecta, trichotillomenia, delusion of parasitosis and others. These cases are not uncommon problems seen in daily clinical practice.

Self-inflicted dermatosis induced by kerosene is not well documented in Iraqi medical literatures, but during Iran-Iraq war 1980-1988, cases of intradermal kerosene injection are practiced by soldiers during the army attacks in order to have sick leave [14] [15]. It is well known that children may ingest kerosene instead of water, while adults may burn themselves by bathing with kerosene [7] [13]-[16].

In the last ten years cases of intradermal kerosene injection had been seen as a part of emotional problems but unfortunately all cases are misdiagnosed initially as most doctors are not aware of this problem.

So the aim of the present report is to present the clinical picture of these cases to encourage doctors to have right initial diagnosis.

In conclusion self-induced panniculitis by intradermal kerosene injection is a distinctive entity that should be managed early to have right treatment and to avoid future complications. Psychological evaluation should be carried out in all cases.

## Disclosure

This study was an independent study and not funded by any drug companies.

## References

[1]    Rice, R.H. and Mauro, T.M. (2008) Toxic Responses of the Skin. In: Casarett, L.J., Ed., *Casarett and Doull's Toxicology: The Basic Science of Poisons*, 7th Edition, McGraw-Hill, New York, 143-518.

[2]    Baynes, R.E., Brooks, J.D., Budsaba, K., Smith, C.E. and Riviere, J.E. (2001) Mixture Effects of JP-8 Additives on the Dermal Disposition of Jet Fuel Components. *Toxicology and Applied Pharmacology*, **175**, 269-281.
http://dx.doi.org/10.1006/taap.2001.9259

[3]    Nixon, S.A. (1985) Kerosene Induced Abscesses. *Archives of Internal Medicine*, **145**, 1743.
http://dx.doi.org/10.1001/archinte.1985.00360090219045

[4]    Rao, G.S., Kannan, K., Goel, S.K., Pandya, K.P. and Shanker, R. (1984) Subcutaneous Kerosene Toxicity in Albino Rats. *Environmental Research*, **35**, 516-530.

[5]    Terzi, C., Bacakoglu, A., Unek, T. and Ozkan, M.H. (2002) Chemical Necrotizing Fasciitis Due to Household Insecticide Injection: Is Immediate Surgical Debridement Necessary? *Human Experimental Toxicology*, **21**, 687-690.
http://dx.doi.org/10.1191/0960327102ht308cr

[6]    Enchsen, H. and Lynge, P. (1979) Chemical Inflammation and Subcutaneous Necrosis after Injection of Benzene. *Ugeskrift for Læger*, **141**, 1337.

[7]    Al-Dabbas, M.H. (2006) Deliberate Self-Burning: The Psychosocial and Clinical Patterns among Patients Admitted to Burn Unit in King Hussein Medical Center/Jordan. *The Arab Journal of Psychiatry*, **17**, 253-256.

[8]    Awe, A.J., Soliman, M.A. and Gourdie, R.W. (2003) Necrotizing Fasciitis Induced by Self-Injection of Kerosene. *Annals of Saudi Medicine*, **23**, 388-390.

[9]    Nazar, M. (2012) Mohammad Amin, Nashmeel Rasool Hamah Ameen, Reem Abed, Mohammed Abbas. Self-Burning in Iraqi Kurdistan: Proportion and Risk Factors in a Burns Unit. *International Psychiatry*, **9**, 72-74.

[10]  Apex Oil Company, Inc. (2005) Material Safety Data Sheet, Kerosene: (Straight Run, Hydrodesulfurized, Clear or Dyed). http://www.apexoil.com/msds/kero.pdf

[11]  Wikipedia (The Free Encyclopedia) (2012) History of Petroleum.

[12]  Karam, G.E., Hajjar, R.V. and Salamoun, M.M. (2007) Suicidality in the Arab World Part I: Community Studies. *The Arab Journal of Psychiatry*, **18**, 99-107.

[13]  Hosseinian, A, Mahammad, A.T.J. and Alireza, R. (2009) Clinical Finding and Outcome in Suicidal Attempt Due to

Intravenous Injection of Kerosene. *Pakistan Journal of Biological Sciences*, **12**, 439-442.
http://dx.doi.org/10.3923/pjbs.2009.439.442

[14] Kafaween, H., Rbehat, H. and Hawil, K.N. (2010) Necrotizing Fascitis Induced by Self-Injection of Kerosene, Case Report. *The Middle East Journal of Family Medicine*, **8**, 35-39.

[15] Khammash, M.R., Hussein, A.D. and Musmer, M. (1997) Management of Kerosene Injection in the Upper Limb. *Saudi Medical Journal*, **18**, 188-190.

[16] Younis, M.S. (2012) Self-Mutilation by Subcutaneous Injection of Kerosen: Report from Iraq. 12*th Pan Arab Psychiatric Conference*, 29-30 November-1 December 2012.

[17] Hassan, H.S. (1999) Self Mutilation. *The Arab Journal of Psychiatry*, **10**.
http://www.arabjpsychiat.com/index.php?option=com_content&view=article&id=28:1999vol102november&catid=1:volumes-a-articles&Itemid=2

# 15

# Patient Reported Frequency of Lupus Flare: Associations with Foundation Makeup and Sunscreen Use

Marline L. Squance[1,2,3,4,5*], Glenn E. M. Reeves[1,3,4,5], John Attia[1,4,5]

[1]Faculty of Health and Medicine, University of Newcastle, Callaghan, Australia
[2]Faculty of Science and Information Technology, University of Newcastle, Callaghan, Australia
[3]Autoimmune Resource and Research Centre, New Lambton Heights, Australia
[4]Hunter New England Health District, New Lambton Heights, Australia
[5]Hunter Medical Research Institute, New Lambton Heights, Australia
Email: [*]marline.squance@hnehealth.nsw.gov.au

## Abstract

Objective: To test the hypothesis that usage of foundation makeup (FM) and sunscreen lotion (SS), used individually or in combination, is associated with significant changes in the likelihood of lupus symptom exacerbation. Methods: Self-reported flare days (SRF) and use of FM and SS products, were retrospectively examined in 80 Caucasian Australian women with ACR classified SLE for a year. Negative binomial regression modelled SRF days (outcome) against independent FMSS variable and covariates: age; diagnosis years; outdoor hours; BMI; stress; immune therapy medication (ITM) use. Results: Statistically significant inverse associations between SRF days and FMSS use were found. Protective effects were statistically significant ($p < 0.05$) for combined FMSS exposure days (OR 0.998, CI 0.997 - 1.0) and FM alone (OR 0.603, CI 0.363 - 1.0). Significant associations consistent with increased SRF risk were seen in sub-analysis models for participants taking ITM: univariate model (OR 1.968, $p = 0.03$); multivariate model for FMSS (OR 2.11, CI 1.161 - 3.835); FM days (OR 1.855, CI 1.023 - 3.364). Results show SRF day reduction of 0.15% for each day of product exposure. Conclusion: Study results highlight protective effects of wearing FM with or without SS. This reduction in flare days ultimately has potential to improve quality of life in SLE patients.

## Keywords

Lupus, Patient Perspective, Flare, Makeup, Sunscreen, Photosensitivity, Uv Protection, Immune Therapy Medications

---

[*]Corresponding author.

## 1. Introduction

Systemic Lupus Erythematosus (SLE) is a chronic autoimmune illness characterised by multi-system involvement that can be mild through to life threatening. SLE prevalence worldwide was recently estimated as 32 per 100,000 [1], with potential for underestimation due to milder cases not being diagnosed [2]-[4]. Community burden of SLE, particularly in industrialised western countries and Caucasian populations, is reported to be on the increase, which cannot be attributed to improved diagnostic criteria and investigations alone [4].

Environmental interactions along with intrinsic factors such as genetics, hormones and age have been reported as playing a role in SLE pathogenesis [5]-[7], with a small number of researchers suggesting that environmental exposures have a role in SLE progression and exacerbation patterns of sensitive individuals [5]-[10]. The interplay of endogenous and exogenous factors is thought to stimulate endocrine and immune regulatory systems interfering with immune tolerance [3] [9] [11]-[13], manifesting in either suppression or heightening of immune system responses.

The illness commonly exhibits periods of symptom quiescence and exacerbation (flare events). The unpredictable nature of SLE flares reduces quality of life and has the capacity to reduce functional ability [13]. The numbers of SLE specific risk assessment studies investigating relationships between illness exacerbation and everyday products are limited. Stimuli such as UV exposure, certain pharmaceutical compounds, hormones, infection and stress are the most researched and accepted triggers of flares [8] [14] [15]; however, in the majority of individuals, reasons for why and when flares occur remain unclear. Exposure to environmental agents including personal hygiene and grooming products, which regularly contain solvents, phthalates, parabens, perfumes, UV filters and pigments [16] [17], is suggested as potential flare triggers.

This study assesses the hypothesis that the use of common makeup products of foundation (FM) and sunscreen lotion (SS), used individually or in combination, is associated with significant changes in the likelihood of self-reported flares (SRF) of lupus symptoms.

## 2. Patients and Methods

This study was a retrospective analysis of a cohort of 80 Caucasian female SLE patients as defined by the American College of Rheumatology (ACR) classification criteria for SLE [18]. Participants completed study specific questionnaires and interview to examine their flare experience and exposure to environmental products within daily living practices as part of a wider pilot study, "The Environmental Determinants of Lupus Flare (EDOLF)". Data were of a self-reported nature over a 12 month study period capturing a full seasonal cycle.

Methods have been reported previously in detail [19] and are briefly summarized here with methods specific to exposure and usage of foundation makeup (FM) and sunscreen (SS) outlined. Ethical review and approval according to Declaration of Helsinki 2008 [20] was granted from the University of Newcastle and Hunter New England Health Human Research Ethics Committees.

### 2.1. Study Population

Participants were recruited through the Autoimmune Resource and Research Centre (ARRC) and private Immunology clinics in the Hunter/Central Coast region of New South Wales, Australia. SLE diagnosis was confirmed through a health record audit to establish SLE diagnosis adhered to the ACR SLE Classification guidelines [18]. Due to minimal numbers of males meeting the ACR criteria, the final study cohort was limited to females only. The population was of a homogeneous Caucasian background.

### 2.2. Data Collection

Participants completed study specific questionnaires for assessment of medical history, home environment, and lifestyle practices as part of the wider EDOLF study. Of particular interest were participant patterns of commercial product usage associated with personal hygiene and household cleaning practises. Participants also attended the ARRC for a clinical appointment where standard measures of health and their SLE flare history experience (SRF) were documented.

#### 2.2.1. Product Exposure Assessment
Participants completed a Home Cleaning and Maintenance Product list (HCMPL) documenting all products used

within their home for cleaning and for personal care. The HCMPL collected the following product information: product type description, intended purpose of use, brand names and product usage over the study year. Exposure was calculated by combining count values of self-reported use of each product within a scale of "daily", "weekly", "monthly", "yearly" and "don't know".

The study goal was to examine common product use patterns and flare events; therefore, the developed methods did not direct participants to particular products or product categories. The HCMPL instructed participants to document all products used and stored within cupboards in various housing rooms (bathroom, kitchen, laundry, garages, etc.). Participants self-selected the products they documented without independent visual confirmation that all products had been documented.

Product groups were categorised based on intended purpose of named product. The product category of "makeup" (FMSS) consisted of topical lotions of FM and SS only. Other makeup products such as lipsticks, eye shadow, mascara and colouring agents such as blush were self-reported by a small number of participants only, so they were not included within this analysis. As a crosscheck technique for products of specific interest, participants were asked questions within the primary study questionnaire regarding FM and SS and their regime of use.

Days of FMSS exposure was calculated for each participant as a total exposure day count by collating self-reported product/chemical exposure activity information and the specific product question responses from the primary study questionnaire. Duplication of individual products and usage day counts was avoided by cross-checking data from each source.

### 2.2.2. Patient Reported Flare Outcomes

Flare assessment processes were not administered by a physician within a clinical review appointment, therefore traditional tools for assessing disease activity (e.g., SLEDAI) could not be used. To capture the lived experience of lupus, study flare event history was taken directly from the individual participant perspective and used standardisation scripted structured flare history interview [19] inclusive of a novel flare definition. The flare event definition chosen reflected a chronic autoimmune illness characterised by relapsing and remitting flare patterns whilst also incorporating the concept of symptom stability, punctuated by sustained exacerbation.

An exacerbation is defined as: The appearance of a new clinical sign/symptom or the clinical worsening of a previous sign/symptom that had been stable for at least the previous 30 days and which persisted for a minimum of 24 hours [21].

SRF days were a calculation of self-reported number and average length of SRF events reported in the study period. Final analysis did not include participants that reported a "constant" state of flaring.

### 2.2.3. Risk Factors

Study specific questionnaires completed included information on participant demographic, medical history, general health and wellbeing. Each participant nominated an approximate date of their SLE diagnosis which was crosschecked within the health record audit phase of the study. Participant self-assessment of their socio economic status (SES) of "Above Australian Average", "Australian Average" and "Below Australian Average" were recorded. Stress levels were recorded via a visual analogue scale (VAS) of 0-100 with end points of "Not stressed at all" and "Highly stressed". Participant body mass index (BMI) was calculated and coded according to Australian Government Health Guidelines categories of "underweight (<18.5)", "normal weight (18.5 - 24.99)", "overweight (25 - 29.99)" and "Obese (>30)". Study period hours spent outdoors were calculated from participants' nominated hours for each weekday and weekend day. Current smoking status was captured as a dichotomised "yes", "no" response.

Immune modulating and suppressant medications (immune therapy medications, ITM): Methotrexate, Hydroxychloroquine, Prednisolone, Azathioprine, intravenous immunoglobulin, Dapsone and Mycophenolate were categorised as a single group to examine effect on SRF history in relation to FMSS use. Vitamin D supplementation, whilst considered by many to have properties of immune modulation [22]-[25], was considered separately.

### 2.3. Statistical Methods

Due to over dispersion, a negative binomial regression model was used to assess the relationship between SRF days and FMSS usage days. Covariates considered were: participant age; diagnosis years; outdoors hours; SES;

BMI; stress; Vitamin D, hormones and ITM use.

Initially, all variables of interest were included in the model with a backward stepwise approach to identify the best possible multivariate model. Interactions were tested for SRF days and covariates with significant effects at the <0.05 level retained in the model. All normality assumptions were verified by inspection of probability plots and histograms of residuals. Associations were expressed as odds ratios with 95% confidence intervals. All analyses were performed with the use of STATA v11.0 (StataCorp LP, College Station, Texas, USA).

## 3. Results

A total of 159 personal health records were audited to confirm a SLE diagnosis based upon documented evidence of the 11 ACR classification criteria [18]. Of these, 83 participants met the classification criterion of ≥4 out of 11, and completed all components of the study. The structured interview process resulted in 3 participants reporting a SRF history of "constant flaring"; therefore these participants were excluded from final analysis. Health record audit showed a broad representation of SLE clinical manifestations with clinical features of malar rash, photosensitivity, arthritis, and presence of antinuclear antibodies being frequently documented.

**Table 1** represents the distribution of characteristics across the final 80 SLE participants. Participants' mean age was 47.69 years and diagnosed with SLE for approximately 2 - 38 years (mean 7.7 years). The participant

**Table 1.** Demographic characteristics.

|  | n | Mean | SD | Range | 95% CI | |
|---|---|---|---|---|---|---|
| Age (Years) | 80 | 47.7 | 13.6 | 19 - 77 | 44.7 | 50.7 |
| Diagnosis (Years) | 77 | 7.7 | 6.3 | 2 - 38 | 6.3 | 9.1 |
| Current health score (VAS scale)[a] | 80 | 54.2 | 22.6 | 0 - 98 | 49.2 | 59.2 |
| Stress score (VAS scale)[b] | 80 | 50.8 | 27.4 | 0 - 100 | 44.7 | 56.9 |
| Outdoor hours (Year) | 80 | 490.6 | 433.2 | 0 - 2044 | 394.2 | 587.0 |

| n = 80 | n | % | n = 80 | n | % |
|---|---|---|---|---|---|
| **Comorbidity** | | | **Body mass index** | | |
| Autoimmune Illness not SLE | 43 | 53.8 | Underweight | 2 | 2.5 |
| Other illness not autoimmune | 50 | 62.5 | Normal | 21 | 26.25 |
| **Ethnic background** | | | Overweight | 33 | 41.25 |
| Caucasian | 70 | 87.5 | Obese | 24 | 30.0 |
| **Educational background** | | | **Smoking status** | | |
| Year 9 (15 years) | 8 | 10.0 | Current smoker | 6 | 7.5 |
| School leaving certificate | 24 | 30.0 | Past smoker | 30 | 37.5 |
| Higher school certificate | 2 | 2.5 | Use ITM | 66 | 82.5 |
| Apprenticeship | 4 | 5.0 | Use Vitamin D supplement | 24 | 30.0 |
| Tertiary (University/College) | 36 | 45.0 | Use hormone supplement | 30 | 37.5 |
| Postgraduate studies | 6 | 7.5 | Regular sun | 39 | 48.8 |
| **Clinical SLE features** | | | Regular sun + Sunscreen | 30 | 76.9 |
| Malar rash | 57 | 71.3 | **Socio economic status** | | |
| Discoid rash | 3 | 3.8 | Above average | 15 | 18.8 |
| Photosensitivity | 43 | 53.8 | Average | 56 | 70.0 |
| Oral/nasal ulcers | 29 | 36.3 | Below average | 9 | 11.3 |
| Arthritis | 63 | 78.8 | **ACR SLE classification criteria** | | |
| Serositis | 20 | 25.0 | 4 criteria | 26 | 32.5 |
| Renal disorder | 37 | 46.3 | 5 criteria | 24 | 30.0 |
| Neurological disorder | 33 | 41.3 | 6 criteria | 17 | 21.25 |
| Haematological disorder | 39 | 48.8 | 7 criteria | 7 | 8.75 |
| Immunologic disorder | 27 | 33.8 | 8 criteria | 4 | 5.0 |
| Antinuclear antibody | 73 | 91.3 | 9 criteria | 2 | 2.5 |
| +ve response to pharmaceutics | 75 | 93.8 | | | |

[a]Visual Analogue Scale Score of 0 - 100—Current Health (0) Extremely Poor—(100) Excellent; [b]Stress (0) Not stressed at all—(100) Highly stressed.

inclusion criteria did exclude persons with a diagnosis history less than 2 years duration. Over 62.5% of participants self-reported comorbidities. The majority of participants were not current smokers (92.5%) however, a larger number reported being past smokers (37.5%). Current smoking status was confirmed by serum cotinine assay and showed concordant results with self-report.

The analysis also included data on the usage of ITM as well as supplementation of Vitamin D and hormonal treatments. Participant use of ITM was common (82.5%) with many being prescribed 2 or more ITMs. No assessment of individual participant medication compliance was undertaken.

**Table 2** represents data in specific reference to SRF events and makeup product usage. Tabulated results showed that participants experienced a mean of 6.8 SRF events within the study year ranging from 0 flare events to 1 event per week. Counts of SRF days ranged 0 - 240 days with a mean count of 29.2 SRF days. Three participants reported single events that equated to 60 - 90 SRF day counts. FM was used by 73.75% of the cohort and SS was used by 77.5%. Many participants used more than one FMSS product each day. SS usage in regards to regular sun exposure was explored with 49% reporting regular sun exposure (**Table 1**) and of those 76.9% responded as always wearing SS when in the sun. A range of 0 - 1223 (mean 291) total exposure days for overall FMSS category indicates multiple individual product usage within the study year.

Negative binomial regression was used to model SRF days (outcome) against independent FMSS product variables as well as social, lifestyles and illness variables with results summarised within **Table 3**. Statistically

**Table 2.** Self-reported flare (SRF) and makeup product (FMSS) usage.

|  | $n$ | Mean | SD | Range | 95% CI | |
|---|---|---|---|---|---|---|
| SRF no. (Year) | 80 | 6.8 | 9.7 | 0 - 52 | 4.6 | 8.9 |
| SRF days (Year) | 80 | 29.2 | 39 | 0 - 240 | 20.5 | 37.9 |
| FMSS exposure days | 80 | 291.1 | 214.2 | 0 - 1223 | 243.4 | 338.7 |
| FMSS product count | 80 | 1.6 | 0.9 | 0 - 7 | 1.4 | 1.8 |
| $n = 80$ | $n$ | % |  |  |  |  |
| Use of FM | 59 | 73.8 |  |  |  |  |
| Use of SS | 62 | 77.5 |  |  |  |  |

**Table 3.** Negative binomial regression for flare days (Fc) and independent variables.

|  | OR | p > \|Z\| | 95% CI | |
|---|---|---|---|---|
| **Univariate model (Fc)** | | | | |
| FMSS product days | 0.998 | **0.01** | 0.998 | 1.0 |
| Immune therapy medications | 1.968 | **0.03** | 1.088 | 3.56 |
| FM | 0.58 | **0.04** | 0.35 | 0.96 |
| SS | 0.79 | 0.43 | 0.45 | 1.40 |
| Vitamin D | 1.51 | 0.10 | 0.93 | 2.45 |
| Hormone treatment | 1.22 | 0.39 | 0.78 | 1.94 |
| Age | 0.99 | 0.06 | 0.97 | 1.00 |
| Years of diagnosis | 0.97 | 0.07 | 0.93 | 1.00 |
| Body mass index | 1.23 | 0.78 | 0.28 | 5.41 |
| Smoking | 1.61 | 0.27 | 0.69 | 3.73 |
| Stress | 1.00 | 0.63 | 0.99 | 1.01 |
| Outdoor hours | 1.0 | 0.10 | 1.0 | 1.00 |
| Regular sun | 0.93 | 0.74 | 0.59 | 1.45 |
| **Multivariate model (Fc)** | | | | |
| FMSS product days | 0.998 | **0.00** | 0.997 | 1.0 |
| Immune therapy medication | 2.11 | **0.01** | 1.161 | 3.835 |
| FM days | 0.603 | **0.05** | 0.363 | 1.0 |
| Immune therapy medication | 1.855 | **0.04** | 1.023 | 3.364 |

significant associations for independent variables were found for FMSS product days, ITM and FM use; but not for SS as a sub group analysis of the FMSS product days. The analysis was adjusted for age, diagnosis years, SES, BMI, smoking, stress, therapeutic supplements of vitamin D and hormone treatments, sunburn events, and outdoor hours in the study year. No confounding effect was found for any of these factors.

Protective effects, as demonstrated by odds ratio values, were statistically significant on both univariate and multivariate analysis of FMSS product exposure days (OR 0.998, CI 0.997 - 1.0) and FM usage (OR 0.603, CI 0.363 - 1.0). Surprisingly, significant associations consistent with increased SRF risk were seen in a univariate model for participants undertaking ITM (OR 1.968, p = 0.03). This ITM association was also retained within multivariate models for FMSS product days (OR 2.11, CI 1.161 - 3.835) and the sub analysis of FM days (OR 1.855, CI 1.023 - 3.364). This is likely a reflection of selection bias in that those with more severe SLE are more likely to be prescribed ITM.

Participant total SRF days as a function of FMSS exposure (with 95% CI) within the study year for participants undertaking ITM and also for those that are not on ITM are presented in **Figure 1**. A reduction of SRF days with usage of FMSS products was demonstrated, and was consistent regardless of the participant taking ITM or not. There were significantly more SRF days in individuals on ITM (p = 0.01) however overall reduction of SRF days with increased chemical exposure was not contingent upon ITM therapy. The model estimates that an SLE patient on ITM can potentially have reduction in SRF days experienced within a year by a factor of 0.0015 (0.15%) with each day of increasing FMSS product exposure. Absolute FMSS product exposure ranges from 0 to ~600 exposure days: for every 100 days of additional FMSS product exposure, the lupus SRF incidence rate drops by 14%. Across the exposure range, the risk drops by 59%-putting this in terms of risk reduction, the SRF incidence rate for FMSS exposure level equal to 600 days is over half that observed with an exposure level equal to 0.

## 4. Discussion

This study found a statistically significant inverse association between SRF days and exposure to FMSS products defined as FM and SS. Results show those SRF days were reduced by a factor of 0.15% for each day of FMSS product exposure over the study year, indicating a protective component to FMSS product usage. The sub analysis of FMSS category with ITM usage indicates that the reduction of SRF days was not contingent on ITM use. This reduction in symptom exacerbation days ultimately has potential to improve quality of life in SLE patients.

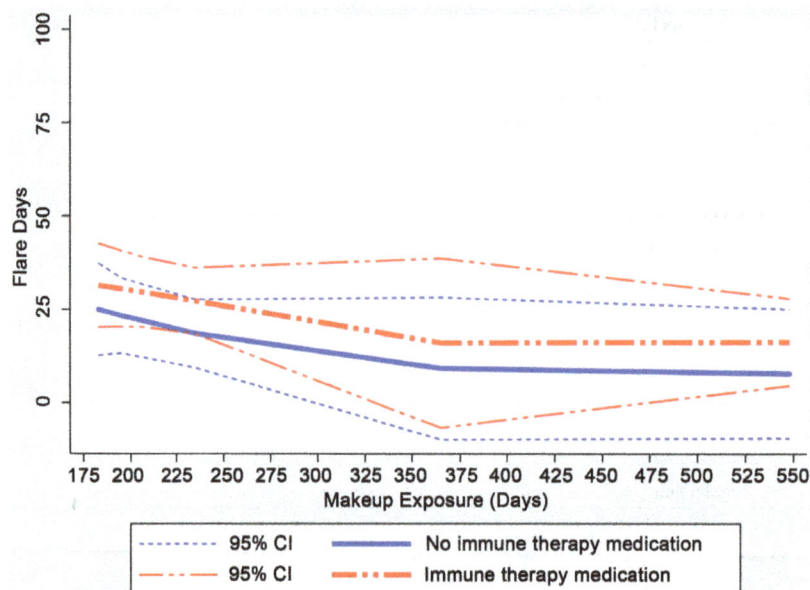

**Figure 1.** Self-reported flare (SRF) day events as a function of FMSS exposure days and immune therapy medication use for the study year, together with 95% confidence bands.

SLE flare days within this study were calculated from the lived health experience of the individual participant rather than clinical markers of symptom exacerbation. Total flare days were calculated using the number and average length of SRF in days. No assessments of SRF severity in regards to health and quality of life impacts were made; however, 3 participants recalled long periods of symptom activation and recovery of 60 - 90 days. Due to the retrospective nature of reporting, symptom exacerbation characteristics specific to a reported single SRF were not explored. However, the reported tendency of lupus patients to inaccurately attribute symptom fluctuations to flare events [26]-[29] would tend to create bias against detection of a significant association with product exposure.

Within the study group, symptoms of malar and body rash, photosensitivity, joint pain and fatigue were widely reported as common flare symptoms (**Table 1**) and they also had a high impact on quality of life and body self-image. The health record audit found that the commonest symptoms included joint involvement (arthritis 78.75%), malar rash (71.25%) and photosensitive reactions (54%). These rates are similar to other studies examining epidemiology of SLE and symptom exacerbation [2] [6] [14] [30] [31]; however, the reported rates of malar rash within these studies are lower than that found within our Australian study population. This could be a result of the study involving a homogeneous Caucasian population; UV exposure intensity within the Australian environment; and the high prescribed usage of a known photosensitizing pharmaceutical, Hydroxychloroquine, as a primary treatment within the study population.

ITM usage (82.5%) was considered a potential confounder of the impact of FMSS product use; unexpectedly, our results indicate that ITM use presented an elevated risk of SRF activity (OR 2.11). It is likely that this is a reflection of selection bias in that those with more severe SLE illness experience more flare days as a result of flare frequency and intensity, requiring a management regime involving one or more ITM.

SLE skin symptoms of malar rash, scarring and photosensitive reactions result as either an illness manifestation or pharmaceutical therapy side effect [32]. To better manage these symptoms and their impacts, clinicians and health educators offer self-management advice to adopt lifestyle practices that focus on sun protection measures [30] [33]-[35] and, if necessary, masking of skin irregularities through the application of physical disguises such as makeup [36] [37]. Advice on reduction of UV exposure includes avoidance of long periods of UV exposure, wearing hats and sun protective clothing and regular topical application of physical and chemical UV filters and barriers in the form of lotions.

Adherence to the use of sun protection in the form of SS use has been widely examined and it has been argued to be a sometimes ineffective sun protective measure due to the practise of selective use only when significant exposure activity is planned. This sporadic use can in fact lead to higher UV exposure [38] [39] from prolonged time periods spent within direct sunlight and other UV sources in living and work environments. Repeated mini exposures to UV radiation occurring from sunlight sources and from internal lighting systems of modern homes, offices and places of daily activity, has been estimated at as much as 80% of total lifetime exposure [32] leaving a photosensitive person vulnerable to adverse effects. The amount of incidental lifetime UV exposure indicates that daily application of visually appealing products containing UV protection capabilities as a prophylactic measure of UV protection may be more effective particularly in a photosensitive population.

Vila *et al.* [35], in a SLE and sunlight exposure study, found many clinical outcomes significantly improved with use of photo protection measures. Specifically, patients who adhered to UV protective regimes had significantly lower renal involvement, thrombocytopenia, hospitalisations, and reduced requirement for either increased dosage or additional ITM. Our study, whilst not finding a significant association with the use of SS alone and SRF, did find health improvements in the form of reduced SRF days, with the use of FM alone as well as FMSS as a combined product group.

SS use within the study group was reported at 77.5% which is double that of reported rates of use within the Australian NSW Health adult female population (34.6%) [40]. Comparison rates for the use of FM and SS across other SLE studies was limited due to the small number of studies; however, there are reported rates of 50% SS use within SLE patients in Puerto Rico [35], and 54.7% SS and 60.4% cosmetic use in a US based general population birth mothers study [41]. These rates suggest that our study population was more compliant with sun protection measures than the general Australian population or other international study populations.

Commercial personal product manufacturers have increased the use of UV protective chemicals and physical barriers to improve product saleability and acceptability [30] [42]. UV protectors in products are commonly in the form of organic and physical inorganic chemicals such as Titanium Dioxide ($TiO_2$), Zinc oxides (ZnO) and mineral pigments including mica and other oxides, which act to either block, reflect or scatter UVA and UVB radiation limiting penetration. A wide range of personal care products label these agents within their product ingredients. Everyday products of shampoos, shower gels, face moisturisers, soaps, clothing, cleaning agents as well as common makeup products such as foundation makeup, contain at least one UV protective agent [31] [43].

The NHANES study reports that 96.8% of randomly selected urine samples were found to contain a UV protective chemical, Benzophenone-3, indicating widespread exposure to UV protectors as a result of daily activities. It is possible that the protective and significant association with FM and SS found in our study could be associated with the individual participant's chemical use of other commercial agents, including undisclosed personal cosmetic and cleansing products. The ubiquitous use of UV filters and UV protection chemicals in everyday cleaning and personal products could also result in additional unintentional UV protection via daily chores and hygiene habits [44].

It is also proposed that the reported positive self-image that occurs with cosmetic coverage of disfiguring symptoms, such as malar rash, scarring and photosensitivity [30] [36] [37] [45] could also have resulted in improved psychological wellbeing and quality of life within those participants and therefore reduced impacts of SLE symptoms and recorded flare days.

## Study Strengths and Weaknesses

This study demonstrated that SRF day was reduced in this SLE cohort with exposure to FMSS products of FM and SS. This apparent protective aspect of FMSS product use was detected regardless of whether they were taking ITM as part of their illness management regime. The study provides pilot data within the context of a retrospective study that relies on self-reported participant assessment of exposure and flare events in a Caucasian population. The capacity to assess individual measures of actual exposure or day counts of symptom exacerbation as defined as a "flare" event was not possible at this time. The lack of ethnic diversity within our Australian study population would reduce the capacity for extrapolation of results to the wider, more diverse international SLE population.

Flare assessment was undertaken from a patient perspective with adherence to a strict protocol for documentation; however, confirmation from clinical data did not occur. Hence, flare days were estimated across the study year based upon participant self-report and this may have resulted in an overestimation of actual days. However, this overestimation would be expected to create a bias against detection of a significant association with product exposure.

Measurement bias within the assessment of product exposure process was minimised by adopting a process of crosschecking reported usage within two separate data collection tools (HCMPL and study specific questionnaire). The FMSS product category did not include other cosmetic and personal products that may contain sunscreen agents, so it is possible that the effect we are noting within our study could be attributed in part to other products used routinely. It is unlikely that the reported findings represent recall bias as patients were asked about FM and SS use in the context of a long list of products with no indication of associations being tested.

## 5. Conclusions

This study has examined the effects of FMSS exposure and exacerbation of SLE symptoms as defined by "SRF days". The study results have highlighted a protective effect of wearing FMSS products, in particular FM with or without additional SS products. However, this study has not demonstrated a conclusive link to any particular product chemical component due to the inability to refine: individual product chemical content or concentrations, or the potential effects of product chemical admixing.

The study results indicate that the investigation of SLE illness behaviour in respect to everyday beauty products needs further exploration. Formulations and concentrations of product chemical components change readily to meet consumer and commercial demands reducing capacity for researchers to gauge exact causation links between chemical exposure and health risk.

## Acknowledgements

This study forms part of the Environmental Determinants of Lupus Flare (EDOLF) PhD study, University of Newcastle. The authors would like to thank Associate Professor Howard Bridgman for his guidance in the writing of this paper, the study participants and also Dr. Patrick McElduff, Dr. Maya Guest and Dr. May Boggess for their help with statistical analysis and graphing methods.

The study was supported by the Autoimmune Resource Research Centre (Not-for-profit charity www.autoimmune.org.au), and the Val Badham Research Scholarship for Immunology, University of Newcastle Foundation. The Authors declare that there is no conflict of interest.

## References

[1]    Hayter, S.M. and Cook, M.C. (2012) Updated Assessment of the Prevalence, Spectrum and Case Definition of Auto-immune Disease. *Autoimmunity Reviews*, **11**, 754-765. http://dx.doi.org/10.1016/j.autrev.2012.02.001

[2]    Danchenko, N., Satia, J.A. and Anthony, M.S. (2006) Epidemiology of Systemic Lupus Erythematosus: A Comparison of Worldwide Disease Burden. *Lupus*, **15**, 308-318. http://dx.doi.org/10.1191/0961203306lu2305xx

[3]    Cooper, G.S. and Stroehla, B.C. (2003) The Epidemiology of Autoimmune Diseases. *Autoimmunity Reviews*, **2**, 119-125. http://dx.doi.org/10.1016/S1568-9972(03)00006-5

[4]    Jacobson, D.L., Gange, S.J., Rose, N.R. and Graham, N.M. (1997) Epidemiology and Estimated Population Burden of Selected Autoimmune Diseases in the United States. *Clinical Immunology and Immunopathology*, **84**, 223-243. http://dx.doi.org/10.1006/clin.1997.4412

[5]    Pons-Estel, G.J., Alarcon, G.S., Scofield, L., Reinlib, L. and GS, C. (2010) Understanding the Epidemiology and Progression of Systemic Lupus Erythematosus. *Seminars in Arthritis and Rheumatism*, **39**, 257-268. http://dx.doi.org/10.1016/j.semarthrit.2008.10.007

[6]    Dooley, M.A. and Hogan, S.L. (2003) Environmental Epidemiology and Risk Factors for Autoimmune Disease. *Current Opinion in Rheumatology*, **15**, 99-103. http://dx.doi.org/10.1097/00002281-200303000-00002

[7]    Foster, M.W. and Aston, C.E. (2003) A Practice Approach for Identifying Previously Unsuspected Environmental Contributors to Systemic Lupus Erythematosus and Other Complex Diseases. *Environmental Health Perspectives*, **111**, 593-597. http://dx.doi.org/10.1289/ehp.5665

[8]    Zandman-Goddard, G., Solomon, M., Rosman, Z., Peeva, E. and Shoenfeld, Y. (2012) Environment and Lupus-Related Diseases. *Lupus*, **21**, 241-250. http://dx.doi.org/10.1177/0961203311426568

[9]    Mayes, M.D. (1999) Epidemiologic Studies of Environmental Agents and Systemic Autoimmune Diseases. *Environmental Health Perspectives*, **107**, 743-748. http://dx.doi.org/10.1289/ehp.99107s5743

[10]   Hess, E.V. (1999) Are There Environmental Forms of Systemic Autoimmune Diseases? *Environmental Health Perspectives*, **107**, 709-711. http://dx.doi.org/10.1289/ehp.99107s5709

[11]   Cooper, G.S., Gilbert, K.M., Greidinger, E.L., James, J.A., Pfau, J.C., Reinlib, L., *et al.* (2008) Recent Advances and Opportunities in Research on Lupus: Environmental Influences and Mechanisms of Disease. *Environmental Health Perspectives*, **116**, 695-702. http://dx.doi.org/10.1289/ehp.11092

[12]   Gourley, M. and Miller, F.W. (2007) Mechanisms of Disease: Environmental Factors in the Pathogenesis of Rheumatic Disease. *Nature Reviews Rheumatology*, **3**, 172-180. http://dx.doi.org/10.1038/ncprheum0435

[13]   Cooper, G.S., Treadwell, E.L., St. Clair, E.W., Gilkeson, G.S. and Dooley, M.A. (2007) Sociodemographic Associations with Early Disease Damage in Patients with Systemic Lupus Erythematosus. *Arthritis Care and Research*, **57**, 993-999. http://dx.doi.org/10.1002/art.22894

[14]   Cooper, G.S., Wither, J., Bernatsky, S., Claudio, J.O., Clarke, A., Rioux, J.D., *et al.* (2010) Occupational and Environmental Exposures and Risk of Systemic Lupus Erythematosus: Silica, Sunlight, Solvents. *Rheumatology (Oxford)*, **49**, 2172-2180. http://dx.doi.org/10.1093/rheumatology/keq214

[15]   Hess, E.V. (2002) Environmental Chemicals and Autoimmune Disease: Cause and Effect. *Toxicology*, **181-182**, 65-70.

[16]   Dodson, R.E., Nishioka, M., Standley, L.J., Perovich, L.J., Brody, J.G. and Rudel, R.A. (2012) Endocrine Disruptors and Asthma-Associated Chemicals in Consumer Products. *Environmental Health Perspectives*, **120**, 935-943. http://dx.doi.org/10.1289/ehp.1104052

[17]   Altman, R.G., Morello-Frosch, R., Brody, J.G., Rudel, R., Brown, P. and Averick, M. (2008) Pollution Comes Home and Gets Personal: Women's Experience of Household Chemical Exposure. *Journal of Health and Social Behavior*, **49**, 417-435. http://dx.doi.org/10.1177/002214650804900404

[18]   Rheumatology ACo (2005) 1997 Update of the 1982 American College of Rheumatology Revised Criteria for Classification of Systemic Lupus Erythematosus. Classification Criteria for Diagnosis of Systemic Lupus Erythematosus.

[19]   Squance, M.L., Guest, M., Reeves, G., Attia, J. and Bridgman, H. (2014) Exploring Lifetime Occupational Exposure and SLE Flare: A Patient-Focussed Pilot Study. *Lupus Science & Medicine*, **1**, e000023.

[20]   Association, W.M. (2008) World Medical Association Declaration of Helsinki. 59*th WMA General Assembly*, Seoul,

October 2008. www.wma.net/en/30publications/10policies/b3/17c.pdf

[21]  Poser, C.M., Paty, D.W., Scheinberg, L., McDonald, W.I., Davis, F.A., Ebers, G.C., *et al.* (1983) New Diagnostic Criteria for Multiple Sclerosis: Guidelines for Research Protocols. *Annals of Neurology*, **13**, 227-231. http://dx.doi.org/10.1002/ana.410130302

[22]  Borges, M.C., Martini, L.A. and Rogero, M.M. (2011) Current Perspectives on Vitamin D, Immune System, and Chronic Diseases. *Nutrition*, **27**, 399-404. http://dx.doi.org/10.1016/j.nut.2010.07.022

[23]  Guillot, X., Semerano, L., Saidenberg-Kermanac'h, N., Falgarone, G. and Boissier, M.C. (2010) Vitamin D and Inflammation. *Joint Bone Spine*, **77**, 552-557. http://dx.doi.org/10.1016/j.jbspin.2010.09.018

[24]  Parravicini, V. and Caserta, S. (2010) The Immunomodulatory Roles of Vitamin D: New Tricks for an Old Dog. *Molecular Interventions*, **10**, 204-208. http://dx.doi.org/10.1124/mi.10.4.3

[25]  Zhang, H.L. and Wu, J. (2010) Role of Vitamin D in Immune Responses and Autoimmune Diseases, with Emphasis on its Role in Multiple Sclerosis. *Neuroscience Bulletin*, **26**, 445-454. http://dx.doi.org/10.1007/s12264-010-0731-8

[26]  Carr, F.N., Nicassio, P.M., Ishimori, M.L., Moldovan, I., Katsaros, E., Torralba, K., *et al.* (2011) Depression Predicts Self-Reported Disease Activity in Systemic Lupus Erythematosus. *Lupus*, **20**, 80-84. http://dx.doi.org/10.1177/0961203310378672

[27]  Griffiths, B., Mosca, M. and Gordon, C. (2005) Assessment of Patients with Systemic Lupus Erythematosus and the Use of Lupus Disease Activity Indices. *Best Practice & Research Clinical Rheumatology*, **19**, 685-708. http://dx.doi.org/10.1016/j.berh.2005.03.010

[28]  Leong, K.P., Chong, E.Y., Kong, K.O., Chan, S.P., Thong, B.Y., Lian, T.Y., *et al.* (2010) Discordant Assessment of Lupus Activity between Patients and Their Physicians: The Singapore Experience. *Lupus*, **9**, 100-106. http://dx.doi.org/10.1177/0961203309345748

[29]  Yen, J.C., Abrahamowicz, M., Dobkin, P.L., Clarke, A.E., Battista, R.N. and Fortin, P.R. (2003) Determinants of Discordance between Patients and Physicians in Their Assessment of Lupus Disease Activity. *The Journal of rheumatology*, **30**, 1967-1976.

[30]  Obermoser, G. and Zelger, B. (2008) Triple Need for Photoprotection in Lupus Erythematosus. *Lupus*, **17**, 525-527. http://dx.doi.org/10.1177/0961203308089440

[31]  Wang, J., Kay, A.B., Fletcher, J., Formica, M.K. and McAlindon, T.E. (2008) Is Lipstick Associated with the Development of Systemic Lupus Erythematosus (SLE)? *Clinical Rheumatology*, **27**, 1183-1187. http://dx.doi.org/10.1007/s10067-008-0937-6

[32]  Ting, W.W. and Sontheimer, R.D. (2001) Local Therapy for Cutaneous and Systemic Lupus Erythematosus: Practical and Theoretical Considerations. *Lupus*, **10**, 171-184. http://dx.doi.org/10.1191/096120301667674688

[33]  Ilchyshyn, L., Hawk, J.L. and Millard, T.P. (2008) Photoprotection: Does It Work? *Lupus*, **17**, 705-707. http://dx.doi.org/10.1177/0961203308093924

[34]  Kuhn, A., Gensch, K., Haust, M., Meuth, A.M., Boyer, F., Dupuy, P., *et al.* (2011) Photoprotective Effects of A Broad-Spectrum Sunscreen in Ultraviolet-Induced Cutaneous Lupus Erythematosus: A Randomized, Vehicle-Controlled, Double-Blind Study. *Journal of the American Academy of Dermatology*, **64**, 37-48. http://dx.doi.org/10.1016/j.jaad.2009.12.053

[35]  Vila, L.M., Mayor, A.M., Valentin, A.H., Rodriguez, S.I., Reyes, M.L., Acosta, E., *et al.* (1999) Association of Sunlight Exposure and Photoprotection Measures with Clinical Outcome in Systemic Lupus Erythematosus. *Puerto Rico Health Sciences Journal*, **18**, 89-94.

[36]  Boehncke, W.H., Ochsendorf, F., Paeslack, I., Kaufmann, R. and Zollner, T.M. (2002) Decorative Cosmetics Improve the Quality of Life in Patients with Disfiguring Skin Diseases. *European Journal of Dermatology*, **12**, 577-580.

[37]  Shear, N.H. and Graff, L. (1987) Camouflage Cosmetics in Dermatologic Therapy. *Canadian Family Physician*, **33**, 2343-2346.

[38]  Autier, P., Boniol, M. and Dore, J.F. (2007) Sunscreen Use and Increased Duration of Intentional Sun Exposure: Still a Burning Issue. *International Journal of Cancer*, **121**, 1-5. http://dx.doi.org/10.1002/ijc.22745

[39]  Manova, E., von Goetz, N., Hauri, U., Bogdal, C. and Hungerbuhler, K. (2012) Organic UV Filters in Personal Care Products in Switzerland: A Survey of Occurrence and Concentrations. *International Journal of Hygiene and Environmental Health*, **216**, 508-514.

[40]  NSW Government (2011) Research CfEa. New South Wales Population Health Survey 2010. Centre for Epidemiology and Research PHD, NSW Department of Health, Australia.

[41]  Schlumpf, M., Kypke, K., Wittassek, M., Angerer, J., Mascher, H., Mascher, D., *et al.* (2010) Exposure Patterns of UV Filters, Fragrances, Parabens, Phthalates, Organochlor Pesticides, PBDEs, and PCBs in Human Milk: Correlation of UV Filters with Use of Cosmetics. *Chemosphere*, **81**, 1171-1183. http://dx.doi.org/10.1016/j.chemosphere.2010.09.079

[42] Nohynek, G.J., Lademann, J., Ribaud, C. and Roberts, M.S. (2007) Grey Goo on the Skin? Nanotechnology, Cosmetic and Sunscreen Safety. *Critical Reviews in Toxicology*, **37**, 251-277. http://dx.doi.org/10.1080/10408440601177780

[43] NLM (2013) Household Products Database. http://householdproducts.nlm.nih.gov/index.htm

[44] Calafat, A.M., Wong, L.Y., Ye, X., Reidy, J.A. and Needham, L.L. (2008) Concentrations of the Sunscreen Agent Benzophenone-3 in Residents of the United States: National Health and Nutrition Examination Survey 2003-2004. *Environmental Health Perspectives*, **116**, 893-897. http://dx.doi.org/10.1289/ehp.11269

[45] Hale, E.D., Treharne, G.J., Norton, Y., Lyons, A.C., Douglas, K.M., Erb, N., *et al*. (2006) "Concealing the Evidence": The Importance of Appearance Concerns for Patients with Systemic Lupus Erythematosus. *Lupus*, **15**, 532-540. http://dx.doi.org/10.1191/0961203306lu2310xx

# 16

# Preliminary Colorimetric Assessment of Progressive Nonsegmental Vitiligo under Short-Term Intravenous Methylprednisolone Pulse Therapy

Yuiko Nagata*, Atsushi Tanemura*, Emi Ono, Aya Tanaka, Kenichi Kato, Mizuho Yamada, Ichiro Katayama

Department of Dermatology, Integrated Medicine Osaka University Graduate School of Medicine, Suita, Japan
Email: tanemura@derma.med.osaka-u.ac.jp

## Abstract

Although the administration of systemic steroid for nonsegmental vitiligo in the progressive stage is a recommended treatment according to guidelines, the clinical efficacy of this regimen has not been fully established. In this study, we evaluated the clinical efficacy of half-dose steroid treatment and stratified the evidence regarding its usefulness in progressive vitiligo patients. Half-dose steroid pulse therapy (500 mg/day of methylprednisolone for three sequential days) was administered intravenously three times monthly in five vitiligo patients. The visual changes in vitiligo lesions were evaluated on photographs and quantified using a spectrophotometer. As results, all patients completed three cycles of treatment without severe adverse events. Three of the five patients achieved disease arrest with decrease in white contrast. Therefore, short-term and half-dose steroid therapy is well tolerated and effective for achieving disease arrest in progressive nonsegmental vitiligo. The whiteness assessed by a spectrophotometer is possibly associated with therapeutic response to steroid therapy.

## Keywords

Intravenous Methylprednisolone Pulse Therapy, Progressive Nonsegmental Vitiligo, Spectrophotometer

---

*These authors are equally contributed to this study.

# 1. Introduction

The recommended treatment for nonsegmental vitiligo vulgaris includes topical ointments of steroids and tacrolimus, ultraviolet phototherapy, systemic steroids and surgery according to international guidelines [1] [2].

Ultraviolet light therapy such as narrow band UVB has been considered to be the most common modalities in treating cases of disseminated vitiligo. However, narrow band UVB irradiation requires consultations once or twice a week and is mostly refractory in advanced and/or long-lasting cases. Steroid therapy for advanced vitiligo recommended as a class C1 treatment in one set of guidelines [2] is known as fairly effective and has two routes of administration, namely, oral and intravenous. Although oral steroid therapy suggested by Radakovic [3], Kim [4], and Pasricha [5], unacceptable side effects (moon face, exacerbation of diabetes mellitus and hypertension, and so on) were observed in 50% or more of patients due to the long-term administration period. Meanwhile, with respect to intravenous steroid pulse therapy, Seiter obtained disease improvements in pathology in 90% of cases with temporary and reversible side effects [6].

In this preliminary study, we evaluated a therapeutic effect of half-dose methylprednisolone pulse therapy for patients with progressive nonsegmental vitiligo based on ocular inspection and unique objective calculation of white contrast and redness and supposed the future position of this treatment on guidelines in reference with previous literatures.

# 2. Methods

Five nonsegmental vitiligo patients in a state of progression were enrolled in this study; their demographic characteristics are summarized in **Table 1**. All patients had noticed lesion enlargement with no improvement six months before their first visit.

## Quantitative Evaluation of Color Changes

We used a spectrophotometer, an apparatus used to digitize three elements of color: hue (color, such as red, blue, etc.), brightness (degree of brightness) and chroma (degree of saturation). The L, a, and b scores represent skin whiteness, erythematous changes and bluntness, respectively. The delta L score represents a white contrast as difference of the degree between lesional minus perilesional skin. The target lesions were arbitrarily assigned for assessment, and the color scores were calculated using a spectrophotometer for an objective color evaluation (CD-2600d, Konica Minorta, Japan) both before and after treatment. The assigned sites did not change throughout the study. The mean of three calculated scores was used as representative data.

The paired $t$-test was used for the analysis of differences in color tone before and after treatment. A value of p < 0.05 (two-tailed) was considered to be statistically significant. All statistical analyses were performed using the Prism software program, version 5 (GraphPad Software Inc., La Jolla, CA, USA).

# 3. Cases and Results

## Representative Case

A 62-year-old Japanese female noticed depigmented macules on her frontal chest four years ago and subsequently suffered from progressive depigmentation on the buttock and lower extremities as well as perilesional hyperpigmentation, regardless of treatment with narrowband UVB phototherapy. A screening examination did not detect any complications associated with nonsegmental vitiligo treatment that are expected to be exacerbated by the use of systemic steroids, such as infective disease, hypertension or diabetes mellitus. After the first cycle of steroid half-pulse therapy, most of the depigmented macules became blurred and stopped expanding. After the third cycle of therapy, the depigmented lesions, particularly those on the cubital fossa and lower extremities, decreased in size (**Figure 1(a)**). No exacerbation or recurrence of the lesions were detected for 12 months after the three cycles of half-pulse therapy, and the patient felt good about clinical outcome in the series of half-pulse therapy treatments.

In this study, each lesion was compared using routine photographs of the whole body. Three of the five patients achieved disease arrest. One patient exhibited enlargement of the lesions, particularly on the lower extremities. As to adverse events, a slight increase in the white blood cell count and temporal insomnia were noted in three and two patients, respectively. The trend of delta L scores before and after treatment was significantly

**Table 1.** Patients' demographics and disease outcome.

| | Patient' characteristics | | | | | Disease outcome after intervention | | | | | | |
|---|---|---|---|---|---|---|---|---|---|---|---|---|
| Patient | Age (years) | Sex | Duration of disease (years) | Treatment history | Complications | Period of intervention | Disease arrest | Boarder blurring | Repigmentation | Assinged site | Adverse effect | Period of follow up |
| 1 | 68 | M | 20 | Topical corticosteroid vitamin D$_3$ | N.P. | Aug. to Mar. | No | No | No | Back of neck | N.P. | 1 year 4 months |
| 2 | 17 | M | 5 | Topical corticosteroid tacrolimus vitamin D$_3$ | N.P. | Aug. to Apr. | No | No | Follicular repigmentation but recurrented | Left forearm, right lower leg | N.P. | 1 year 4 months |
| 3 | 71 | F | 35 | Topical corticosteroid vitamin D$_3$ oral corticosteroid | Sjögren's syndrome | Dec. to Mar. | Yes | Yes | Peripheral repigmentation | Each cheek, fprehead | Temporal insomnia | 1 year 3 months |
| 4 | 71 | M | 2 | Topical corticosteroid vitamin D$_3$ UV | N.P. | Nov. to Jan. | Yes | Yes | Peripheral repigmentation | Left lower abdomen, left lower leg | Temporal insomnia | 1 year 4 months |
| 5 | 64 | F | 4 | Topical corticosteroid UV | N.P. | Apr. to Jan. | Yes | Excellent | Peripheral repigmentation | Back of neck, anterior chest | Temporal insomnia | 2 year 3 month |

N.P.: not particular.

separated between the patients with and without disease arrest (**Figure 1(b)**). Once the a score tended to increase in all patients after study, maybe reflecting on steroid-induced telangiectasia, each p-value of the a or b score was not significant (**Figure 1(c)**; the b scores not shown).

## 4. Discussion

Short term intravenous steroid half-pulse therapy was applied in five progressive nonsegmental vitiligo patients refractory to other treatments, and disease arrest and/or slurred lesions were observed in three of the five patients. It is very important to inhibit disease progression in cases of nonsegmental vitiligo in the progressive stage because, once they develop, vitiligo lesions are difficult to cure. Although we were unable to measure the exact percentage of lesions with repigmentation in the patients with lesion obscureness, the outcomes were highly valued by the patients due to the remarkable improvement in their appearance. No severe adverse events were observed for at least six months after the initial treatment, except for temporary insomnia. In the present study, there was high number of lesions in which the border was notably altered to be more obscure; therefore, most patients reported being satisfied with the treatment outcomes.

The efficacy of short-term systemic steroid therapy is supported by growing evidence as well as the results of the present study and previous publications [3]-[9]. Seiter *et al.* applied treatment with 8 mg/kg body weight of steroids three times for three consecutive days, similar to our regimen, and observed a rate of repigmentation of 71% among patients with progressive vitiligo, whereas no improvements were noted in those with stable vitiligo [6]. In contrast, a long-term oral steroid regimen comprising the administration of 10 mg of dexamethasone for two days followed by five days off for 24 weeks has also been found to be effective for achieving disease arrest, although mild to moderate side effects were reported in 69% of patients [4]. In addition, combination therapy consisting of high-dose intravenous prednisolone and PUVA has been shown to be highly effective in treating patients with generalized vitiligo [9]. It is conceivable that short-term treatment induces less frequent and milder adverse events than the long-term administration of steroid.

We used a spectrophotometer to measure the color changes determined according to the Lab score before and after the administration of steroid therapy. The device was useful to calculate the white contrast when we compared therapeutic effect between narrowband UVB and sun irradiation in addition to topical tacalcitol [10]. The delta L score exhibited a tendency to decrease after treatment in the patients who achieved disease arrest not disease progression or recurrence, as expected. However, sun exposure on measurement and seasonal changes both of which can affect the scores should be considered to prevent data deviation and variation.

Corticosteroids are known to enhance melanogenesis in an endogenous and/or exogenous manner [11] [12]. In murine melanoma cell lines, diethylstilbestrol induces melanin synthesis via the activation of the cAMP-PKA signaling pathway followed by the upregulation of tyrosinase and MITF [11]. In general, corticosteroids bind to

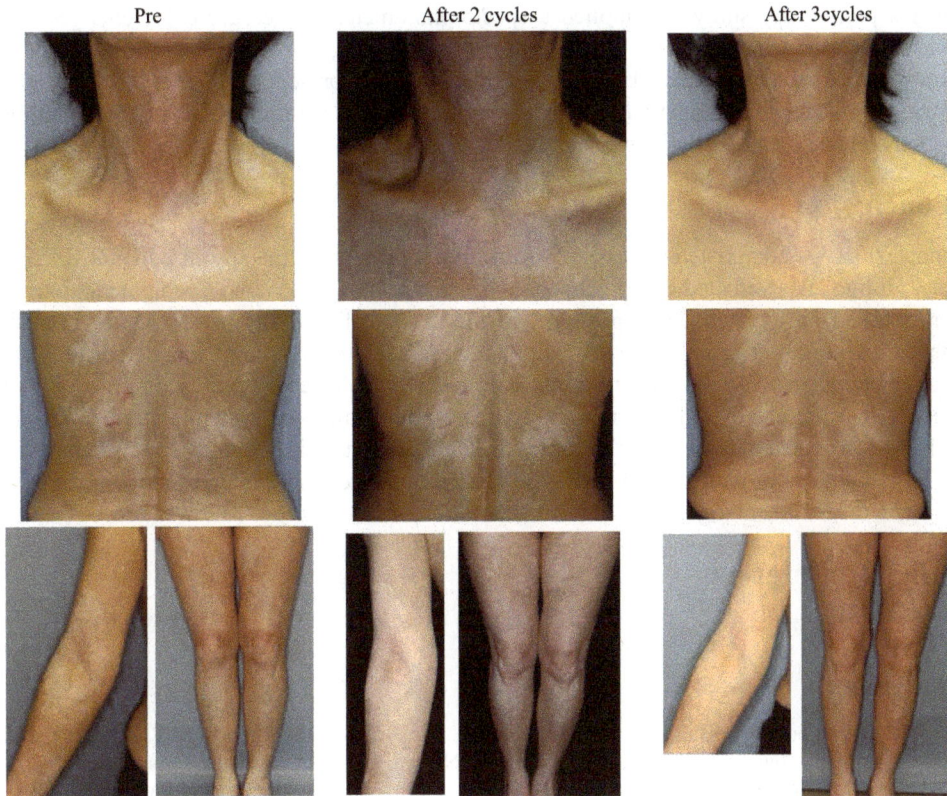

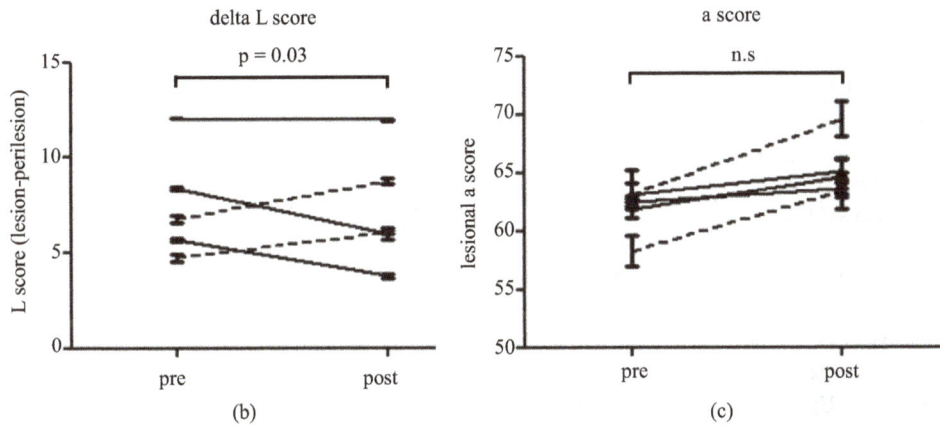

**Figure 1.** (a) Clinical appearance of a representative case before (left) and after 2 (middle) and 3 cycles (right) of half-pulse therapy. The views of front neck, middle back, and extremities are placed on upper, middle, and lower panels, respectively; (b) The change of delta L score before and after treatment was compared between the patients with and without disease arrest. The score change on lesions with and without disease arrest are shown by a solid and dotty lines, respectively. Notably, decrease in delta L score was more evident in patients with disease arrest, indicating that the change of delta L score reflected on therapeutic response; (c) The change of a score before and after treatment was compared between patients with and without disease arrest.

their receptors, thus forming a homodimer, and move into the nucleus where they upregulate the expression of MITF and downregulate the expression of inflammatory cytokines, such as IL-1, 2, 6 and TNF-$\alpha$ transcription factors [12]. A decreased cytokine expression can inhibit lymphocyte infiltration in the skin. In view of physiological effects of corticosteroids on melanogenesis and inflammation, it is believed that systemic corticosteroid therapy is valuable for treating vitiligo patients without complete melanocyte loss.

In this preliminary study, we applied a spectrophotometer to measure color changes and quantify the improvements in the vitiligo lesions. However, the L and delta L scores did not significantly decrease, even in the patients with diffuse repigmentation, as described in the representative case. The side effects of short-term treatment were minimal compared to that of long-term, low-dose oral steroids, which can induce osteoporosis, hypertension and increased carbohydrate tolerance.

## 5. Conclusion

In conclusion, we administered the short-term mini-pulse steroid therapy in patients with progressive nonsegmental vitiligo and evaluated the effectiveness of this regimen in achieving repigmentation and improving color contrast based on both ocular inspection and the results of a spectrometer. More than 50% of the patients achieved disease arrest and obscureness, with a high social value on the final appearance. The delta L score is an objective parameter of lesion whiteness and improvements in disease severity. In view of current stratified data, including that presented in the current study, the administration of systemic steroids instead of phototherapy should be considered in patients with progressive nonsegmental vitiligo in early stage. Further controlled studies with large numbers of patients and variety in the treatment regimen are needed to establish the proper position and line in the treatment algorithm for this disease.

## Conflicts of Interest

None.

## References

[1]  Taieb, A., Alomar, A., Bohm, M., Dell'Anna, M.L., De Pase, A., Eleftheriadou, V., Ezzedine, K., Gauthier, Y., Gawkrodger, D.J., Jouary, T., Leone, G., Moretti, S., Nieuweboer-Krobotova, L., Olsson, M.J., Parsad, D., Passeron, T., Tanew, A., van der Veen, W., van Geel, N., Whitton, M., Wolkerstorfer, A. and Picardo, M. (2013) Guidelines for the Management of Vitiligo: The European Dermatology Forum Consensus. *British Journal of Dermatology*, **168**, 5-19. http://dx.doi.org/10.1111/j.1365-2133.2012.11197.x

[2]  Oiso, N., Suzuki, T., Wataya-Kaneda, M., Tanemura, A., Tanioka, M., Fujimoto, T., Fukai, K., Kawakami, T., Tsukamoto, K., Yamaguchi, Y., Sano, S., Mitsuhashi, Y., Nishigori, C., Morita, A., Nakagawa, H., Mizoguchi, M. and Katayama, I. (2013) Guidelines for the Diagnosis and Treatment of Vitiligo in Japan. *Journal of Dermatology*, **40**, 1-11. http://dx.doi.org/10.1111/1346-8138.12099

[3]  Radakovic-Fijan, S., Fürnsinn-Friedl, A.M., Hönigsmann, H. and Tanew, A. (2001) Oral Dexamethasone Pulse Treatment for Vitiligo. *Journal of American Academy of Dermatology*, **44**, 814-817. http://dx.doi.org/10.1067/mjd.2001.113475

[4]  Kim, S.M., Lee, H.S. and Hann, S.K. (1999) The Efficacy of Low-Dose Oral Corticosteroids in the Treatment of Vitiligo Patients. *International Journal of Dermatology*, **38**, 546-550. http://dx.doi.org/10.1046/j.1365-4362.1999.00623.x

[5]  Pasricha, J.S. and Khaitan, B.K. (1993) Oral Mini-Pulse Therapy with Betamethasone in Vitiligo Patients Having Extensive or Fast-Spreading Disease. *International Journal of Dermatology*, **32**, 753-757. http://dx.doi.org/10.1111/j.1365-4362.1993.tb02754.x

[6]  Seiter, S., Ugurel, S., Tilgen, W. and Reinhold, U. (2000) Use of High-Dose Methylprednisolone Pulse Therapy in Patients with Progressive and Stable Vitiligo. *International Journal of Dermatology*, **39**, 624-627. http://dx.doi.org/10.1046/j.1365-4362.2000.00006.x

[7]  Hertz, K.C., Gazze, L.A., Kirkpatrick, C.H. and Katz, S.I. (1977) Autoimmune Vitiligo: Detection of Antibodies to Melanin-Producing Cells. *New England Journal of Medicine*, **297**, 634-637. http://dx.doi.org/10.1056/NEJM197709222971204

[8]  Barret, D.F. and Lee, H.A. (1982) Corticosteroid Pulse Therapy in Dermatology. *British Journal of Dermatology*, **107**, 31.

[9]  Lee, Y., Seo, Y.J., Lee, J.H. and Park, J.K. (2007) High-Dose Prednisolone and Psoralen Ultraviolet A Combination Therapy in 36 Patients with Vitiligo. *Clinical and Experimental Dermatology*, **32**, 499-501. http://dx.doi.org/10.1111/j.1365-2230.2007.02387.x

[10] Tanemura, A., Takahashi, A., Ueki, Y., Murota, H., Yamaguchi, Y. and Katayama, I. (2012) Therapeutic Comparison between Sun Irradiation vs. Narrowband UVB Phototherapy along with Topical Tacalcitol for Vitiligo Vulgaris. *Journal of Cosmetics, Dermatological Sciences and Applications*, **2**, 88-91. http://dx.doi.org/10.4236/jcdsa.2012.22020

[11] Jian, D., Jiang, D., Su, J., Chen, W., Hu, X., Kuang, Y., Xie, H., Li, J. and Chen, X. (2011) Diethylstilbestrol Enhances

Melanogenesis via cAMP-PKA-Mediating Up-Regulation of Tyrosinase and MITF in Mouse B16 Melanoma Cells. *Steroids*, **76**, 1297-1304. http://dx.doi.org/10.1016/j.steroids.2011.06.008

[12] Birlea, S.A., Costin, G.E. and Norris, D.A. (2009) New Insights on Therapy with Vitamin D Analogs Targeting the Intracellular Pathways That Control Repigmentation in Human Vitiligo. *Medicinal Research Reviews*, **29**, 514-546. http://dx.doi.org/10.1002/med.20146

# 17

# Isolation of Anti Ageing Molecules Secreted by Human Gingival Stem Cells. Protection of Collagen and Elastic Networks

**Hafida Chérifi**[1,2,3,4], **Adrien Naveau**[1,2,3,4], **Ludwig Loison Robert**[1,2,3,4], **Bruno Gogly**[1,2,3,4]

[1]Dental Department, A. Chenevier-H. Mondor Hospital, Créteil, France
[2]UMR S872, Université Paris Descartes, Sorbonne Paris Cité, France
[3]UMR S872, Centre de Recherche des Cordeliers, Université Pierre et Marie Curie, Paris, France
[4]INSERM U872, Paris, France
Email: bruno.gogly@ach.aphp.fr

## Abstract

Skin aging results in an imbalance between synthesis and degradation of the extracellular matrix. Overproduction of degradative enzymes (MMPs) and oxygen free radicals during chronological and photo-induced aging leads a degradation of the network and elastic skin collagen. Our previous work demonstrated that a culture supernatant of gingival stem cells had anti-aging activities *in vitro*, *ex vivo* and *in vivo* in humans. However, this culture medium is very complex and currently not responding to the European cosmetics regulation. After the analysis of the culture medium we have isolated 4 molecules interesting in terms of skin anti-aging activity: TIMP1, Selenium, Folic Acid and Glycin (TSAG). After the study of the most efficiency concentration of each molecule, the composition of TSAG is tested on irradiated UVA human dermal fibroblast and human skin. TSAG preserves the elastin and collagen network and inhibits the MMP1, MMP3 and MMP9 activities. The advantage of this mimetic solution of stem cells is to be stable, easily reproducible and non-human origin. The outlook for cosmetology seems interesting.

## Keywords

Human Gingival Stem Cell, MMPs, Collagen, Elastin

## 1. Introduction

Skin aging is associated with an increase in the number and depth of wrinkles as a result of the degradation of macromolecules of the dermis with collagen and elastin. In the dermis, the overproduction of MMPs that is involved in chronological aging and induces by solar radiation is stimulated by the overproduction of oxygen free radicals [1]. This is particularly true in the sun-exposed areas, such as facial skin; where the deleterious effects of ultraviolet radiation: collagen imperfect synthesis, skin pigmentation and solar elastolysis result in degradation of skin elastic network. Our previous work has shown that the culture supernatant of human gingival fibroblasts, that have exceptional healing capacity, inhibits the degradation of human skin subjected to UV exposure [2]. Since this publication in 2010 we have isolated a subpopulation of human gingival stem cells (hGSC) [3]. These cells are extensively studied and have very different perspectives in human cell therapy [4]. However, the culture supernatant of these cells is very complex and also has deleterious components for positive matrix remodeling including MMPs and pro-inflammatory cytokines. Currently, European regulations cosmetology no longer allows the use of products of human origin. The use of human products may cause contaminations. Moreover the composition of a cell culture supernatant may vary depending on the cell line. It seems interesting to realize that a combination of active product that is reproducible, stable and contains the most interesting of these supernatant molecules in terms of skin anti-aging activity. We therefore cultured human gingival fibroblasts and human gingival stem cells to study the composition of the culture media and observe any differences in the culture medium. After a careful analysis of the cell culture supernatant, four molecules found in the supernatant have a major activity in skin aging. These molecules are known for their antioxidant, anti-free radicals and anti MMPs. They stimulate the synthesis of macromolecules including collagen and elastin. These molecules are selenium, folic acid, glycin and the TIMP1. We found in our experiments the optimal concentrations of four molecules in terms of inhibition of MMP activity and protection of collagen and elastic networks. The active substance is a mixture of TIMP1, Selenium, Folic Acid and Glycin was called TSAG. TSAG product has been tested *in vitro* on skin fibroblasts and *ex vivo* human skin biopsies irradiated with ultraviolet A.

## 2. Material and Methods

### 2.1. *In Vitro* Experiences

#### 2.1.1. Obtaining Cells (hGF, hGSC and hDF)

Five Human gingival fibroblast (hGF) cultures were obtained from gingival explants of healthy patients with no periodontitis history. Five Human dermal fibroblast (hDF) cultures were obtained from skin biopsies of normal subjects after aesthetic or reconstructive surgery (the same biopsies as those used for organotypic studies). All patients (20 - 30 years old) gave their informed consent according to the Helsinki Declaration (1975) and denied having recently taken drugs that could affect connective tissue metabolism. The tissue samples were divided into two parts: one for a histologic analysis and the other for a cell culture. The serial gum tissue sections were stained with hematoxylin and eosin for assessing of the tissue quality and the absence of inflammatory infiltrates in the gingiva. Only the histological healthy tissue was used for experiments.

The primary cultures were established in 25 cm$^2$ culture flasks from explants and used from passage 3 to 5. The monolayer cultures were maintained during 3 weeks in Dulbecco's modified Eagle's medium (DMEM, Invitrogen-Life Technologies, Cergy Pontoise, France) with Knock-Out Serum Replacement (SFm, Serum Free medium) (KOSR, Invitrogen-Life Technologies) at 37°C in a 5% $CO_2$ and 95% $O_2$ atmosphere. The Serum-free medium (SFm) developed in our study consisted of DMEM supplemented with 20% KOSR. The SFm was optimized with 1 mM L-Glutamine and 1% non-essential amino acids. The SFm required supplementation with basic Fibroblast Growth Factor (b-FGF, 1 ng/mL, human recombinant; Invitrogen-Life Technologies) for long term culture, and insulin (5 μg/mL, human recombinant; Invitrogen-Life Technologies) for facilitating cell cycle progression [5].

The cell culture medium was changed every 72 hours. After the first passage, cells were routinely maintained either in SFM.

#### 2.1.2. Obtention and Characterization of HGSC Are Largely Described in Our Publication [3]

In short, after two weeks, the gingival fibroblasts were trypsinised and single cell suspension were seeded at very low concentration (concentration ≤ 100 cellules/cm$^2$; medium DMEM 10% of FCS with 50 μg/mL of ascorbic acid) after having checked the absence of aggregates of cells to avoid false-positives. After 14 days of culture, the colony-forming units of fibroblasts (CFU-F) were counted under a microscope. Only aggregates of more than 50 cells are regarded as colonies. The CFU-F was then transferred and gathered into a 25 cm$^2$ flask and cultivated in DMEM 10% supplemented with 50 μg/mL of ascorbic acid. The characterization of the hGSC was confirmed by osteoblastic cellular differentiation carried out using specific media of induction. Differentiation in osteoblasts was induced in a medium DMEM including 10% FCS, 50 μg/mL of ascorbic acid, 100 nM dexamethasone and 20 mM $\beta$-glycerophosphate [3].

### 2.1.3. Preparation of hGF and hGSC Conditioned Medium (hGFm and hGSCm)

The culture medium from 75 cm$^2$ flasks of confluent hGF or hGSC cultures was discarded. 24 mL of SFm was then added and retrieved 24 hours later. The conditioned medium was then freezed at −80°C until analyse.

### 2.1.4. Analysis of hGFm and hGSCm

Analysis of cell culture supernatant is carried out by various medical laboratories using HPLC techniques, spectrometry, ELISA and biological techniques. The analysis can show the presence of four molecules that play a major role in skin aging: TIMP1, selenium, folic acid and glycine.

For to determine the concentration of TIMP1 of the future composition, a first series of experiments aimed for optimal inhibition of MMPs activity induced by UVA irradiation of human dermal fibroblasts (classical model of aging *in vitro* [2]).

### 2.1.5. Inhibition of MMPs Secreted by the Irradiated hDF (hDFi) by UVA—Preparation of hDF

Two 24-well plates (Nunc) of each culture were cultured with hDF from a 25 cm$^2$ flask. When confluence is reached (75 000 cells per well), hDF plate is irradiated with UVA 15 Joules/cm$^2$ (hDFi) [2], the second plate is used as a control to verify the absence of MMP-9 in the absence of irradiation. The culture media are changed after irradiation. In the hDFi cultures the following solutions are added: PBS only in 4 wells (500 μL per well), PBS 20 pg/mL TIMP1 in 4 wells (500 μL per well), PBS 80 pg/mL TIMP1 in 4 wells (500 μL per sinks), PBS 160 pg/mL TIMP1 in 4 wells (500 μL per well), PBS 320 pg/mL TIMP1 in 4 wells (500 μL per well). Culture media are then collected 24 hours later, aliquoted and stored at −80°C for analysis of MMPs.

The optimum concentration of TIMP1 is also determined (80 pg/mL) and the solution TSAG is prepared.

### 2.1.6. Preparation of the Active Solution TSAG: TIMP1/Selenium/Folic Acid/Glycine (TSAG)

After to have determined the optimum concentration of TIMP1, 3 other molecular solutions are added at the same concentration as they are secreted by the "embryo-like" cells: selenium (10 ng/mL), folic acid (4 μg/mL) and glycine (30 μg/mL) (**Table 1**).

### 2.1.7. Anti MMPs Activity of TSAG Solution on hDFi

hDFi 4 wells are grown 24 h with a solution of PBS + TSAG. After 24 hours the cell culture supernatant is analyzed.

### 2.1.8. Protein Analysis of Cellular Culture Media

MMP-1 (DMP100), MMP-3 (DMP300), MMP-9 (DMP900), TIMP-1 (DTM100), were analysed by ELISA (R&D Systems) according to the recommendations of the manufacturer.

The statistical analysis was made using Wilcoxon and Mann-Whitney tests. Please note that the isoforms of these molecules are much conserved between the various species: it enabled the use of human ELISA kits for a human supernatant immunodetection.

## 2.2. Organotypical *ex Vivo* Experiment

Five human skin biopsies cultures were obtained from normal subjects after aesthetic or reconstructive surgery. All biopsies were rinsed with a Hank's solution. Each of the five skins samples was split up into fragments of 5 mm with a trocar, each fragment was weighed and UVA-irradiated or not at 15 Joules/cm$^2$ (Si$_{15}$) and then cultivated in a collagen with or without TSAG for seven days.

In a 10 mL Erlenmeyer, 6 mL of serum free medium (SFm) or 6 mL of SFm containing TSAG (see the paragraph *in vitro* cellular experiments), 3.4 mL of rat type I collagen (Jacques Boy Institute, 2 mg/mL, ref: 207050257) and 600 μL filtered NaOH 0.1 N (to neutralize the acid collagen solution) were mixed. Then a skin fragment was deposited in the prepared solution and carefully homogenized with the solution. Lastly, the whole was placed in a 60 mm Petri dish and in an incubator at 37°C/5% CO$_2$.

**Table 1.** Composition of the supernatant of HGF and HGSC in culture. The concentrations are in mg/L.

| Components | Concentration (mg/L) | |
|---|---|---|
| Amino acids | hGFm | hGSCm |
| Glycine | 28 | 27 |
| L-arginine hydrochloride | 79 | 79 |
| L-cystine 2HCI | 56 | 55 |
| L-glutamine | 540 | 532 |
| L-histidine hydrochloride-$H_2O$ | 38 | 38 |
| L-isoleucine | 99 | 92 |
| L-leucine | 104 | 96 |
| L-lysine hydrochloride | 135 | 134 |
| L-methionine | 30 | 29 |
| L-phenylalanine | 64 | 58 |
| L-serine | 37 | 35 |
| L-threonine | 84 | 76 |
| L-tryptophan | 12 | 12 |
| L-tyrosine | 66 | 62 |
| L-valine | 94 | 90 |
| Vitamins | | |
| Choline chloride | 4 | 3,8 |
| D-calcium panthonetate | 4 | 3,8 |
| Folic acid | 4 | 4 |
| i-inositol | 7.2 | 7 |
| Niacinamide | 4 | 3,5 |
| Pyridoxine hydrochloride | 4 | 3,2 |
| Riboflavin | 0.4 | 0,3 |
| Thiamine hydrochloride | 4 | 3 |
| Inorganic salts | | |
| Calcium chloride ($CaCl_2$-$2H_2O$) | 260 | 245 |
| Ferric nitrate ($Fe(NO_3)_3$-$9H_2O$) | 0.1 | 0,1 |
| Magnesium sulfate ($MgSO_4$-$7H_2O$) | 192 | 187 |
| Potassium chloride (KCI) | 304 | 258 |
| Sodium bicarbonate ($NaHCO_3$) | 3204 | 2468 |
| Sodium chloride (NaCI) | 5279 | 4981 |
| Sodium phosphate monobasic ($NaH_2PO_4$-$2H_2O$) | 124 | 114 |
| Other components | | |
| D-glucose (dextrose) | 3900 | 3820 |
| Sodium pyruvate | 106 | 104 |
| MMP1 | $24 \times 10^{-6}$ | $17 \times 10^{-6}$ |
| MMP2 | $31 \times 10^{-6}$ | $24 \times 10^{-6}$ |
| MMP3 | $21 \times 10^{-6}$ | $17 \times 10^{-6}$ |
| TIMP1 | $86 \times 10^{-6}$ | $72 \times 10^{-6}$ |
| TIMP2 | $68 \times 10^{-6}$ | $64 \times 10^{-6}$ |
| IL1$\beta$ | $113 \times 10^{-6}$ | $94 \times 10^{-6}$ |
| IL4 | $321 \times 10^{-6}$ | $221 \times 10^{-6}$ |
| IL6 | $18 \times 10^{-6}$ | $18 \times 10^{-6}$ |
| TGF$\beta$ | $412 \times 10^{-6}$ | $370 \times 10^{-6}$ |
| Concentration of trace components | | |
| $Ag^+$ | 0.00009 | 0.00001 |
| $AI^{3+}$ | 0.0001 | 0.0001 |
| $Ba^{2+}$ | 0.001 | 0.0006 |
| $Cd^{2+}$ | 0.005 | 0.0004 |
| $Co^{2+}$ | 0.0005 | 0.0005 |
| $Cr^{3+}$ | 0.00004 | 0.00003 |
| $Ge^{4+}$ | 0.0005 | 0.00005 |
| $Se^{4+}$ | 0.007 | 0.0075 |
| $Br^{3+}$ | 0.00006 | 0.00004 |
| I | 0.0001 | 0.00009 |
| $Mn^{2+}$ | 0.00006 | 0.00006 |
| F | 0.002 | 0.0015 |
| $SI^{4+}$ | 0.02 | 0.003 |
| $V^{5+}$ | 0.00038 | 0.00038 |
| $Mo^{6+}$ | 0.0007 | 0.0007 |
| $NI^{2+}$ | 0.00003 | 0.000024 |
| $Rb^+$ | 0.0008 | 0.0006 |
| $Sn^{2+}$ | 0.00003 | 0.00002 |
| $Zr^{4+}$ | 0.0001 | 0.0001 |

Five control collagen lattices were cultivated without skin fragments, in order to test whether bioactive molecules within the collagen gel and the culture medium would contribute to the results.

The cultures were maintained for a week and analysed at day 1, 3 and 7. At each point of experimentation 3 mL of supernatant were collected and stored at −80°C for further analysis of the secreted proteins.

### Histological Analysis by Computerized Image Analysis

The skin biopsies (control at day 0) and their surrounding collagen lattices were collected at 7 days, rinsed with PBS 1× and fixed in Paraformaldehyde 4%/PBS during 48 hours. They were then dehydrated with alcohol 70%, then 95%, then 100% and finally in a toluene before a paraffin inclusion. Sections (7 μm) were stained using three different specific protocols.

Hemalun/eosin protocol: after rehydration, the sections were covered with hemalun during five minutes before using with tap water, then with eosin during 1 minute.

Sirius Red protocol (collagen network): after rehydration, the sections were covered with Sirius Red during 30 minutes. The quantification of collagen density was performed within 2 steps. Firstable, the color image was transformed into monochrome with a 255 level gray scale. Thereafter, we evaluated the relative number of pixels classified as red by adjusting the threshold permitting a binary analysis. The measurements were performed in three independent fields by slide.

Orcein protocol (elastin network): after partial rehydration (stopped with alcohol 95%), the sections were immersed into an orcein solution during half an hour. A fast rinsing with alcohol 95% (with 2 hydrochloric acid drops added) was then carried out. Slides were lastly rinsed with distilled water before dehydratation and final assembling. The elastin density was quantified similarly as the collagen density.

## 3. Results

1) Isolation and characterization of HGSC (**Figure 1**)

For each of the five cultures of gingival fibroblasts we isolated by the limiting dilution technique cell clones (**Figure 1(a)**). To verify that these clones were well made of HGSC we have oriented towards a pathway of osteoblast differentiation. We then proceeded to staining by Alizarin Red the bone material secreted by the osteoblasts (**Figure 1(b)**) [3]. The HGSC isolated and characterized were cultured in the same manner that hGF which they are derived.

2) Analysis and hGFm hGSCm (**Table 1**) (TSAG isolated molecules)

Culture media of 5 hGF are mixed to achieve an average products secretion of five cellular cultures. A similar operation is performed with the 5 cultures of hGSC. Analysis of culture media of hGF and hGSC show little differences in composition. This first experiment shows that there are no significant differences between the secretions and hGF hGSC. For the following experiments hGSCm only are used.

3) Determination of the concentration of TIMP1 of TSAG on hDFi cultures: anti-metalloproteases activities (**Figure 2**)

After the hDF irradiation amount of MMP1 and MMP3 secreted by the cells are multiplied by 6 (respectively

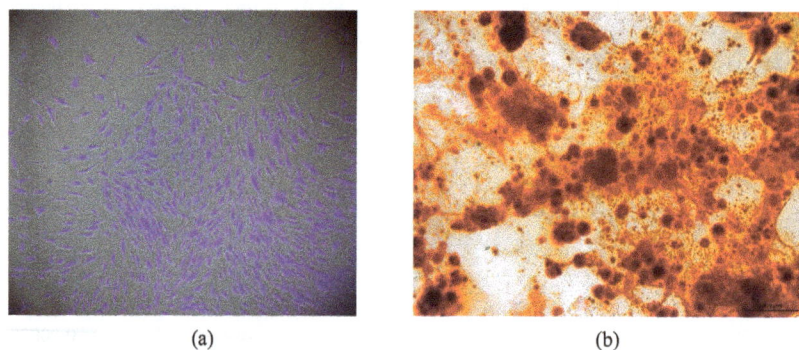

(a)  (b)

**Figure 1.** Isolation and characterization of hGSC. (a) Colony forming at low density of hGSC. The stem cells are colored with Trypan blue. (b) The osteogenic differentiation is characterized by the secretion of extra cellular mineral matrix colored with Alizarin red.

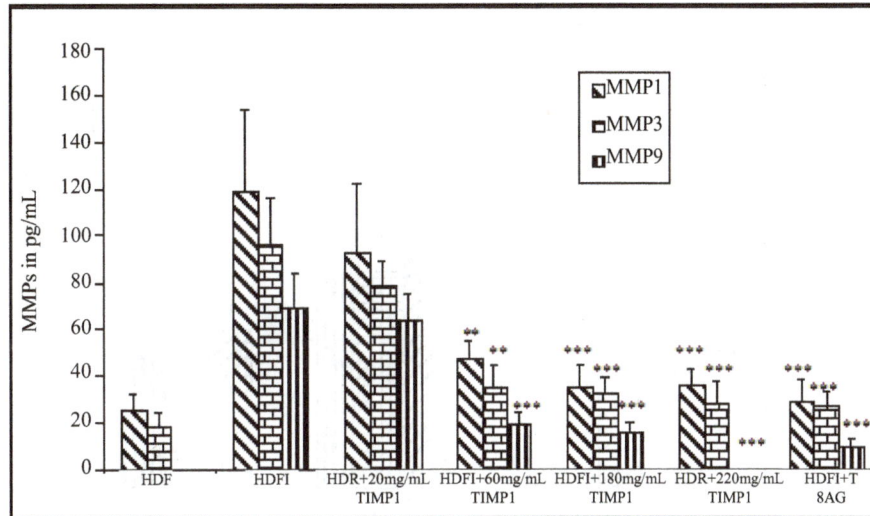

**Figure 2.** Determination of the optimal concentration of TIMP1 (80 mg/mL) for inhibition of MMPs secreted by the irradiated hDF (hDFi) by UVA. Effect of the composition of TSAG on hDFi.

25 and 18 to 119 pg/mL and 96 pg/mL). The hDF cultures do not secrete MMP9, while after irradiation; the concentration of MMP9 is 69 pg/mL. The addition of 20 pg/mL of TIMP1 in the culture medium of irradiated cells allows a non significant reduction of MMP activity. At 80 pg/mL, TIMP1 induces a significant reduction of the activity of MMP1 (119 to 47 pg/mL, $p < 0.05$), of MMP3 (96 to 35 pg/mL, $p < 0.01$) and of MMP9 (69 to 19 pg/mL, $p < 0.01$). A 160 pg/mL, TIMP1 inhibition of MMP activity is very similar to 80 pg/mL. A TIMP1 320 pg/mL of inhibition of the activity of MMP1 and MMP3 is the same as the concentration of 80 pg/mL and MMP9 activity becomes undetectable like to the cultures of unirradiated skin cells. The concentration of 80 pg/mL of TIMP1 is the most effective on the activity of MMPs. This concentration of TIMP1 is used for the composition of the active product TSAG. The 3 others molecules are added at the same concentration as they are secreted by the "embryo-like" cells hGCS: selenium (10 ng/mL), folic acid (4 µg/mL) and glycine (30 µg/mL). The product composition TSAG is thus determined. On irradiated cells, TSAG composition greatly reduces the activity of MMP-1 (119 to 41 pg/mL), MMP3 (96 to 34 pg/mL) and MMP9 (69 to 12 pg/mL) and statistically highly significant ($p < 0.01$).

4) Effect of TSAG on the activity of MMP-1, 3, 9 secreted by irradiated human skin (**Figure 3**)

The solution inhibits TSAG the activity of MMPs secreted by human skin biopsies irradiated with UVA. After 48 hours of cultures, MMP1 activity decreases by 35% ($p < 0.01$), that of MMP3 by 42% ($p < 0.05$) and MMP9 activity decreases by 52% ($p < 0.01$).

5) Protection of the elastic an collagen network by TSAG on irradiated human skin (**Figure 4**)

After 7 days of culture, the solution TSAG limits the degradation of the elastic and collagen networks of the irradiated skin. However, this observed inhibition does not completely inhibit the effect of the irradiation. Thus the loss of the elastic network of the irradiated skin was 58% compared to the control and only 17% in the presence of TSAG (**Figure 4(a)**). In a comparable manner, the loss of collagen network of the irradiated skin was 33% compared to the control and only 9% in the presence of TSAG (**Figure 4(b)**).

## 4. Discussion

Our previous work demonstrated that a culture supernatant of neurectodermic stem cells had anti-aging activities *in vitro*, *ex vivo* and *in vivo* in humans: preservation of elastic networks collagen and inhibiting the activity of MMP's responsible for the degradation of the dermal extracellular matrix. However, this culture medium is very complex and currently not responding to the European cosmetics regulation, which prohibits the use of products of human origin. It seems that interesting to make a composition that is reproducible and that reproduces the molecules of this supernatant the most interesting in terms of skin anti-aging activity. 4 molecules found in the culture medium are known for their antioxidant effects, anti-free radical, anti MMPs and enter the synthesis of

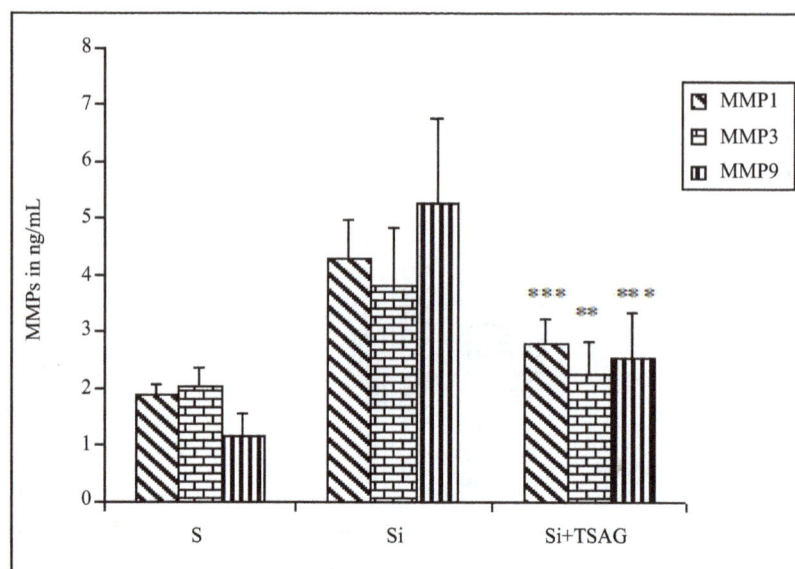

**Figure 3.** Evaluation of the anti MMPs activity of TSAG on human skin irradiated in organotypic cultures.

macromolecules including collagen and elastin: the TIMP1, selenium, and folic acid Glycine (TSAG). We therefore performed a molecular composition of these 4 products by determining the optimal concentration of each. TSAG product thus prepared showed skin anti-aging activities of particular interest. Each component of TSAG is individually known as active cosmetic product. The originality of this work is to combine these components whose concentrations are similar to those produced by human stem cells and thus achieve a stable, reproducible active composition and meet regulatory requirements.

The TMP1 is the tissue inhibitor of key enzymes responsible for the destruction of the dermal extracellular matrix including MMP1, MMP3 and MMP9 [6]. These three enzymes are involved in the degradation of collagen, elastin, proteoglycans and glycoproteins. These enzymes are overexpressed by dermal fibroblasts under UV stimulation and oxygen free radicals [7]. Many substances which inhibit MMPs are currently used against skin aging. They help to inhibit the degradation of the extracellular matrix induced by the sun and oxygen free radicals. The TIMP1, an inhibitor of these enzymes is a natural protector of the skin extracellular matrix.

Selenium is found in trace amounts in the body, where it belongs to the family of trace elements. By 1969, many epidemiological studies have demonstrated the preventive action of selenium in cancer development. As such, the selenium is not an antioxidant: in fact it is unable to interact with activated oxygen species (AOS) as are vitamins C and E and beta-carotene. Selenium is an essential micronutrient required for at least two types of enzymes involved in defence against oxidative stress [8] [9]. These enzymes, glutathione peroxidase and thioredoxin reductase, are an important part of the cell's defences against oxidative stress and are essential to maintaining a stable redox balance. In enzymes, selenium is present as selenocysteine [10]. The selenium has a protective effect against the damage induced by UV whose cytotoxicity [11] [12] the oxidation of the DNA, the expression of interleukin 10 [13] and lipid peroxidation [14]. Oral intake of sodium selenite protects against UV-induced erythema in mice against the appearance of skin pigmentation [15] and the development of skin cancers [16] [17]. His skin anti-aging effect is related is its powerful indirect antioxidant effect [18] [19]. Its use in cosmetology appears to be very promising.

Folic acid is a vitamin that belongs to the group of vitamin B. This water soluble vitamin is also known as vitamin B9, vitamin M or folacin rarely. Remember that the human body is unable to synthesize vitamins and therefore they must be supplied through diet or supplementation. As a precursor to methionin (essential amino acid which the body can not synthesize), folic acid plays a role in the synthesis of DNA and RNA and thus in cell renewal. The role of folic acid is essential when a cell in the body requires a rapid renewal (blood cells, stomach, intestine, mouth, skin). Topical application of folic acid significantly improves the *in vivo* skin firmness. *In vitro*, the secretion of collagen by dermal fibroblasts is stimulated by acid folic, suggesting that the *in vivo* anti-wrinkle effects are based on the stimulation of collagen metabolism [20].

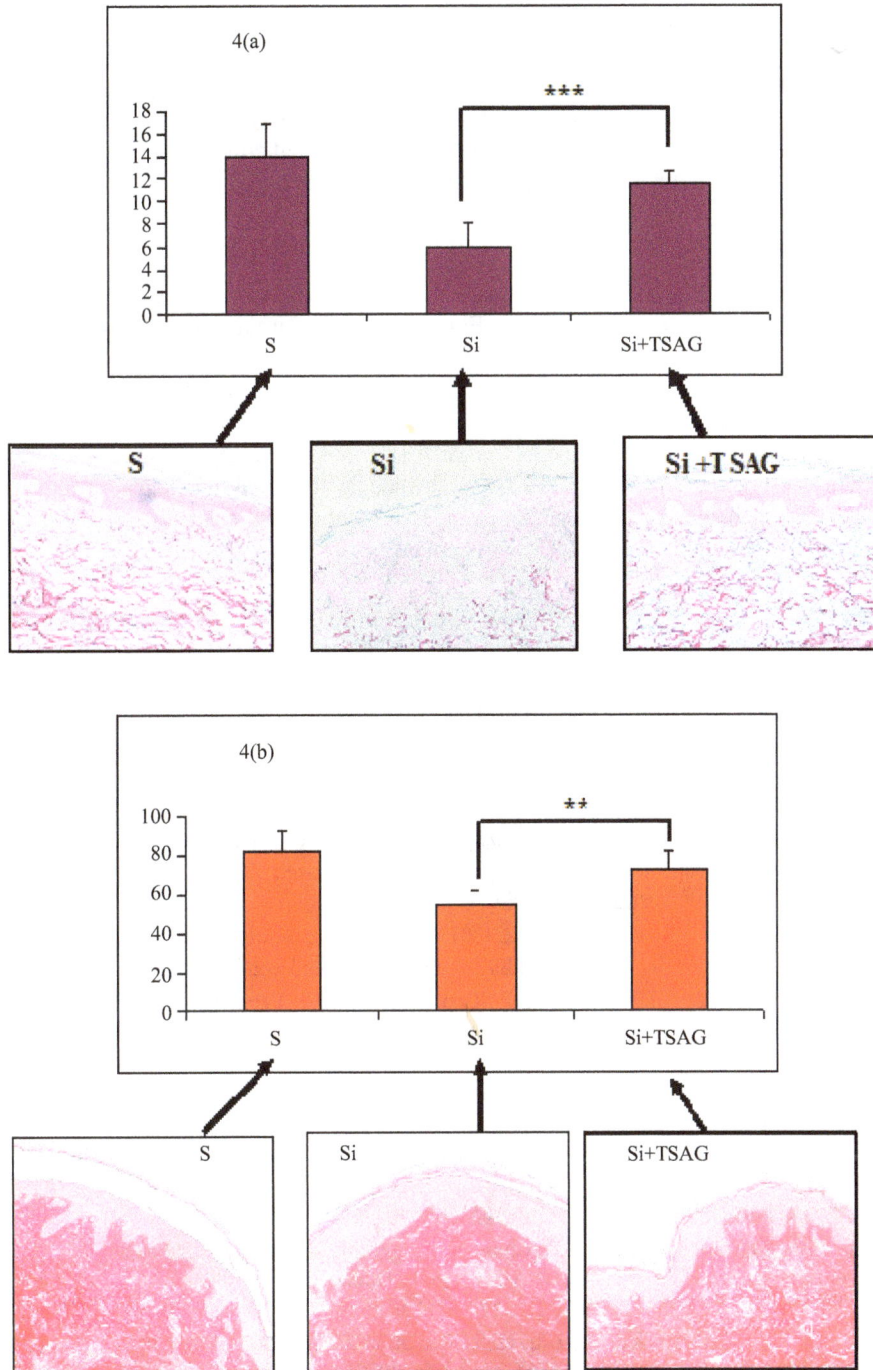

**Figure 4.** Evaluation of the protective effect of the elastic and collagen networks by TSAG in irradiated human skin in organotypical culture.

Glycine, formerly called glycine or amino acetic acid, is a non-essential amino acid α said because it can be produced by the body from other amino acids. This is the simplest amino acid and represents more than 30% of the amino acids used in the formation of fibrillar collagens including collagen I, collagen main skin. Collagen I is composed of a sequence of amino acid triplet Gly-X-Y, and its synthesis is essential for skin repair. Degradation is major in the phenomena of aging and is responsible for the appearance of wrinkles [2] [21]. Glycine is also the main constituent of elastin with prolin. Collagen and elastin are essential to maintaining the mechanical properties of the skin and target molecules are many anti aging assets.

The originality of this research is associated 4 molecules of skin network in a new molecular composition whose concentrations are those secretions from stem cells in culture. The molecular composition is perfectly reproducible and does not have the disadvantages of a variable cell secretion and which contains many deleterious molecules skin (inflammatory cytokines, proteolytic enzymes, possible contamination). The composition TSAG shows *in vitro* and *ex vivo* a major protective effect of elastic and collagen network and inhibits the enzymes responsible for the degradation of the entire dermal extracellular matrix.

## 5. Conclusion

In the first study published in 2011, we showed that the supernatant of cultures of gingival stem cells exhibited anti-aging activity in humans. Currently the European regulation on cosmetic products prohibits the use of human origin substances. We have studied the composition of the culture supernatant to determine the molecules responsible for the anti-aging activity. Four molecules which were widely used in cosmetics are present in the culture medium. We therefore carried out a solution with precise concentrations of these four molecules and tested this solution on human skin models *in vitro* and *ex vivo*. It appears that this composition called TSAG outperforms the supernatant of stem cells from our models of skin aging. The advantage of the solution is to be stable, easily reproducible and non-human origin. The outlook for cosmetology seems interesting and will be evaluated on an anti wrinkle 6-month study in humans.

## References

[1]    Rafferty, T.S., Green, M.H., Lowe, J.E., Arlett, C., Hunter, J.A., Beckett, G.J. and McKenzie, R.C. (2003) Effects of Selenium Compounds on Induction of DNA Damage by Broadband Ultraviolet Radiation in Human Keratinocytes. *British Journal of Dermatology*, **148**, 1001-1009. http://dx.doi.org/10.1046/j.1365-2133.2003.05267.x

[2]    Gogly, B., Ferré, F., Cherifi, H., Naveau, A. and Fournier, B. (2011) Inhibition of Elastin and Collagen Networks Degradation in Human Skin by Gingival Fibroblast. *In Vitro, ex Vivo* and *in Vivo* Studies. *Journal of Cosmetics, Dermatological Sciences and Applications*, **1**, 4-14.

[3]    Fournier, B., Ferré, F., Couty, L., Lataillade, J.J., Gourven, M., Naveau, A., Coulom, B., Lafont, A. and Gogly, B. (2010) Multipotent Progenitor Cells in Gingival Connective Tissue. *Tissue Engineering Part A*, **16**, 2891-2899. http://dx.doi.org/10.1089/ten.tea.2009.0796

[4]    Fournier, B., Larjava, H. and Hakkinen, L. (2013) Gingiva as a Source of Stem Cells with Therapeutic Potential. *Stem Cells and Development*, **22**, 3157-3177. http://dx.doi.org/10.1089/scd.2013.0015

[5]    Naveau, A., Lataillade, J.J., Fournier, B.P., Couty, L., Prat, M., Ferré, F.C., Gourven, M., Durand, E., Coulomb, B., Lafont, A. and Gogly, B. (2010) Phenotypic Study of Human Gingival Fibroblasts in a Medium Enriched with Platelet Lysate. *Journal of Periodontology*, **82**, 632-641. http://dx.doi.org/10.1902/jop.2010.100179

[6]    Hornebeck, W. (2003) Down-Regulation of Tissue Inhibitor of Matrix Metalloprotease-1 (TIMP-1) in Aged Human Skin Contributes to Matrix Degradation and Impaired Cell Growth and Survival. *Pathologie Biologie*, **51**, 569-573. http://dx.doi.org/10.1016/j.patbio.2003.09.003

[7]    Rittié, L. and Fisher, G.J. (2002) UV-Light-Induced Signal Cascades and Skin Aging. *Ageing Research Reviews*, **1**, 705-720. http://dx.doi.org/10.1016/S1568-1637(02)00024-7

[8]    Emonet-Piccardi, N., Richard, M.J., Ravanat, J.L., Signorini, N., Cadet, J. and Béani, J.C. (1998) Protective Effects of Antioxidants against UVA-Induced DNA Damage in Human Skin Fibroblasts in Culture. *Free Radical Research*, **29**, 307-313. http://dx.doi.org/10.1080/10715769800300341

[9]    McKenzie, R.C. (2000) Selenium, Ultraviolet Radiation and the Skin. *Clinical and Experimental Dermatology*, **25**, 631-636. http://dx.doi.org/10.1046/j.1365-2230.2000.00725.x

[10]   Stadtman, T.C. (2000) Selenium Biochemistry. Mammalian Selenoenzymes. *Annals of the New York Academy of Sciences*, **899**, 399-402. http://dx.doi.org/10.1111/j.1749-6632.2000.tb06203.x

[11]   Emonet, N., Leccia, M.T., Favier, A., Beani, J.C. and Richard, M.J. (1997) Thiols and Selenium: Protective Effect on Human Skin Fibroblasts Exposed to UVA Radiation. *Journal of Photochemistry and Photobiology B*, **40**, 84-90. http://dx.doi.org/10.1016/S1011-1344(97)00041-9

[12]   Rafferty, T.S., McKenzie, R.C., Hunter, J.A., Howie, A.F., Arthur, J.R., Nicol, F. and Beckett, G.J. (1998) Differential Expression of Selenoproteins by Human Skin Cells and Protection by Selenium from UVB-Radiation-Induced Cell Death. *Biochemical Journal*, **332**, 231-236.

[13]   Rafferty, T.S., Walker, C., Hunter, J.A., Beckett, G.J. and McKenzie, R.C. (2002) Inhibition of Ultraviolet B Radiation-Induced Interleukin 10 Expression in Murine Keratinocytes Byselenium Compounds. *British Journal of Dermato-*

*logy*, **146**, 485-489. http://dx.doi.org/10.1046/j.1365-2133.2002.04586.x

[14] Moysan, A., Morlière, P., Marquis, I., Richard, A. and Dubertret, L. (1995) Effects of Selenium on UVA-Induced Lipid Peroxidation in Cultured Human Skin Fibroblasts. *Skin Pharmacology and Physiology*, **8**, 139-148. http://dx.doi.org/10.1159/000211337

[15] Thorling, E.B., Overvad, K. and Bjerring, P. (1983) Oral Selenium Inhibits Skin Reactions to UV Light in Hairless Mice. *Acta Pathologica et Microbiologica Scandinavica A*, **91**, 81-83.

[16] Overvad, K. (1998) Selenium and Cancer. *Bibliotheca Nutritio et Dieta*, **54**, 141-149.

[17] Reid, M.E., Duffield-Lillico, A.J., Slate, E., Natarajan, N., Turnbull, B., Jacobs, E., Combs Jr., G.F., Alberts, D.S., Clark, L.C. and Marshall, J.R. (2008) The Nutritional Prevention of Cancer: 400 mcg per Day Selenium Treatment. *Nutrition and Cancer*, **60**, 155-163. http://dx.doi.org/10.1080/01635580701684856

[18] Pinnell, S.R. (2003) Cutaneous Photodamage, Oxidative Stress, and Topical Antioxidant Protection. *Journal of the American Academy of Dermatology*, **48**, 1-19. http://dx.doi.org/10.1067/mjd.2003.16

[19] Puizina-Ivić, N., Mirić, L., Carija, A., Karlica, D. and Marasović, D. (2010) Modern Approach to Topical Treatment of Aging Skin. *Collegium Antropologicum*, **34**, 1145-1153.

[20] Fischer, F., Achterberg, V., März, A., Puschmann, S., Rahn, C.D., Lutz, V., Krüger, A., Schwengler, H., Jaspers, S., Koop, U., Blatt, T., Wenck, H. and Gallinat, S. (2011) Folic Acid and Creatine Improve the Firmness of Human Skin *in Vivo*. *Journal of Cosmetic Dermatology*, **10**, 15-23. http://dx.doi.org/10.1111/j.1473-2165.2010.00543.x

[21] Pickart, L. (2008) The Human Tri-Peptide GHK and Tissue Remodeling. *Journal of Biomaterials Science, Polymer Edition*, **19**, 969-988. http://dx.doi.org/10.1163/156856208784909435

# 18

# Evaluation of Self-Treatment of Acne Using Silk'n Blue Phototherapy System

Judith Hellman*, Cielo A. Ramirez

Mt. Sinai Hospital, New York, USA
Email: *jhderm@gmail.com

## Abstract

**Background: At-home phototherapy devices for the treatment of acne have emerged as an appealing treatment option and as an effective adjunct treatment to existing modalities. The principal goal of the study was to determine the changes in the number of inflammatory lesions in acne patients. Methods: Patients received instruction for daily at-home use of Silk'n Blue device for 12 weeks. Follow-up visits were conducted at 1 and 3 months to collect data. Results: Fifteen subjects with mild to severe cases experienced improvement over the course of the trial. The decrease in mean inflammatory acne counts (from 41.26 to 24.46) and mean percent reduction (41.8%) were statistically significant ($p < 0.001$). Some participants experienced percent reductions as great as 67%. No adverse events were recorded. Conclusions: The Silk'n Blue device is a safe and effective modality for at-home treatment of mild, moderate, and severe inflammatory acne vulgaris with proper use.**

## Keywords

**Acne, Blue Light Therapy, LED Phototherapy**

## 1. Introduction

Acne vulgaris affects 80% - 90% of people during their adolescence, and half continue to experience symptoms into adulthood [1]-[3]. The condition is moderate-to-severe in 15% - 20% of people in their late teens [4]. It is characterized by noninflammatory open or closed comedones, and by inflammatory papules, pustules, and cysts. Secondary scarring may also result. The disfigurement caused by severe acne and acne scars can have negative psychological and psychosocial effects [5]. These include stigmatization from peers, lower self-esteem, interpersonal difficulties, anxiety, depression, and higher unemployment rates [6].

---

*Corresponding author.

The treatment of acne is directed towards four known pathogenic factors. These are the plugging of the follicle, excess sebum production, the presence and activity of the bacteria *Propionibacterium acnes* (*P. acnes*), and inflammation of the skin [7]. Existing pharmacotherapeutic options are topical comedolytics, topical and systemic antibiotics, hormonal manipulations, and oral retinoids. Procedural treatments include manual extraction of comedones, intralesional steroid injections, and superficial glycolic or salicylic acid peels.

Despite a wide variety of treatment options, there is a growing demand among both patients and practitioners for fast, safe, and side-effect-free interventions [8]. Various forms of phototherapy with visible light have been shown to be effective in the treatment of acne vulgaris [9]. Treatments using light within the blue range have been found to be particularly effective in the selective destruction of *P. acnes* bacterium. The bacteria produce and store endogenous porphyrins, absorbing light energy at the near-UV and blue light spectrum [9]. Absorption of the appropriate wavelength of light energy causes the creation of a highly reactive free radical species leading to the destruction of the bacterial cell wall [10]. Infrared laser light selectively targets the dermal layer where sebaceous glands are located [8]. The heat from the absorbed energy creates thermal injury and alters the structure of the sebaceous glands. Reduction in size of sebaceous glands and sebum output also results in acne improvement.

The objective of this open-label study was to evaluate the safety, efficacy, and usage compliance of the FDA-approved Silk'n Blue system for the self-treatment of mild to severe acne. The primary goal of the study was to determine the changes in the number of inflammatory lesions.

## 2. Materials and Methods

### 2.1. Study Design

This study was a 12-week, open-label, prospective cohort study carried out in New York, NY, USA between June and October 2013. Patients were instructed to treat themselves at home daily for 12 weeks. Follow-up visits to evaluate the results were scheduled at 1 and 3 months following the last treatment. Each patient served as its own control by comparing the acne count at base-line to the follow-up results.

During the first visit, each patient received verbal instruction of treatment guidelines and was instructed on how to turn on the Silk'n Blue device and to hold the applicator against the skin. Patients were to hold the Blue applicator on the skin without moving the device for 3 minutes on a section of the affected area, repeating until the entire affected area had been treated. Treatment time could be increased to 5 minutes as tolerated per actively treated area.

Inflammatory lesion counts were conducted at baseline, at 1 month, and at 3 months, using individual lesion counts of the entire face, ranging from hairline to jawline. Standardized digital photographs were taken at all three visits. A subject questionnaire on response to treatment and discomfort was completed at each follow-up visit.

### 2.2. Subjects

Written informed consent was obtained from all subjects prior to enrollment. Fifteen participants aged 17 - 31 years with Fitzpatrick skin types I-VI (12 women and 3 men) were enrolled. Mild acne was graded as the presence of a small number of inflammatory papules. Moderate acne was graded as a greater number of papules, pustules, and some inflammatory cysts. Severe acne was characterized by a greater number of papules, pustules, and inflammatory cysts, as well as the presence of inflamed acne scars.

The inclusion criterion for participants was the presence of persistent inflammatory acne. Patients were allowed to continue using prescribed topical acne treatments. Participants were required to refrain from using systemic oral treatments or undergoing laser treatments during this period of time or the 6 months preceding participation in this clinical trial.

### 2.3. Light Source

The Silk'n Blue (Home Skinovations, Yokneam, Israel) is a rechargeable hand-held device for patient-controlled application of blue light therapy and an infrared heating. An array of 24 LEDs produces blue-violet light of wavelengths in the 405 - 460 nm range. The light is emitted in a uniform distribution to avoid hot spots. A proximity sensor causes the lights to turn on only with skin contact to the light head. The device features a temperature sensor that turns the device off when the skin temperature reaches 41°C to prevent overheating of the skin.

## 2.4. Statistics

One-tailed student's t tests were used to determine the statistical significance for a non-normal distribution with large variation.

# 3. Results

## 3.1. Acne Counts

Inflammatory lesion counts were significantly reduced by blue light LED treatments after one month of treatment (41.7% reduction, from a mean of 40.26 to 26.33, $p < 0.001$) (see **Figure 1(a)** and **Figure 1(b)**). The greatest decrease occurred during the first month, and this significant improvement was sustained over the course of the study. At 3 months, the mean percent reduction from baseline was 41.8% (from a mean of 41.26 to 24.46, $p < 0.001$). Representative clinical photographs are shown in **Figure 2(a)** and **Figure 2(b)**.

At 3 months, fourteen of the fifteen participants showed a decrease in total lesions from baseline. Two participants experienced percent reductions in inflammatory lesions of 61% and 67%. Eleven patients experienced further improvement after the first month of treatment. Three participants experienced an increased lesion count after the first month, and one patient returned to baseline results at 3 months. These results demonstrate short-term efficacy in the reduction of lesions for all participants and a long-term maintenance of improved outcomes for the majority of patients with continued use.

## 3.2. Patient Subjective Assessment

The subjective surveys elicited some important information. Two participants of Fitzpatrick skin type IV experienced slight pain and tenderness for 10 - 15 minutes after treatments. In both cases, these symptoms subsided after one week of continued use. Eight subjects reported that they "liked" the device and found it to be effective. Four subjects said that they "loved" the treatment system and expressed a commitment to continued use. Only one participant did not see noticeable improvement and stopped consistent use of the device after breaking out during the fourth week of the trial. Four participants expressed some difficulty in maintaining a consistent schedule, but reported that they were overall pleased with the results.

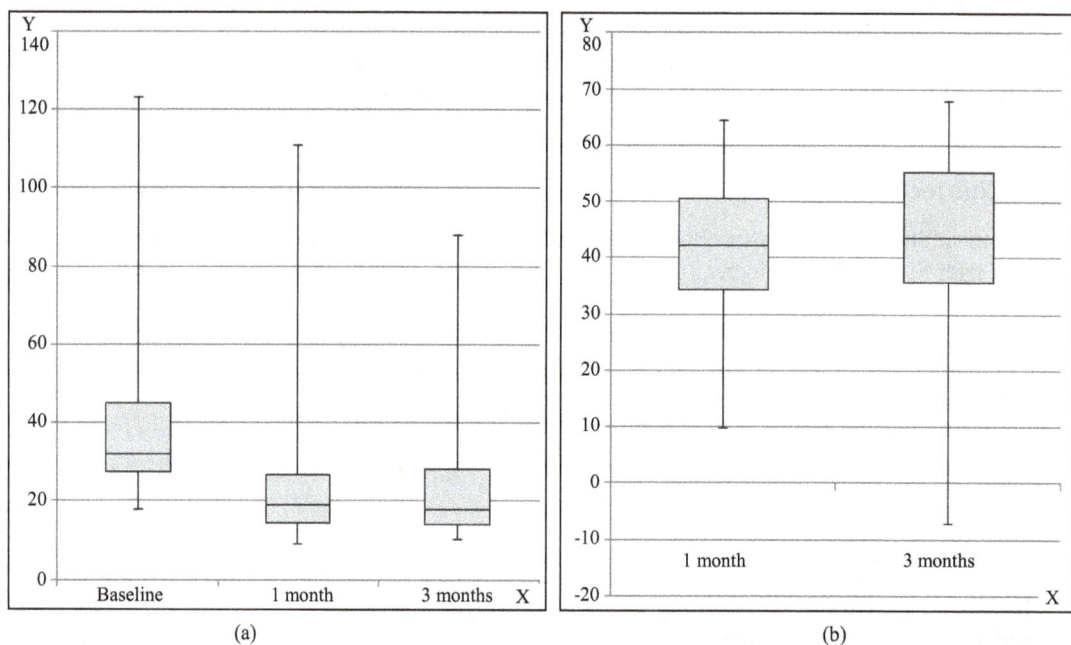

**Figure 1.** (a) Inflammatory acne lesion counts; (b) Percent improvement in lesion count. X = time, Y = lesion count (a); % improvement (b).

**Clinical Photographs**

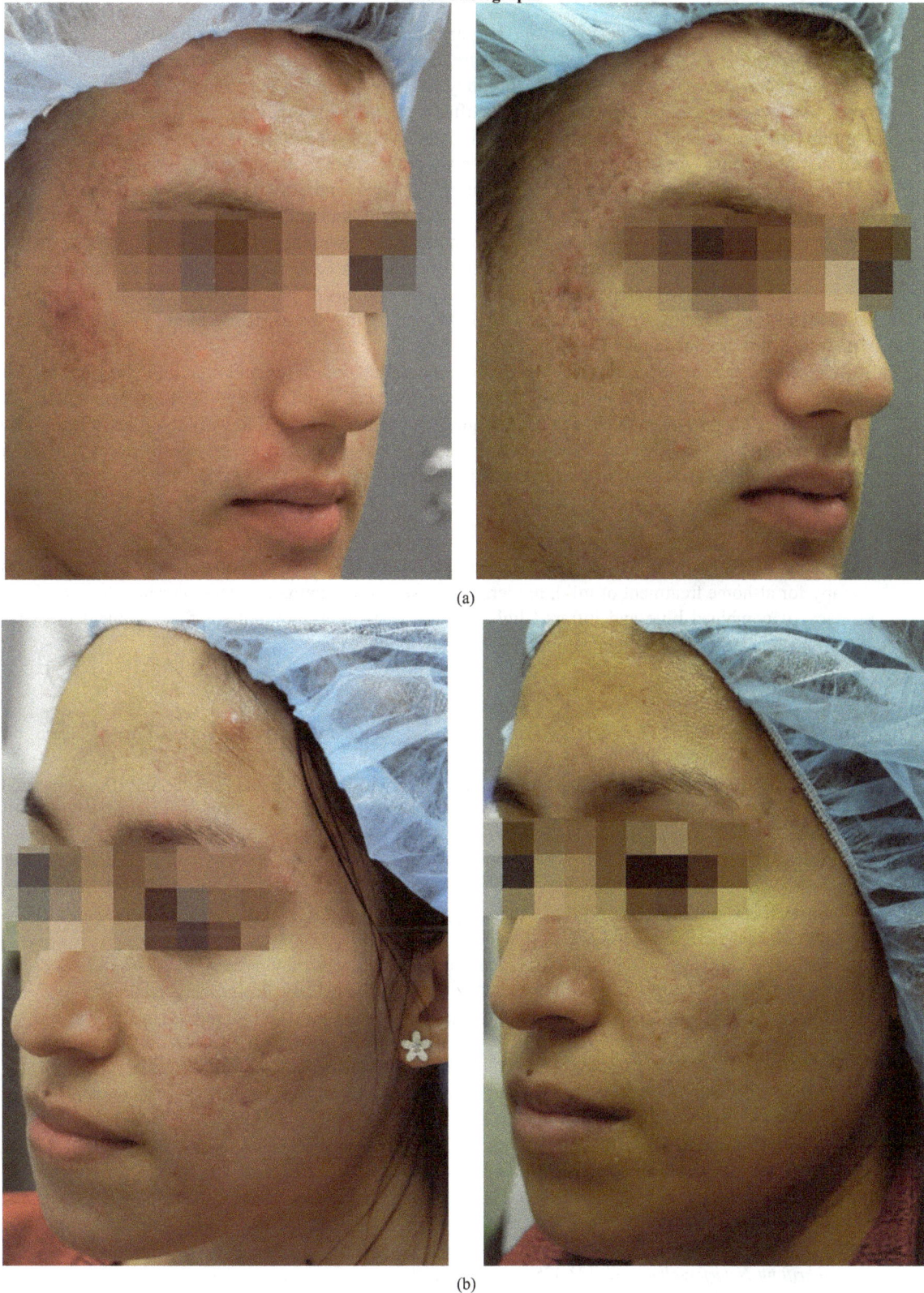

(a)

(b)

**Figure 2.** (a) Male, 19 yo, Fitzpatrick skin type II. Left: baseline, right: 3 months follow-up; (b) Female, 24 yo, Fitzpatrick skin type IV. Left: baseline, right: 3 months follow-up.

## 4. Discussion

Inflammatory lesions counts decreased for all participants during the first month. The majority of participants were significantly satisfied with their overall trend towards clearer skin. They found that they were able to maintain and improve upon the progress that they had made into the third month of treatment. Four of the 15 participants experienced an increase in lesions after 4 weeks, which may be explained by a decrease in novelty and motivation to uphold usage compliance as directed. Nearly all patients stated that integrating the Silk'n Blue treatment system into their daily routine had been a worthy use of their time and efforts.

This is the second open-label study investigating the safety and efficacy of the Silk'n Blue device [11]. This trial evaluated the device's at-home efficacy in reducing inflammatory lesion counts for a sample group with greater variation in acne severity. The similarity in results between these two trials indicates that the Silk'n Blue system is suitable for patients who may prefer self-treatment or have decreased access to regular in-office treatments. The results of the present study support previous findings of blue and infrared light therapy as a suitable stand-alone treatment for Acne vulgaris. This light therapy may be as, if not more, effective in combined use with modalities that only a doctor can provide a patient.

Related studies have found that devices that use a combination of red and blue light are similarly effective in decreasing the amount of *P. acnes* and inflammation in treated skin [12]. Red light can penetrate to the level of the sebaceous glands and may have anti-inflammatory properties related to cytokine release from macrophages [9]. A comparative study between the effectiveness of blue light therapy versus combination blue-red light therapy is our recommendation for further research in this field.

## 5. Conclusion

The results of this study suggest that the Silk'n Blue device may be a safe and effective blue and infrared light therapy for at-home treatment of mild, moderate, and severe inflammatory acne. Further study of the safety and efficacy of combined blue and infrared light therapy systems is required for the treatment of different acne symptoms in a larger set of patients with longer follow-up periods.

## References

[1]   Yentzer, B.A., Hick, J., Reese, E.L., Uhas, A., Feldman, S.R. and Balkrishnan, R. (2010) Acne Vulgaris in the United States: A Descriptive Epidemiology. *Cutis*, **86**, 94-99.

[2]   Law, M.P., Chuh, A.A., Lee, A. and Molinari, N. (2010) Acne Prevalence and Beyond: Acne Disability and Its Predictive Factors among Chinese Late Adolescents in Hong Kong. *Clinical and Experimental Dermatology*, **35**, 16-21. http://dx.doi.org/10.1111/j.1365-2230.2009.03340.x

[3]   Yahya, H. (2009) Acne Vulgaris in Nigerian Adolescents—Prevalence, Severity, Beliefs, Perceptions, and Practices. *International Journal of Dermatology*, **48**, 498-505. http://dx.doi.org/10.1111/j.1365-4632.2009.03922.x

[4]   Bhate, K. and Williams, H.C. (2013) Epidemiology of Acne Vulgaris. *British Journal of Dermatology*, **168**, 474-485. http://dx.doi.org/10.1111/bjd.12149

[5]   Niemeier, V., Kupfer, J. and Gieler, U. (2006) Acne Vulgaris—Psychosomatic Aspects. *Journal der Deutschen Dermatologischen Gesellschaft*, **4**, 1027-1036. http://dx.doi.org/10.1111/j.1610-0387.2006.06110.x

[6]   Mulder, M.M., Sigurdsson, V., van Zuuren, E.J., Klaassen, E.J., Faber, J.A., de Wit, J.B. and van Vloten, W.A. (2001) Psychosocial Impact of Acne Vulgaris. Evaluation of the Relation between a Change in Clinical Acne Severity and Psychosocial State. *Dermatology*, **203**, 124-130. http://dx.doi.org/10.1159/000051726

[7]   Harper, J.C. (2004) An Update on the Pathogenesis and Management of Acne Vulgaris. *Journal of the American Academy of Dermatology*, **51**, S36-S38. http://dx.doi.org/10.1016/j.jaad.2004.01.023

[8]   Elman, M. and Lebzelter, J. (2004) Light Therapy in the Treatment of Acne Vulgaris. *Dermatologic Surgery*, **30**, 139-146. http://dx.doi.org/10.1111/j.1524-4725.2004.30053.x

[9]   Rai, R. and Natarajan, K. (2013) Laser and Light Based Treatments of Acne. *Indian Journal of Dermatology, Venerology, and Leprology*, **79**, 300-309. http://dx.doi.org/10.4103/0378-6323.110755

[10]  Melo, T.B. (1987) Uptake of Protoporphyrin and Violet Light Photodestruction of Propionibacterium Acnes. *Zeitschrift für Naturforschung*, **42**, 123-128.

[11]  Gold, M.H., Biron, J.A. and Sensing, W. (2013) Clinical and Usability Study to Determine the Safety and Efficacy of the Silk'n Blue Device for the Treatment of Mild to Moderate Inflammatory Acne Vulgaris. *Journal of Cosmetic and Laser Therapy*. http://dx.doi.org/10.3109/14764172.2013.854638

[12] Kwon, H.H., Lee, J.B., Yoon, J.Y., Park, S.Y., Ryu, H.H., Park, B.M., Kim, Y.J. and Suh, D.H. (2013) The Clinical and Histological Effect of Home-Use, Combination Blue-Red LED Phototherapy for Mild-to-Moderate Acne Vulgaris in Korean Patients: A Double-Blind, Randomized Controlled Trial. *British Journal of Dermatology*, **168**, 1088-1094. http://dx.doi.org/10.1111/bjd.12186

# 19

# Umbrella with Ultraviolet Radiation Protection

Kasama Vejakupta, Montree Udompataikul

Skin Centre, Srinakarinwirot University, Bangkok, Thailand
Email: iweevy@gmail.com

## Abstract

Background: Ultraviolet radiation (UVR) causes harm to the eye and skin in human. There are many ways to protect one from UVR. Umbrella is widely used due to its convenience as well as its ability to protect one from rain. However, there are limited numbers of studies on UVR protection of different types of umbrellas. Objective of study: To determine UVR protection efficacy of different umbrella designs. Methods: The experimental study was performed on five sunny days. Six manikins were placed in an open area, five of which were equipped with five different types of black canopy umbrellas. One manikin was placed without an umbrella as a control sample. Polysulfone film badges were attached in six different areas in each manikin for measuring the UVR from 10 am - 3 pm Results: All types of umbrellas provides 64.5% - 92.3% UVR photo protection efficacy. An umbrella with UV-filter coating on the inner surface provides maximum UVR photo protection efficacy. However, UVR proto protection efficacies of an umbrella with UV-filter coating on the inner surface and one with UV-filter coating on the outer surface and one without UV-filter coating are not statistically significant (p-value = 0.37). Umbrellas with a diameter of 122 cm and 152 cm provide comparable UVR photo protection efficacy while an umbrella with a diameter of 112 cm provides the least UVR photo protection efficacy. However, UVR photo protection efficacies of umbrellas with different diameter are not statistically significant (p-value = 0.36). The area of the body that received the most UVR photo protection is the forehead which is statistically significant when compared with other areas of the body (p-value < 0.001). The areas of the body that received the least UVR photo protection are the left ear and the back of the neck, which are statistically significant when compared with other areas of the body (p-value < 0.001). Conclusion: All types of umbrellas provide UVR photo protection efficacy. The study shows that umbrellas with different canvas material including both the UV-filter coating and different diameter of umbrellas could effectively protect the user from UVR without significant group difference in this study.

## Keywords

Umbrella, Ultraviolet, Protection, Filter Coating, Radius

# 1. Introduction

Ultraviolet radiation (UVR) is an electromagnetic wave [1] [2]. It is originated from the sun and travels to the surface of the Earth. While UVR is vital to human, it can also cause harm especially to the eye and skin such as burn, hyperpigmentation, photoaging skin, keratoconjunctivitis, stimulation of photodermatoses and cutaneous cancer [1]-[3]. For this reason, there are several ways to protect one from UVR [4] which can be categorized into two methods namely Chemical protection (Sunscreen) and Physical protection such as using hats [5], garments [6], sunglasses [7]. Umbrella is one of the ways to protect one from UVR [8] due to its convenience, availability as well as its ability to protect one from rain. Nevertheless, there are only few studies on UVR protection efficacy of different types of umbrellas [8]-[13] and no clear conclusions can be drawn.

# 2. Objective of Study

The objective of this study is to evaluate UVR photoprotection efficacies of umbrellas with different canvases (umbrellas with UVR-filter coating on the inner surface of the canvas, umbrellas with UVR-filter coating on the outer surface of the canvas and umbrellas with plain canvas) as well as umbrellas with different diameters (112 cm, 122 cm and 152 cm).

# 3. Methods

This study was an *in-vitro* experimental study. Five types of black umbrellas were selected—canopy umbrella with diameter of 122 cm and UV-filter coating on the inner surface of the canvas, canopy umbrella with diameter of 122 cm and UV-filter coating on the outer surface of the canvas, canopy umbrella with diameter of 122 cm without UV-filter coating on the canvas, canopy umbrella with diameter of 112 cm and UV-filter coating on the inner surface of the canvas, canopy umbrella with diameter of 152 cm and UV-filter coating on the inner surface of the canvas. Aluminium paste is used as UV-filter coating on the umbrella's canvas. All 5 umbrellas had exactly the same thickness and tightness of weave from the same company (Thai Ocean Industrial company limited). Each of the first five manikins was equipped with an umbrella and one manikin was placed without an umbrella. All six manikins were set facing north. The efficacy of UVR protection was measured by using Polysulfone film badges [14]. All Polysulfone film badges were standardized and UVR exposed film badges were sent to Manchester University, UK for readings of UVR exposure using CECIL CE292 Spectrophotometer and their readings were recorded in Standard Erythemal Dose unit (SED; 1 SED = 100 Joules/m$^2$). Six Polysulfone film badges were placed at various anatomical areas of each manikin; forehead, nose, left ear, right ear, occiput and the back of the neck (**Figure 1**). The experiment was performed in an open area of Srinakarinwirot University's arena (SWU), Bangkok, Thailand (Latitude 13.75, Longitude 100.57) during 10.00 am - 3.00 pm in five clear sky days in November, 2013.

UVR exposure data in Standard Erythemal Dose unit of Polysulfone film badges recorded in those five days were analyzed. Two analyses were performed.

## 3.1. Fundamental Analysis

Differences in UVR exposure were calculated against control sample data using the following formula:

$$\text{UVR different} = \text{UVR control} - \text{UVR umbrella} \tag{1}$$

UVR control = UVR exposure of control sample (manikin without an umbrella)
UVR umbrella = UVR exposure
UVR different = Amount of UVR protection (difference in UVR exposure)
UVR protection data were then calculated in percentage using the following formula:

$$\frac{\text{UVR different}}{\text{UVR control}} \times 100 \tag{2}$$

## 3.2. Statistical Analysis

Two groups of data were analyzed:
1) Compare UVR exposure of manikins under 122 cm diameter umbrellas with different types of canvas

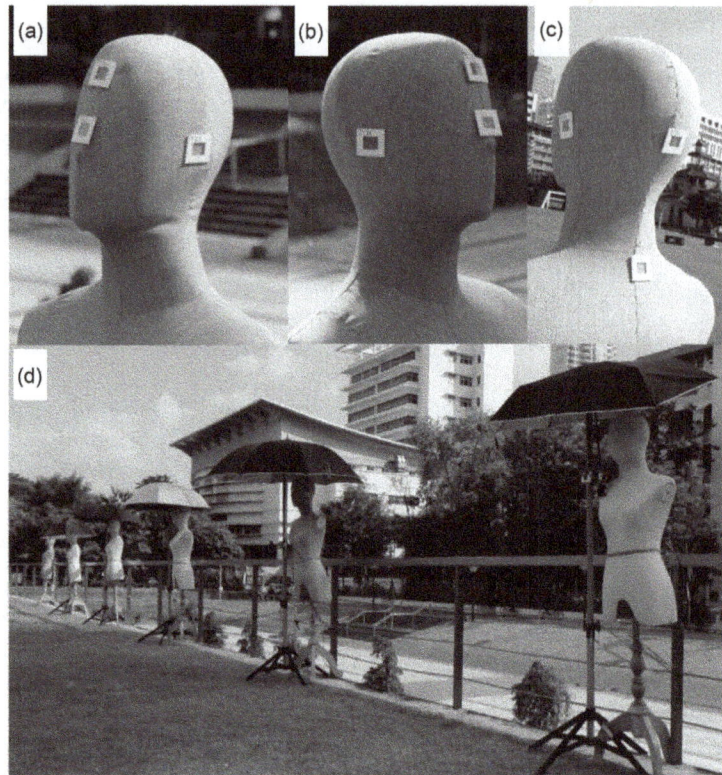

**Figure 1.** (a)-(c) showed the polysulfone film badges on the manikins; (d) showed all the manikins were set with umbrellas in the experiment.

materials (UV-filter coating on the inner surface of the canvas, UVR-filter coating on the outer surface of the canvas, and canvas with no UV-filter coating).

2) Compare UVR exposure of manikins under umbrellas with different radii (canopy umbrellas with UV-filter coating on the inner surface of the canvas with diameter of 112 cm, 122 cm and 152 cm)

With more than two groups of samples, ANOVA test and Bonferrini test were used.

## 4. Results

During the second day of the experiment, some of the manikins fell over. The amount of UVR exposure readings from these manikins significantly differed from other groups of samples. Therefore, results from the second day of the experiment were discarded and only data from four other days of experiments were used in the analysis.

Fundamental data analysis showed that average UVR exposure readings from four days of experiments were calculated (**Table 1**). Average UVR protection data (in percentage) from four days of experiments were also calculated (**Table 2**). The results showed that average UVR protection efficacies of all five umbrellas were in the range of 64.5% - 92.3%.

Statistical analysis showed that canopy umbrellas with UV-filter coating on the inner surface provided the most UVR photo protection efficacies (81.6%) but is statistically insignificant (p-value = 0.37) when compared with that of canopy umbrellas with UVR-filter coating on the outer surface (UVR photo protection efficacies of 77%) and that of canopy umbrellas without UV-filter coating (UVR photo protection efficacies of 76.5%) as shown in **Table 3**. In addition, canopy umbrellas with diameter of 122 and 152 cm provided UVR photo protection efficacies of 81.6% and 81.4% respectively while canopy umbrellas with radiii of 22 inches provided the least UVR photo protection efficacies (77.2%). However, UVR photo protection efficacies of canopy umbrellas with diameter of 112, 122 and 152 cm were statistically insignificant (p-value = 0.36) as shown in **Table 4**.

While umbrellas with different canvas types and their radii showed insignificant differences in UVR photo protection efficacies, data from **Table 2** were analyzed further to see how well different parts of the body are

**Table 1.** The fundamental data of the mean UVR values[a] of different areas and different types of umbrella.

|  | Control | 122 cm, UV-filter inner | 122 cm, No UV-filter | 122 cm, UV-filter outer | 112 cm, UV-filter inner | 152 cm, UV-filter inner |
|---|---|---|---|---|---|---|
| Forehead | 5.9 (0.3) | 0.5 (0.1) | 0.8 (0.8) | 0.6 (0.8) | 0.5 (0.1) | 0.5 (0.1) |
| Nose | 5.9 (0.6) | 0.5 (0.1) | 1.5 (1.1) | 0.8 (0.8) | 0.9 (0.4) | 0.7 (0.3) |
| Left ear | 2.7 (0.4) | 0.8 (0.1) | 0.9 (0.4) | 1.0 (0.5) | 1.0 (0.5) | 0.7 (0.1) |
| Right ear | 5.9 (0.5) | 0.8 (0.4) | 1.1 (0.4) | 1.1 (0.8) | 0.9 (0.4) | 1.0 (0.4) |
| Occiput | 6.0 (1.8) | 1.3 (0.5) | 1.4 (0.6) | 1.9 (1.4) | 1.7 (1.1) | 1.4 (0.6) |
| Upper back | 10.1 (0.8) | 2.9 (1.0) | 2.7 (1.4) | 3.0 (2.2) | 3.6 (1.7) | 2.6 (0.9) |

[a]Unit in Standard Erythemal Dose (SED; 1 SED = 100 Joules/metre$^2$).

**Table 2.** The UVR values and photoprotection efficacy of various types of umbrella on different anatomical sitestype styles.

|  |  | Control | 122 cm, UV-filter inner | 122 cm, No UV-filter | 122 cm, UV-filter outer | 112 cm, UV-filter inner | 152 cm, UV-filter inner |
|---|---|---|---|---|---|---|---|
| Forehead | Percent |  | 91.1 (1.0) | 86.5 (11.8) | 89.9 (11.7) | 91.0 (2.2) | 92.3 (1.9) |
|  | Different | 5.9 | 0.5 | 0.8 | 0.6 | 0.5 | 0.5 |
| Nose | Percent |  | 91.7 (1.7) | 75.1 (18.0) | 87.3 (11.9) | 85.6 (6.3) | 88.6 (4.1) |
|  | Different | 5.9 | 0.5 | 1.5 | 0.8 | 0.9 | 0.7 |
| Left ear | Percent |  | 69.6 (3.7) | 66.6 (11.7) | 64.5 (12.8) | 65.8 (15.4) | 72.7 (2.5) |
|  | Different | 2.7 | 0.8 | 0.9 | 1 | 1 | 0.7 |
| Right ear | Percent |  | 86.9 (6.2) | 81.3 (7.1) | 80.9 (12.9) | 84.1 (15.9) | 83.8 (6.5) |
|  | Different | 5.9 | 0.8 | 1.1 | 1.1 | 0.9 | 1 |
| Occiput | Percent |  | 78.0 (9.0) | 76.1 (10.2) | 70.1 (18.5) | 72.3 (15.4) | 76.9 (8.9) |
|  | Different | 6 | 1.3 | 1.4 | 1.9 | 1.7 | 1.4 |
| Upper back | Percent |  | 71.9 (8.4) | 73.2 (13.5) | 69.6 (23.1) | 64.2 (17.8) | 73.8 (10.1) |
|  | Different | 10.1 | 2.9 | 2.7 | 3 | 3.6 | 2.6 |

**Table 3.** It showed mean percentage of UVR protection in various canopy types.

| Canopy type (122 cm) | Mean (SD) | p-Value |
|---|---|---|
| Inner UV-filter | 81.6 (10.5) |  |
| No UV-filter | 76.5 (12.8) | 0.37 |
| Outer UV-filter | 77.0 (17.0) |  |

**Table 4.** It showed mean percentage of UVR protection in various diametres.

| Diameter (inner UV-filter) | Mean (SD) | p-Value |
|---|---|---|
| 112 cm | 77.2 (14.9) |  |
| 122 cm | 81.6 (10.5) | 0.36 |
| 152 cm | 81.4 (9.5) |  |

protected from UVR as shown in **Table 5**. It was found that differences in UVR photo protection for six different parts of the body are statistically significant. The results showed that the area of the body that received the most UVR photo protection is the forehead which is statistically significant when compared with other areas of the body (UVR photo protection efficacy of 90.2% with p-value <0.001). The areas of the body that received the least UVR photo protection are the left ear and the back of the neck, which are statistically significant when compared with other areas of the body (UVR photo protection efficacy of 67.8% with p-value <0.001 and UVR photo protection efficacy of 70.6% with p-value <0.001 respectively).

## 5. Discussion

Based on the results of this research, differences in UVR photo protection efficacies of umbrellas with different

**Table 5.** Showed mean percentage of UVR protection in various anatomical sites.

| Anatomical site | Mean (SD) | p-Value |
|---|---|---|
| Forehead | 90.2 (7.0) | |
| Nose | 80.7 (10.8) | |
| Left ear | 67.8 (9.8) | <0.001 |
| Right ear | 83.4 (7.6) | |
| Occiput | 74.6 (11.9) | |
| Upper back | 70.6 (14.2) | |
| Compare forehead with other sites | | |
| Forehead | 90.2 (7.0) | <0.001 |
| Other sites | 76.4 (12.9) | |
| Compare left ear with other sites | | |
| Left ear | 67.8 (9.8) | <0.001 |
| Other sites | 80.9 (12.7) | |
| Compare occiput with other sites | | |
| Occiput | 74.6 (11.9) | <0.001 |
| Other sites | 80.3 (12.4) | |

canvas types were statistically insignificant. It might be possible that black nylon canvas could effectively absorb UVR. Thus, additional UVR photo protection of umbrella canvas with UVR-filter coating was only marginal. That differences in UVR photo protection efficacies of umbrellas with diameter between 112 - 152 cm were statistically insignificant may be explained by the fact that Polysulfone film badges were placed at manikins near the center of the umbrella. More Polysulfone film badges placed further away from the center of the umbrella may give significantly different results. Umbrellas with wider range of diameter may also give significantly different results.

With regards to different areas where Polysulfone film badges were placed, the reason why the forehead received the most UVR photo protection might be for the fact that it is the closest to the center of the umbrella and to the umbrella canopy. However, the fact that the left ear received the least UVR photo protection might be for the fact that the manikins were facing slightly North-east, the left ears of all manikins were facing North-west and the experiments were conducted in November from 10 am - 3 pm when the sun was slightly towards the South, making the North-west less exposed to the sun light and all the center of the umbrellas were on the right side of manikin, making unequal angles on the umbrella and both ears. Therefore, the UVR exposure readings on the left ear were much lower than those in other areas of the manikins and resulted in low UVR protection efficacies. The fact that the back of the neck received significantly low UVR protection might be explained by additional UVR reflected from white canvases that were placed behind each manikin compared with UVR reflected from the yard at the front.

There are other factors that the researcher did not study due to some limitations such as Solar Zenith Angle which might affect UVR photo protection. This is because the fact that the duration of the experiments expanded over five hours resulted in different Solar Zenith Angle. Additional comparison on the ground, reflected UVR, colour of umbrella canvas, canvas materials and other different areas of the body, especially both cheeks, chin, shoulders and arms of the manikins might be helpful.

## 6. Conclusion

All types of umbrellas in this study provided UVR photo protection efficacy in the range of 64.5% - 92.3%. Canopy umbrellas with UVR-filter coating on the inner surface provided the most UVR photo protection efficacies. Canopy umbrellas with diameter of 122 and 152 cm provided the most UVR photo protection efficacies. However, differences in UVR photo protection efficacies of umbrellas with different canvas types and diameters are statistically insignificant. The area of the body that received the most UVR photo protection is the forehead which is statistically significant while the areas of the body that received the least UVR photo protection are the left ear and the back of the neck, which are statistically significant. Therefore, it can be included that the type of umbrella canvas and the radius of the umbrella are not significant factor in UVR photo protection efficacy and that the forehead receives the most protection from UVR. Additional means of UVR protection for the back of the neck should also be considered.

## Acknowledgements

This research paper is made possible through the help and support from everyone; please allow me to dedicate my acknowledgment of gratitude toward the following significant advisors and contributors:

First and foremost, I would like to thank Dr. Ann Webb and Dr. Richard Kift, University of Manchester, for the Polysulfone film badges.

Second, I would like to thank Dr. Sumaman Buntung, Silpakorn University, Thailand, for precious and valuable advice and Dr. Natta Rajatanavin for advice and recommendations for the experiments.

Third, I would like to thank Mr. Touchapong Taksinvarajarn and Miss. Chayaporn Vasinchatchawal, Medical students of SWU for helping with manikins/umbrellas setting and Vinzenta Company Limited for supporting the manikins.

Fourth, I would like to thank Mr. Petch Aekviriyavanich, my friend for valuable support me in English translation.

Finally, I sincerely thank to my parents, family, and friends, who provide the advice and financial support. The product of this research paper would not be possible without all of them.

## References

[1]     Kochevar, I.E., Taylor, C.R. and Krutmann, J. (2012) Fundamental of Cutaneous Photobiology and Photoimmunology. In: *Fitzpatrick's Dermatology in General Medicine*, The McGraw Hill Companies, New York, 1031-1048.

[2]     Rünger, T.M. (2012) Ultraviolet Light. In: *Dermatology*, Elsevier Limited, China, 1455-1465.

[3]     Vandergriff, T. and Bergstresser, P. (2012) Abnormal Response to Ultraviolet Radiation: Idiopathic, Problably Immunologic, and Photoexacerbated. In: *Fitzpatrick's Dermatology in General Medicine*, The McGraw Hill Companies, New York, 1049-1065.

[4]     Tuchinda, C., Srivannaboon, S. and Lim, H.W. (2006) Photoprotection by Window Glass, Automobile Glass and Sunglasses. *Journal of the American Academy of Dermatology*, **54**, 845-854. http://dx.doi.org/10.1016/j.jaad.2005.11.1082

[5]     Hatch, K.L. and Osterwalder, U. (2006) Garments as Solar Ultraviolet Radiation Screening Materials. *Dermatologic Clinics*, **24**, 85-100. http://dx.doi.org/10.1016/j.det.2005.09.005

[6]     Diffey, B.L. and Cheeseman, J. (1992) Sun Protection with Hats. *British Journal of Dermatology*, **127**, 10-12. http://dx.doi.org/10.1111/j.1365-2133.1992.tb14816.x

[7]     Cheng, S., Lian, S., Hao, Y., *et al.* (2010) Sun-Exposure Knowledge and Protection Behavior in a North Chinese Population: A Questionnaire-Based Study. *Photodermatology*, *Photoimmunology* & *Photomedicine*, **26**, 177-181. http://dx.doi.org/10.1111/j.1600-0781.2010.00513.x

[8]     McMichael, J.R., Veledar, E. and Chen, S.C. (2013) UV Radiation Protection by Handheld Umbrellas. *JAMA Dermatology*, **149**, 757-758.

[9]     Turnbull, D.J. and Parisi, A.V. (2003) Spectral UV in Public Shade Settings. *Photochemistry and Photobiology*, **69**, 13-19. http://dx.doi.org/10.1016/S1011-1344(02)00387-1

[10]    Turnbull, D.J. and Parisi, A.V. (2005) Increasing the Ultraviolet Protection Provided by Shade Structures. *Photochemistry and Photobiology*, **78**, 61-67. http://dx.doi.org/10.1016/j.jphotobiol.2004.09.002

[11]    Utrillas, M.P., Martinez-Lozano, J.A. and Nuñez, M. (2012) Ultraviolet Radiation Protection by Beach Umbrella. *Photochemistry and Photobiology*, **86**, 449-456. http://dx.doi.org/10.1111/j.1751-1097.2009.00677.x

[12]    Grifoni, D., Carreras, G., Sabatini, F. and Zipoli, G. (2005) UV Hazard on a Summer's Day under Mediterranean Conditions, and the Protective Role of a Beach Umbrella. *International Journal of Biometeorology*, **50**, 75-82. http://dx.doi.org/10.1007/s00484-005-0278-y

[13]    Diffey, B.L. (2002) Sources and Measurement of Ultraviolet. *Methods*, **28**, 4-13. http://dx.doi.org/10.1016/S1046-2023(02)00204-9

[14]    Sliney, D.H. (1995) UV Radiation Ocular Exposure Dosimetry. *Photochemistry and Photobiology*, **31**, 61-77.

# 20

# Nano-Patterning of Diffraction Gratings on Human Hair for Cosmetic Purposes

**Khawar Abbas[1], Drew F. Goettler[1], Bruce C. Lamartine[2], Zayd C. Leseman[1]**

[1]Mechanical Engineering Department, University of New Mexico, Albuquerque, USA
[2]Los Alamos National Laboratory, Los Alamos, USA
Email: zleseman@unm.edu

## Abstract

A method is presented for nano-patterning a diffraction grating on human hair with a focused ion beam. Strands of brown hair are patterned with hyperbolas and Archimedean spirals whose pitches range from 540 nm to 1040 nm. Exposure of the hair strands to white light at various incident angles demonstrates that light of varying wavelengths is diffracted by the diffraction gratings. The diffraction causes the brown strands of hair to reflect light from the entire range of visible light.

## Keywords

Diffraction, Hair, Nanopatterning, Focused Ion Beam Milling

## 1. Introduction

The practice of hair dying for cosmetic purposes has been around for several hundred years. Temporary hair dyes are applied on hair to change its appearance hiding graying hair or to stay in line with the latest fashion trends. Greeks and Romans used naturally occurring henna as a temporary hair dye while Arab authors described application of the paste formed by the mixture of PbO and slaked lime ($Ca(OH)_2$) in water on hair [1]. Presently there are numerous commercially available products that are used in highlighting hair strands for cosmetic purposes to brighten and/or create unnatural hair colors for Halloween, football games, etc.

Adverse effects of these synthetic hair dyes often range from skin discoloration and allergic irritations [2] to toxicity and cancer [3] [4]. In this paper we present a technique wherein nano-scale diffraction gratings are patterned on hair and could be used as an alternative to common hair dyeing treatments. Diffraction gratings do occur in nature for color generation [5] [6] and similar techniques are used in optics for color separation. We mimic and adapt nature's color generation/separation technique to human hair as an alternative to chemical dyes. A Focused Ion Beam (FIB) was used to mill nano-scale diffraction gratings on individual strands of brown human hair in order to artificially add color to the hair strands through interference of light. Optical and SEM images were collected to qualitatively and quantitatively examine the effects of nano-patterning of the hair with the FIB (nanoFIBrication). Nano-scale Archimedean spirals and hyperbola patterns are the patterns chosen for this work. Though the technique of writing individual patterns on individual hair strands is not practical for commercial applications, nano-pattern transfer by large area direct embossing of the hair strands, or by a similar embossing of a polymer deposited on the hair, is feasible [7]. Large area nano-pattern embossing is easily accomplished and may ultimately become an alternative for hair and fiber coloration because of attractive complex patterns. Furthermore the present use and disposal of chemical dyes would be avoided.

## 2. Focused Ion Beam Milling

Incident light normal to a diffraction grating will produce a diffraction profile that is governed by the grating equation [8].

$$a \sin \theta_n = n\lambda \qquad (1)$$

where $a$ is the pitch of the diffraction grating, $n$ is the $n^{th}$ bright fringe, $\theta_n$ is the angle corresponding to the $n^{th}$ slit, and $\lambda$ is the wavelength of light incident on the grating. In order for the diffraction grating to work, the pitch of the grating must be on the order of the incident light. The wavelengths in the visible spectrum range between approximately 400 - 700 nm and is the range to be considered for coloring hair. Furthermore, light returned from a diffraction grating is usually directional.

Fabricating nanometer-sized patterns on a rough, curved surface of human hair *in-situ* is not a straightforward task. Most chip manufacturers easily create nanometer-sized patterns today, but the surface the pattern is created on is ideal—flat and smooth. Thus standard photolithographic techniques are not practical. For this work a Focused Ion Beam (FIB) is employed to fabricate nano-scale patterns onto individual hair strands. A FIB is a tool that allows for control of a beam of ions with nanometer precision—nanofabrication [9]. The FIB used in this work utilizes $Ga^+$ ions. These are confined to a Gaussian current density distribution [10] [11] with a full-width-half-maximum (FWHM) beam diameter as small as 7 nm [12]. When the $Ga^+$ ions reach the sample, atoms/molecules from the sample's surface are ejected, or sputtered away. By controlling the location of the ion beam, one can control the removal of material from the sample's surface. In this work a Quanta Dual Beam 3D FEG™ scanning electron microscope by FEI was used to mill diffraction patterns on human hair. The Dual Beam system has the $Ga^+$ ion source mounted 52° from vertical for milling and a scanning electron microscope (SEM) mounted vertically for imaging. Imaging with the SEM rather than FIB after milling ensures that no additional material is removed.

Human hair is not electrically conductive, so charge build-up must be overcome. If charge build-up occurs additional incoming ions will be deflected, thus creating two issues: First, milling requires many ions reach the same spot on the surface. If the incoming ions are deflected, then no milling will occur and no pattern can be generated. Second, charge build-up will distort any image taken with the SEM or FIB. Using a lower accelerating voltage, a reduced current, or a minimal beam dwell time on the SEM will minimize image distortions, but this also degrade image quality. In order to mitigate this issue, a thin layer of carbon was sputtered on to the hair. Depositing a thin (~10 nm) carbon layer to help dissipate charge on non-conducting samples is a common technique for SEM and TEM preparation [13], and this same approach solved both issues.

Patterns were generated by a stream file [14]-[17], which controls the location of the Gaussian Beam of ions. Each line in a stream file has three components; dwell time, x-position, and y-position. Dwell time determines the length of time the FIB is at a particular x-y coordinate and is also roughly proportional to the depth of the pattern at a constant acceleration potential of 30 kV in this work. The beam's diameter is dictated by its current, which varies depending on the requirements of the pattern. Both x and y coordinates correspond to pixels on the screen and the coordinates do not correspond to an absolute dimension.

A given pattern's x-y dimensions, as defined by the stream file, are scaled to the horizontal field width (HFW) specified in the system. For the system used in this work there are 4096 pixels in the horizontal-direction (x-direction). If the HFW = 100 μm, then the spacing between each pixel is 24.4 nm. Similarly, changing the HFW to 150 μm creates 36.6 nm spacing etc. So if the spacing between two mill points is only 10 pixels, the actual spacing could either be 244 nm or 366 nm. All of the stream files used for generating ion beam patterns were calculated and stored using MathCAD routines. All scalar inputs could be declared prior to runtime thus parameterizing any pattern for varying HFWs. In addition all patterns were milled with equal arc-length step segments [18] so that the variation in groove's depth with beam position was minimized.

Two different diffraction patterns were used for this work: an Archimedean spiral and a hyperbola. The Archimedean spiral, **Figure 1**, was created with a 30 kV, 1 nA ion beam (44 nm beam diameter at FWHM), and a 3 μs dwell time per pixel. By cycling through the pattern 1000 times, a mill depth greater than 800 nm was achieved. Two different spiral pitches of 730 nm, and 540 nm were milled using two separate HFWs.

The second pattern, a hyperbola, is shown in **Figure 2**. It was milled at 30 kV, 300 pA current (31 nm beam diameter at FWHM), and a 1 μs dwell time per pixel. Cycling through the pattern 3000 times resulted in a mill depth of approximately 800 nm. Two different HFWs created hyperbolas with pitches of 1040 nm, and 840 nm.

## 3. Optical Observations

An optical microscope was used to image and observe the diffraction changes on the hair specimen. The illumination light (perpendicular incidence) of the microscope was not utilized for these micrographs. Instead an external light source was utilizewd at an oblique angle. The light source used was a halogen bulb without filters. By changing the angle of this incident illumination from the side the changes in the diffracted wavelengths were observed.

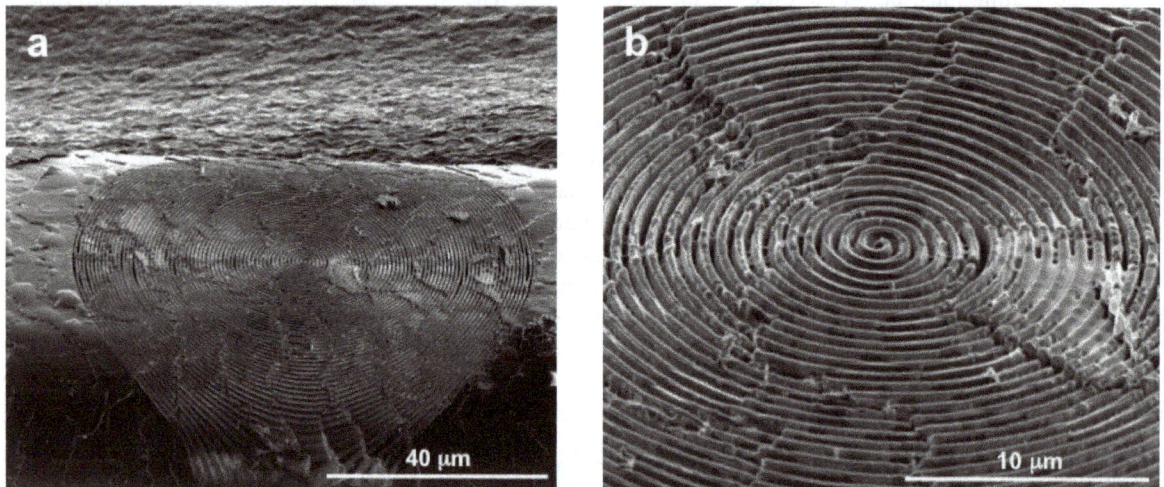

**Figure 1.** Archimedean spiral pattern milled on a strand of brown hair. (a) Overview of entire spiral pattern viewed at an angle of 52˚; (b) Center portion of spiral pattern viewed at an angle of 52˚. The pitch is 730 nm.

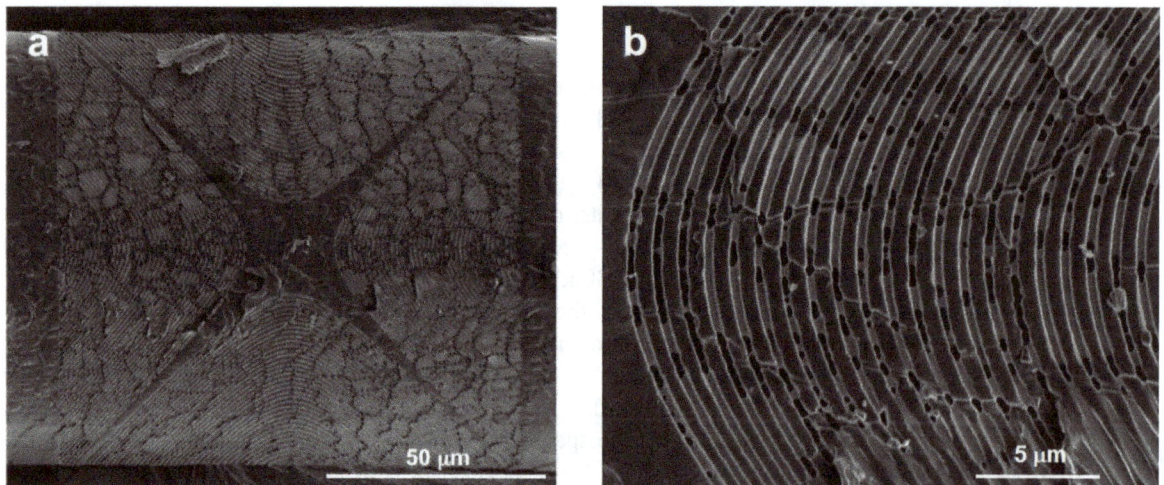

**Figure 2.** Hyperbola pattern milled on strand of brown hair. (a) Overview of entire hyperbola pattern; (b) Center portion of hyperbola pattern. The pitch is 1040 nm.

**Figures 3(a)-3(d)** show the same two hair strands which have been patterned with the Archimedean spirals (top strand) and hyperbola (bottom strand) diffraction gratings. Three Archimedean spirals are patterned on the top strand. From left to right their pitches are 730 nm, 730 nm, and 540 nm. Two hyperbola patterns are patterned on the bottom hair strand. The left hyperbola has a 1040 pitch and the right hand hyperbola has an 840

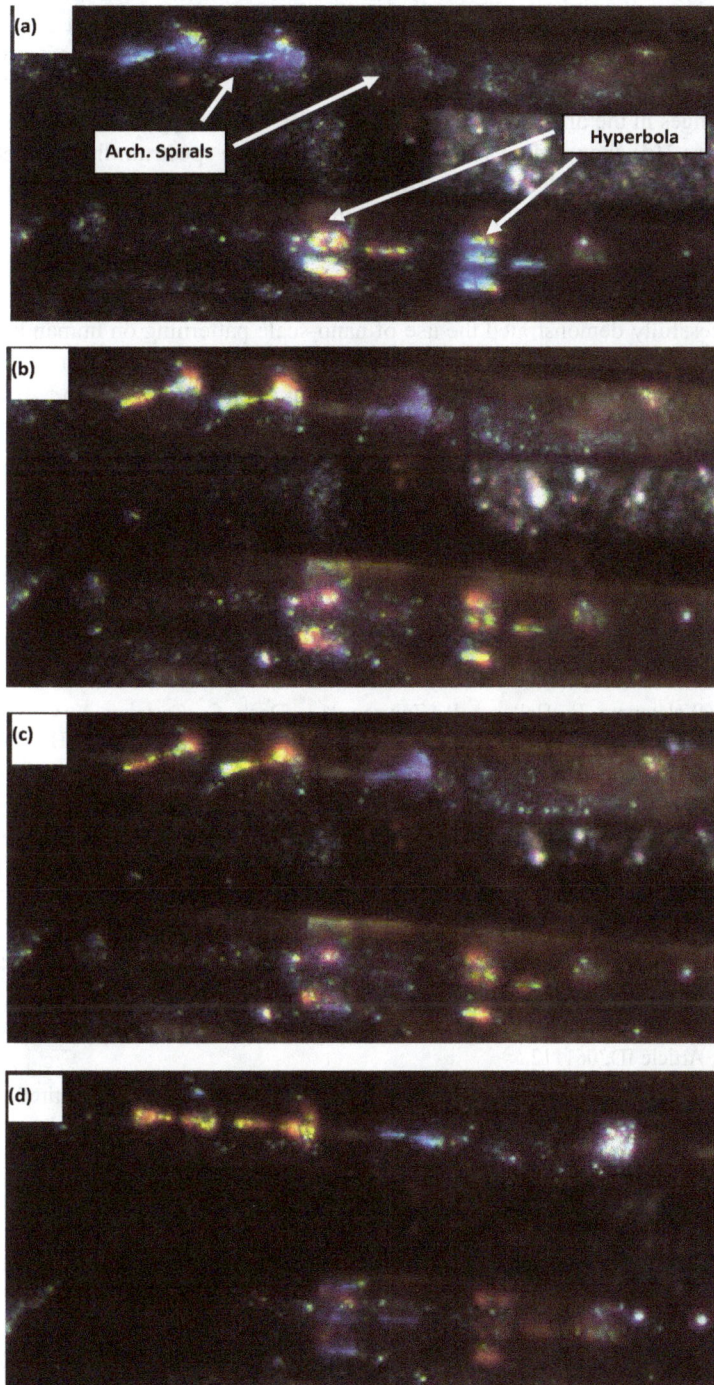

**Figure 3.** Light diffraction from nanoFIBricated patterns at various azimuth angles of incident light. (a) 10°; (b) 20°; (c) 30°; (d) 40°. The pitches on the spirals (left to right) located on the second strand of hair from the top are 730 nm, 730 nm, and 540 nm. The pitches on the hyperbola patterns (left to right) located on the third strand of hair from the top are 1040 nm and 840 nm.

nm pitch. Each successive subfigure in **Figure 3** is the same with the exception that the azimuth angle for the incident light has been rotated in increments of 10°. Specifically, **Figure 3(a)** is for an azimuth of 10°, **Figure 3(b)** is for an azimuth of 20°, etc.

The diffracted wavelengths are the function of the pattern type, pitch of the pattern and angle of the incident light. **Figure 3** shows the transition of the diffracted light on the machined patterns from deep blue hue (**Figure 3(a)**) on Archimedean spiral patterns at the top left corners of the images at 10° azimuth angle of the incident light to green yellow (**Figure 3(b)** azimuth 20°) to yellow-orange (**Figure 3(c)** azimuth 30°) to finally orange-red (**Figure 3(d)** azimuth 40°).

Similarly changes in the diffracted light are also visible on the hyperbola patterns. For example, the hyperbola patterns in **Figure 3(d)** show colors spanning the entire visible spectrum from violet to red. It may also be noted that pitch of the pattern also has an effect on the diffracted patterns. This effect is more pronounced on the hyperbola pattern than on the spiral pattern especially at low azimuthal angles.

## 4. Summary and Conclusion

This work successfully demonstrated the use of nano-scale patterning on human hair for cosmetic purposes. By use of this technique complex patterns could be easily created on human hair to artificially color the hair. Archimedean spirals and hyperbola diffraction patterns with pitches varying from 540 nm - 1040 nm were patterned in this work. Observations of the hair fibers with an optical microscope demonstrated that the diffractions gratings returned light from brown hair that spanned the full color spectrum.

## Acknowledgements

The authors will like to acknowledge the support of Center of Micro-Engineered Materials at the University of New Mexico for this work.

## References

[1]   Walter, P., Welcomme, E., Hallégot, P., Zaluzec, N.J., Deeb, C., Castaing, J., Veyssière, P., Bréniaux, R., Lévêque, J.-L. and Tsoucaris, G. (2006) Early Use of Pbs Nanotechnology for an Ancient Hair Dyeing Formula. *Nano Letters*, **6**, 2215-2219. http://dx.doi.org/10.1021/nl061493u

[2]   Swift, J.A. and Brown, A.C. (1972) The Critical Determination of Fine Changes in the Surface Architecture of Human Hair Due to Cosmetic Treatment. *Journal of the Society of Cosmetic Chemists*, **23**, 695-670.

[3]   Nohyneka, G.J., Fautzb, R., Benech-Kiefferc, F. and Toutaina, H. (2004) Review: Toxicity and Human Health Risk of Hair Dyes. *Food and Chemical Toxicology*, **42**, 517-543. http://dx.doi.org/10.1016/j.fct.2003.11.003

[4]   Thun, M.J., Altekruse, S.F., Namboodiri, M.M., Calle, E.E., Myers, D.G. and Heath, C.W. (1994) Hair Dye Use and Risk of Fatal Cancers in U.S. Women. *Journal of the National Cancer Institute*, **86**, 164-165. http://dx.doi.org/10.1093/jnci/86.3.210

[5]   Sun, C.-H., Jiang, P. and Jiang, B. (2008) Broadband Moth-Eye Antireflection Coatings on Silicon. *Applied Physics Letters*, **92**, Article ID: 061112.

[6]   Wilson, S.J. and Hutley, M.C. (1982) The Optical Properties of "Moth Eye" Antireflection Surfaces. *Journal of Modern Optics*, **29**, 993-1009.

[7]   Lamartine, B.C. and Orler, E.B. (2011) Hair Treatment Process Providing Dispersed Colors by Light Diffraction. Los Alamos National Laboratory Patent.

[8]   Hecht, E. (2002) Optics. 4th Edition.

[9]   Goettler, D.F., Su, M.F., Reinke, C.M., Alaie, S., Hopkins, P.E., Olsson, R.H.I., El-Kady, I. and Leseman, Z.C. (2011) Realization of a 33 GHz Phononic Crystal Fabricated in a Freestanding Membrane. *AIP Advances*, **1**, Article ID: 042001.

[10]  Edinger, K. and Kraus, T. (2001) Modeling of Focused Ion Beam Induced Chemistry and Comparison with Experimental Data. *Microelectronic Engineering*, **57-58**, 263-268. http://dx.doi.org/10.1016/S0167-9317(01)00487-7

[11]  Nassar, R., Vasile, M. and Zhang, W. (1998) Mathematical Modeling of Focused Ion Beam Microfabrication. *Journal of Vacuum Science & Technology B*, **16**, 109-115. http://dx.doi.org/10.1116/1.589763

[12]  (2007) Quanta 3D FEG Datasheet. FEI Company.

[13]  Giannuzzi, L.A. and Stevie, F.A. (1999) A Review of Focused Ion Beam Milling Techniques for Tem Specimen Prep-

aration. *Micron*, **30**, 197-204. http://dx.doi.org/10.1016/S0968-4328(99)00005-0

[14] Lamartine, B.C. (2003) Reflective Diffraction Grating. US 6583933.

[15] Lamartine, B.C. and Stutz, R.A. (1995) Ultrahigh Vacuum Focused Ion Beam Micromill and Articles Therefrom. US 5721687.

[16] Lamartine, B.C. and Stutz, R.A. (1998) Focused Ion Beam Milling and Article Therefrom. US 5773116.

[17] Lamartine, B.C. Direction Aggregate Element Diffraction Patent (daedp). Pending.

[18] Lamartine, B.C. (2010) Angarclen1.Xmcd, an Unpublished MathCAD Program.

# 21

# Anti-Inflammatory Efficacy of Product Containing "Skin Calm Complex" *in Vitro* Reconstructed Epidermis

**María Matabuena de Yzaguirre[1], Gabriela Bacchini[2], Emili Gil Luna[2], Eva Vila-Martínez[2]**

[1]Department of Biology, Faculty of Sciences, Universidad Autónoma de Madrid, Madrid, Spain
[2]Medical Department, Ferrer Health Care, Barcelona, Spain
Email: maria.matabuena@uam.es

## Abstract

Atopic dermatitis is classified as a chronic inflammatory skin disease, which is characterized by alterations in barrier function and immune system of the skin. In a previous study, the efficacy of REPAVAR ATOPIC SKIN BODY CREAM EXTREME (a product containing "SKIN CALM COMPLEX") on the epidermal barrier structure was demonstrated. However, the product has also been formulated to improve inflammation and itching. The aim of this study is to analyze product effectiveness on skin inflammation and itching which is associated with atopic dermatitis, by quantification of IL-1$\alpha$ and IL-8 interleukins secreted by human keratinocytes from reconstructed epidermis by ELISA assay. Mature (aged 17 days) sample tissues were treated with pro-inflammatory agents (PBS 1X and LPS) and with the product containing synergistic mix from plants extracts and Dihydroavenanthramide D, among other ingredients ("SKIN CALM COMPLEX") for 24 hours. Measuring the amounts of interleukins by ELISA assay showed 1) decreased levels of IL-1$\alpha$ and 2) no differences about IL-8 secretion. Product REPAVAR ATOPIC SKIN BODY CREAM EXTREME has an anti-inflammatory effect on the release of pro-inflammatory cytokines, becoming an effective preventive agent on inflammation and itching due to maintenance and improvement of the keratinocyte epidermal structure.

## Keywords

Atopic Dermatitis, Anti-Inflammatory Effect, *In Vitro* Assay

## 1. Introduction

Atopic dermatitis is a chronic inflammatory skin disease, characterized by leukocytes infiltration, alteration of the barrier function of the skin, high rate of water loss, decreased water retention capacity and a lower amount of lipids and ceramides. These events cause uncomfortable symptoms associated with the diseases, such as inflammation and itching, which aggravate the skin condition [1]-[7].

The etiology of this disease includes interactions between genetic, environmental, epithelial barrier, immune factors and stress [8]-[11]. The results are dry skin, cutaneous hyper-reactivity and inflammation due to cytokine release from lymphocytes, Langerhans cells, keratinocytes, mast cells and eosinophils among the most important cells [12]-[14]. There are data about patients with a genetic profile for a vulnerable epithelial barrier, which provokes an altered immune response and inflamed skin. In this context, epidermis plays a fundamental role in the etiology and development of atopic dermatitis. When the epithelial barrier functions are damaged, inflammatory events and sensitization processes IgE mediated occurs. So epidermis is not only a physical barrier, but also a chemical and immune barrier [15]. In addition, itch-scratch cycle exacerbates the epidemic barrier damage, increases water loss, dryness and inflammation, and favors pathogenic infections of the skin [1] [16]. On the other case, in which external factors alter barrier function, a complex process triggers involving resident epidermal cells: keratinocytes, dermal fibroblasts, endothelial cells and leukocytes interacting with each other under the control of cytokine type mediators and lipids. When the epidermal barrier is impaired, keratinocytes secrete IL-$1\alpha$ and pro-inflammatory cytokine that induce production of IL-8 (chemo-attractant cytokine). IL-8 recruits immune system cells which secrete interleukins associated with pruritus and specific inflammation, such as IL-31 in T cells [3] [4] [17] [18].

In a previous study, the efficacy of the REPAVAR ATOPIC SKIN BODY CREAM EXTREME (a product containing "SKIN CALM COMPLEX") on the improving the structure and the epidermal barrier was demonstrated. However, this complex product also contains ingredients to act on inflammation and itching. The study of anti-inflammatory potential was carried out in reconstructed human epithelium model (3D). However, these reconstructed human epithelia lack immune and nervous system cells from human skin [19]. So only the effect of the product on interleukins secreted by keratinocytes was analyzed.

The aim of this work was to confirm the anti-inflammatory action of the REPAVAR ATOPIC SKIN BODY CREAM EXTREME product containing ingredients of the "SKIN CALM COMPLEX" whose effectiveness was demonstrated separately.

## 2. Methods

### 2.1. *In Vitro* Model

*In vitro* Reconstructed Human Epidermis of 0.33 cm$^2$, aged 17 days (28 samples), produced by SkinEthic laboratories (Nice, France) were used (for more information visit SkinEthic website [19]). The tissues were cultured and kept in chemically defined medium, provided by the same laboratory, during the assays. Tissue cultures were performed in an incubator with 5% of $CO_2$ at 37°C. The tissue manipulation process was carried out in sterile conditions.

### 2.2. Treatments

4 samples per group were used: i) Negative control (-SkinEthic Maintenance Medium- SkinEthic laboratories, Nice, France); ii) IL-$1\alpha$ inflammation positive control (phosphate buffered saline, PBS 1X, -HyClone Laboratories, Inc., South Logan, UT-, for 4 hours + maintenance medium for 24 hours); iii) IL-8 inflammation positive control (Escherichia coli LPS 100 μg/ml -Sigma, St. Louis, MO- diluted in maintenance medium, for 24 hours); iv) IL-$1\alpha$ anti-inflammation positive control (PBS 1X, for 4 hours + 10 μM Dexamethasone -Sigma, St. Louis, MO-, diluted in maintenance medium, for 24 hours); v) IL-8 anti-inflammation positive control (LPS 100 μg/ml + 10 μM Dexamethasone, diluted in maintenance medium, for 24 hours); vi) IL-$1\alpha$ inflammation treatment + Product (PBS 1X, for 4 hours + "REPAVAR ATOPIC SKIN BODY CREAM EXTREME", for 24 hours); vii) IL-8 inflammation treatment + Product (LPS 100 μg/ml diluted in maintenance medium + "REPAVAR ATOPIC SKIN BODY CREAM EXTREME", for 24 hours).

### 2.3. MTT Assay

Cellular viability was assessed by MTT (3-[4,5-dimethylthiazol-2-yl]-2,5 diphenyltetrazolium bromide) assay (Sigma, St. Louis, MO), a method based on the activity of mitochondrial dehydrogenases [20]. Stock solution of MTT (5 mg/ml) in PBS, was diluted (1 mg/ml) in SkinEthic culture medium, and then the samples were incubated at 37°C, 5% $CO_2$, 95% humidified atmosphere, for 3 hours. The resulting formazan crystals were dissolved by the addition of isopropanol (Sigma, St. Louis, MO), at room temperature, for 2 hours with gentle agitation. Optical Densities (OD) were measured at 570 nm wavelength.

## 2.4. Immunodetection by ELISA

The release of interleukin in the supernatants from keratinocytes was determined using the ELISA kit for IL-1$\alpha$ (Abcam, Cambridge, UK) and IL-8 (Abcam, Cambridge, UK), following the manufacturer's instructions.

In both cases, the reading of the optical density (OD) was carried out at 450 nm against the blank (diluent).

## 2.5. Statistical Analysis

The statistical analysis was performed using the SPSS 15.0, 1 software (SPSS Inc., Chicago, IL), using Student's t test and analysis of variance (ANOVA), and considering a $p < 0.05$ as statistically significant.

# 3. Results and Discussion

## 3.1. Production of IL-1$\alpha$

IL-1$\alpha$ is a pleiotropic cytokine implicated in inflammation, immune responses and cell differentiation processes, which increases in response to cell damage, inducing apoptosis. In this study, culture maintenance medium was replaced by PBS for 4 hours, to promote disintegration of the epidermal barrier and to check the existence of any relationship between epithelial integrity and swelling.

Standard curve were calculated from DO readings at 450 nm and known protein concentration (pg/ml) (**Figure 1(a)**). Then, production of IL-1$\alpha$ data were calculated for each of the treatment groups.

Means of interleukin release was compared (**Figure 1(b)**) and statistical analysis data showed significant differences ($p < 0.05$) among the negative control group and positive control inflammation (PBS 1X, $p = 0.0268$) and between the negative control and positive control anti-inflammation (PBS 1X + Dexamethasone, $p = 0.0017$), although a notable reduction on IL-1$\alpha$ secretion was detected in this last situation. However, when comparing the groups negative control vs. PBS 1X + Product, p value was >0.05 ($p = 0.1$), indicating that the differences between them are not significant. Therefore, it is confirmed the product "REPAVAR ATOPIC SKIN BODY CREAM EXTREME" effect on inflammation mediated by IL-1$\alpha$, in response to barrier damage.

Extrapolation of inhibiting release of IL-1$\alpha$ in the sample treated with the product "REPAVAR ATOPIC SKIN BODY CREAM EXTREME" was calculated as the percentage of reducing the amount of protein released, relative to positive control anti-inflammatory (PBS 1X + Dexamethasone), having subtracted the value of production of IL-1$\alpha$ negative control. As shown in **Figure 1(c)**, the product "REPAVAR ATOPIC SKIN BODY CREAM EXTREME" seems to prevent the release of IL-1$\alpha$.

## 3.2. Production of IL-8

Since IL-8 is a chemotactic factor, implicated in the attraction and activation of immune cells, produced by keratinocytes in response to inflammatory stimuli, LPS was used to induce the production of this protein.

Following a similar procedure, when comparing LPS positive control group against inflammation treatment IL-8 + Product, p value was >0.05 ($p = 0.15$), indicating that the differences between them are not significant (data not shown). So that, product "REPAVAR ATOPIC SKIN BODY CREAM EXTREME" shows no effect on the release of IL-8.

Analysis of cell viability was included in the experiments as control treatments and data were not shown normally. But in the case of IL-8, surprisingly, meanwhile the positive controls (LPS and LPS + Dexamethasone) showed cell viability values around 80% compared to negative control (maintenance medium), implying the treatments are well tolerated by tissues, the Product-treated sample shows an increase of 35% compared to untreated tissue (negative control), reflecting that effect on epithelial regeneration processes (**Figure 2**).

These results are consistent with data previously obtained [21]. Product "REPAVAR ATOPIC SKIN BODY CREAM EXTREME"-treated tissues showed an increase in the number of cells and an improvement in the epithelial morphology and the expression of structural proteins.

Nowadays, treatments for dermatological diseases characterized by an altered immune response, involving inflammation and itching, as atopic dermatitis, include emollients to increase hydration levels and topical corti-

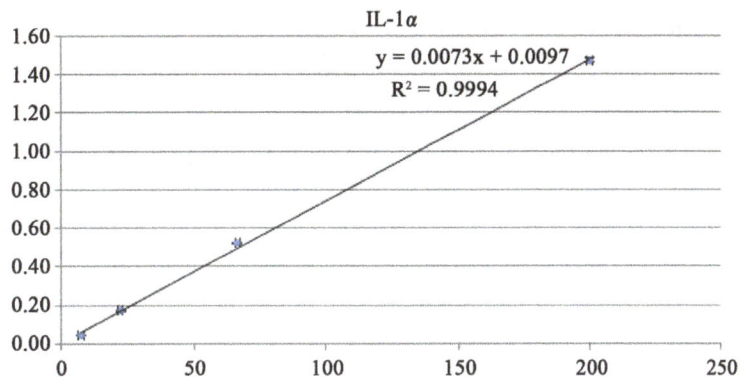

(a)

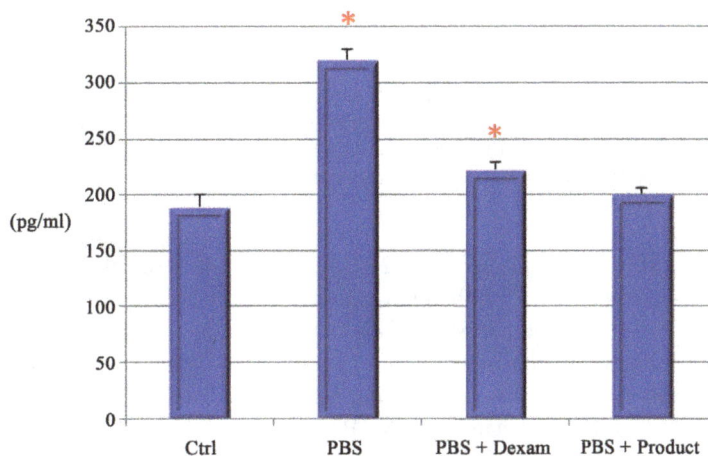

(b)

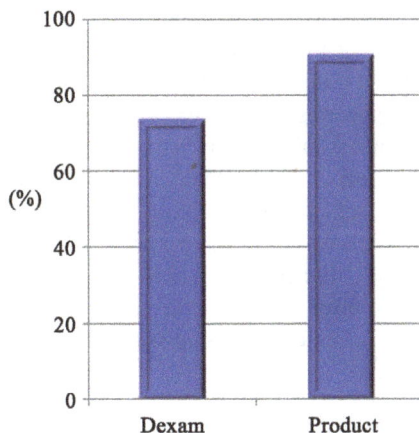

(c)

**Figure 1.** (a) IL-1$\alpha$ Standard Curve. The R value (regression) is reliable, because it is close to X axis, protein concentrations (pg/ml); Y axis, absorbance (450 nm). (b) Release of IL-1$\alpha$. Ctrl, untreated tissues; PBS, positive control inflammation; PBS + Dexamethasone, positive control anti-inflammation; PBS + Product ("ATOPIC SKIN BODY CREAM EXTREME"). The product exerts an anti-inflammatory effect in the case of IL-1$\alpha$. (c) Inhibition of IL-1$\alpha$ induced by Dexamethasone (Dexam) and "ATOPIC SKIN BODY CREAM EXTREME EXTREME BODY CREAM SKIN ATOPIC" (Product). "ATOPIC SKIN BODY CREAM EXTREME EXTREME BODY CREAM SKIN ATOPIC"-treated samples present a 90% of inhibition in IL-1$\alpha$ levels, while the Dexamethasone's efficiency is about 70%.

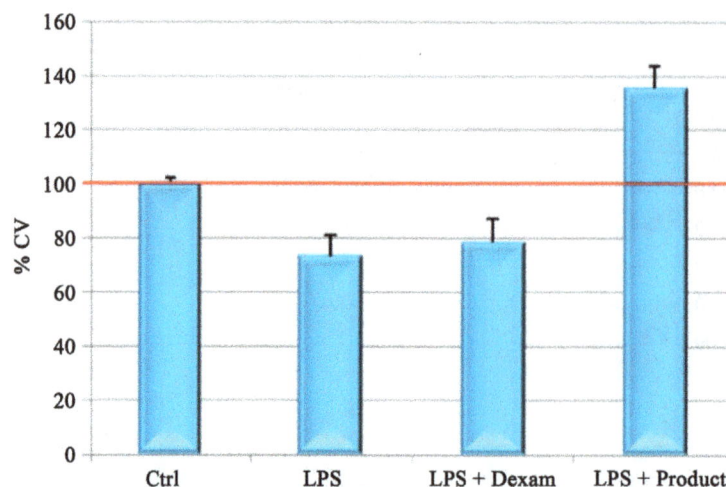

**Figure 2.** Cell viability (% CV). Ctrl, untreated tissues; LPS, positive control of inflammation; LPS + dexamethasone, positive control of anti-inflammation; LPS + Product ("ATOPIC SKIN BODY CREAM EXTREME"). Product-treated sample shows an increase in cell viability of about 35% respecting untreated tissues.

costeroids associated with adverse side effects [22] [23]. At present, research focuses on the search and combination of more effective new agents with the least side effects. The product used in this study ("ATOPIC SKIN BODY CREAM EXTREME") contains "SKIN CALM COMPLEX", which includes, among other ingredients, a multi-herbal complex extracted from seven plants (*Rosemarinus officinalis*, *Matricaria recubita*, *Camellia sinensis*, *Glycyrrhiza glabra*, *Polygonum cuspidatum*, *Scutellaria baicalensis* and *Centella asiatica*) and Dihydroavenanthramide D, synthetic Avenanthramide. Both active ingredients have shown their efficacy in the treatment of atopic dermatitis: i) multicompound herbal preparation showed anti-inflammatory effects by reduction of IL-8 production *in vitro* by lymphocytes and monocytes, and reduction of eczema area severity index (EASI), degree of pruritus and TEWL [24]; ii) keratinocytes treated with Avenanthramides showed a reduction of IL-8 release *in vitro* and topical application in murine models mitigated inflammation and pruritogen-induced scratching [25]. In this study, no effect on the production of IL-8 was found. This fact may be due to the action of Avenanthramides in the product is not as straightforward as when acting in isolation.

However, data obtained from quantization of pro-inflammatory cytokine IL-1$\alpha$, by ELISA assay, demonstrate the anti-inflammatory effect of the product "REPAVAR ATOPIC SKIN BODY CREAM EXTREME" by topical application in reconstructed human epidermis. Other authors postulate thatkeratinocytes aretargets of T lymphocytes infiltrating immune processes, to have an active role in atopic dermatitis. Its role in maintaining homeostasis and proper functionality of the skin is essential not only for the correct expression of proteins that ensure epithelial structure, but for the production of lipids that prevent the loss of water and production of cytokines involved in activation and cell chemotaxis processes (inflammation), in proliferation and differentiation [26] [27].

## 4. Conclusion

This study demonstrates that the product may be highly effective in mild atopic dermatitis and the early stage of a moderate/severe illness. It improves the epidermal barrier effect and prevents inflammation, although studies in patients will be needed to confirm this hypothesis.

## References

[1]   Boguniewicz, M. and Leung, D.Y. (2011) Atopic Dermatitis: A Disease of Altered Skin Barrier and Immune Dysregulation. *Immunological Reviews*, **242**, 233-246. http://dx.doi.org/10.1111/j.1600-065X.2011.01027.x

[2]   Kasraie, S. and Werfel, T. (2013) Role of Macrophages in the Pathogenesis of Atopic Dermatitis. *Mediators of Inflammation*, **2013**, 1-15. http://dx.doi.org/10.1155/2013/942375

[3]   Segre, J.A. (2006) Epidermal Barrier Formation and Recovery in Skin Disorders. *The Journal of Clinical Investigation*, **116**, 1150-1158. http://dx.doi.org/10.1172/JCI28521

[4]   Jensen, L.E. (2010) Targeting the IL-1 Family Members in Skin Inflammation. *Current Opinion in Investigational Drugs*, **11**, 1211-1220.

[5]   Engelhart, K., El Hindi, T., Biesalski, H.K. and Pfitzner, I. (2005) *In Vitro* Reproduction of Clinical Hallmarks of Eczematous Dermatitis in Organotypic Skin Models. *Archives of Dermatological Research*, **297**, 1-9. http://dx.doi.org/10.1007/s00403-005-0575-7

[6]   Tivoli, Y.A. and Rubenstein, R.M. (2009) Pruritus: An Updated Look at an Old Problem. *Journal of Clinical and Aesthetic Dermatology*, **2**, 30-36.

[7]   Steinhoff, M., Bienenstock, J., Schmelz, M., Maurer, M., Wei, E. and Bíró, T. (2006) Neurophysiological, Neuroimmunological, and Neuroendocrine Basis of Pruritus. *Journal of Investigative Dermatology*, **126**, 1705-1718. http://dx.doi.org/10.1038/sj.jid.5700231

[8]   Pastar, Z., Lipozencić, J. and Ljubojević, S. (2005) Etiopathogenesis of Atopic Dermatitis—An Overview. *Acta Dermatovenerologica Croatica*, **13**, 54-62.

[9]   Polo, N. (2003) Dermatitis atópica. JANO, **1.475**, 42-44.

[10]  Novak, N. and Leung, D.Y. (2011) Advances in Atopic Dermatitis. *Current Opinion in Immunology*, **23**, 778-783. http://dx.doi.org/10.1016/j.coi.2011.09.007

[11]  Elias, P.M. (2010) Therapeutic Implications of a Barrier-Based Pathogenesis of Atopic Dermatitis. *Annals of Dermatology*, **22**, 245-254. http://dx.doi.org/10.5021/ad.2010.22.3.245

[12]  Ballona, R. and Ballona, C. (2004) Dermatitis atópica. *Folia Dermatológica Peruana*, **15**, 40-48.

[13]  Theoharides, T.C., Alysandratos, K.D., Angelidou, A., Delivanis, D.A., Sismanopoulos, N., Zhang, B., Asadi, S., Vasiadi, M., Weng, Z., Miniati, A. and Kalogeromitros, D. (2012) Mast Cells and Inflammation. *Biochimica et Biophysica Acta*, **1822**, 21-33.

[14]  Elias, P.M. and Schmuth, M. (2009) Abnormal Skin Barrier in the Etiopathogenesis of Atopic Dermatitis. *Current Allergy and Asthma Reports*, **9**, 265-272. http://dx.doi.org/10.1007/s11882-009-0037-y

[15]  Komine, M. (2009) Analysis of the Mechanism for the Development of Allergic Skin Inflammation and the Application for Its Treatment: Keratinocytes in Atopic Dermatitis—Their Pathogenic Involvement. *Journal of Pharmacological Sciences*, **110**, 260-264. http://dx.doi.org/10.1254/jphs.09R06FM

[16]  Klein, P.A. and Clark, R.A. (1999) An Evidence-Based Review of the Efficacy of Antihistamines in Relieving Pruritus in Atopic Dermatitis. *JAMA Dermatology*, **135**, 1522-1525. http://dx.doi.org/10.1001/archderm.135.12.1522

[17]  Brandt, E.B. and Sivaprasad, U. (2011) Th2 Cytokines and Atopic Dermatitis. *Journal of Clinical & Cellular Immunology*, **2**, 110-123. http://dx.doi.org/10.4172/2155-9899.1000110

[18]  Sonkoly, E., Muller, A., Lauerma, A.I., Pivarcsi, A., Soto, H., Kemeny, L., Alenius, H., Dieu-Nosjean, M.C., Meller, S., Rieker, J., Steinhoff, M., Hoffmann, T.K., Ruzicka, T., Zlotnik, A. and Homey, B. (2006) IL-31: A New Link between T Cells and Pruritus in Atopic Skin Inflammation. *Journal of Allergy and Clinical Immunology*, **117**, 411-417. http://dx.doi.org/10.1016/j.jaci.2005.10.033

[19]  http://www.skinethic.com/RHE.asp

[20]  Merlin, J.L., Azzi, S., Lignon, D., Ramacci, C., Zeghari, N. and Guillemin, F. (1992) MTT Assays Allow Quick and Reliable Measurement of the Response of Human Tumour Cells to Photodynamic Therapy. *European Journal of Cancer*, **28**, 1452-1458. http://dx.doi.org/10.1016/0959-8049(92)90542-A

[21]  Matabuena-de Yzaguirre, M., Bacchini, G., Vila-Martínez, E. and Juarranz, A. (2014) Product Containing "Skin Calm Complex" Improves Barrier Effect *in Vitro*. *Journal of Cosmetics, Dermatological Sciences and Applications*, **4**, 234-243. http://dx.doi.org/10.4236/jcdsa.2014.44032

[22]  Venge, P. (1993) Eosinophil and Neutrophil Granulocytes. *Allergy*, **48**, 39-47. http://dx.doi.org/10.1111/j.1398-9995.1993.tb04697.x

[23]  Hong, J., Buddenkotte, J., Berger, T.G. and Steinhoff, M. (2011) Management of Itch in Atopic Dermatitis. *Seminars in Cutaneous Medicine and Surgery*, **30**, 71-86. http://dx.doi.org/10.1016/j.sder.2011.05.002

[24]  Lee, J., Jung, E., Park, B., Jung, K., Park, J., Kim, K., Kim, K.H. and Park, D. (2005) Evaluation of the Anti-Inflammatory and Atopic Dermatitis-Mitigating Effects of BSASM, a Multicompound Preparation. *Journal of Ethnopharmacology*, **96**, 211-219. http://dx.doi.org/10.1016/j.jep.2004.09.012

[25]  Sur, R., Nigam, A., Grote, D., Liebel, F. and Southall, M.D. (2008) Avenanthramides, Polyphenols from Oats, Exhibit Anti-Inflammatory and Anti-Itch Activity. *Archives of Dermatological Research*, **300**, 569-574. http://dx.doi.org/10.1007/s00403-008-0858-x

[26]  Albanesi, C., Scarponi, C., Giustizieri, M.L. and Girolomoni, G. (2005) Keratinocytes in Inflammatory Skin Diseases.

*Current Drug Target-Inflammation & Allergy*, **4**, 329-334. http://dx.doi.org/10.2174/1568010054022033

[27] Uchiyama, N., Yamamoto, A., Kameda, K., Yamaguchi, H. and Ito, M. (2000) The Activity of Fatty Acid Synthase of Epidermal Keratinocytes Is Regulated in the Lower Stratum Spinousum and the Stratum Basale by Local Inflammation Rather than by Circulating Hormones. *Journal of Dermatological Science*, **24**, 134-141. http://dx.doi.org/10.1016/S0923-1811(00)00088-8

# 22

# Improvement of Scalp Condition and Quality of Life through Proper Skin Care of Dry Scalp

Mika Oshima[1], Maiko Sogawa[1], Hiroshi Matsunaka[2], Yumi Murakami[2], Yumiko Saya[2], Takashi Sugita[3], Yoshihiro Matsudate[1], Nozomi Fukui[1], Kazutoshi Murao[1], Yoshiaki Kubo[1*]

[1]Department of Dermatology, Institute of Health Biosciences, The University of Tokushima Graduate School, Tokushima, Japan
[2]Tokiwa Pharmaceutical Co., Ltd., Tokyo, Japan
[3]Department of Microbiology, Meiji Pharmaceutical University, Tokyo, Japan
Email: [*]kubo@tokushima-u.ac.jp

## Abstract

Introduction: Appropriate skin care for dry scalp includes treatment for dandruff and itchiness. However, little is known about the appropriate washing methods for subjects with dry scalp. Methods: A scalp moisturizing lotion was used for 8 weeks on 30 outpatients at the Tokushima University Hospital who had dry scalp. All subjects were given the same hair shampoo/conditioner and instructions on how to wash their hair. Scalp symptoms were observed before and after the testing period. Indigenous bacteria were collected from the scalp for quantitative assessment. A survey was conducted to assess the quality of life (QOL). Results: All scalp condition items (dryness, scales and desquamation, itchiness, excoriation, and erythema) improved significantly after the testing period; the levels of *Malassezia* and bacterial colonization also decreased significantly. The QOL evaluation indicated significant improvements in "symptoms", "emotions", and "global" measures. A correlation was found between the extent of dryness at the start of the test and the level of *Malassezia* colonization, as well as QOL scores. Conclusion: Using a scalp moisturizing lotion, washing hair with a shampoo and conditioner that cause low irritation levels, and using a hair washing method that avoids irritation led to improvement in scalp condition, QOL, and patient satisfaction.

## Keywords

Atopic Dermatitis, Seborrheic Dermatitis, Moisturizer, *Malassezia*, Bacteria, qPCR

---

[*]Corresponding author.

## 1. Introduction

The scalp is a region where a relatively large number of hair glands exist and the amount of sebum excretion is large [1], making it difficult to dry out. Dry symptoms of the scalp are often triggered, however, due to underlying ailments such as atopic dermatitis, seborrheic dermatitis, or psoriasis vulgaris, as well as low humidity during winter, cooling and heating in highly sealed living environments, or wrong skin care from using an excessive amount of detergent. On the other hand, a rise in sebum excretion induces increased number of indigenous bacteria and changes in bacterial flora [2], resulting in an increased amount of inflammation and desquamation due to dermatitis seborrheica or turnover disorder, which can lead to dryness of the scalp. Therefore, skin problems can readily occur in the scalp, but the awareness about the importance of skin care in this region is low when compared with the face.

In this study, a moisturizing lotion for the scalp was used on test subjects with ailments such as atopic dermatitis, seborrheic dermatitis, and psoriasis vulgaris; the symptoms of these subjects had stabilized because of continuous treatment, but they had dry scalp. Furthermore, their hair shampoo and hair conditioner were replaced with those that had no antibacterial agents or cooling ingredients and cause low skin irritation. The hair washing method used in the present study, which involved brushing through the hair with the fingertips, facilitated improvements with regards to excessive washing or insufficient rinsing. After the testing period, skin findings, the levels of *Malassezia* and bacteria, and patient quality of life (QOL) were assessed, correlations between these parameters were verified, and the clinical efficacy was examined.

## 2. Methods

### 2.1. Subjects

The test was conducted on 30 outpatients of Tokushima University Hospital with ailments such as atopic dermatitis, seborrheic dermatitis, and psoriasis vulgaris; the symptoms of these subjects had stabilized because of continuous treatment, but they had dry scalp. They did not have any severe symptoms of inflammation, papular eruptions, or any serious underlying ailments and were determined to be unsuitable for this study by their physicians-in-charge. They were also provided information about the study before the test was performed, and written informed consent was obtained from those who voluntarily desired to participate in the study.

The following patients were considered eligible for participation: patients with ailments such as atopic dermatitis, seborrheic dermatitis, and psoriasis vulgaris whose symptoms related to their underlying disease had stabilized due to treatment but who had dry scalp; outpatients who were able to wash their hair once a day as a general rule (in case of those whose customary frequency of washing hair was once every 2 days prior to participation in this study, the frequency was set to once every 2 days); and subjects 20 years of age or older, irrespective of gender.

The exclusion criteria were as follows: skin symptoms such as contact dermatitis from formulation ingredients of the product under study, or similar constituents; severe inflammation or rash on the scalp, which would have made the use of the product under study inappropriate; underlying disease symptoms that had not been stabilized; inability to attend follow-up examination 8 weeks later; hair washing frequency of less than once every 2 days; pregnancy or lactation; and other reasons for which patients were deemed unsuitable for participation in this study by their physician-in-charge.

### 2.2. Implementation Period and Implementation Facility

Eight consecutive weeks were set for each patient from April 2013 to October 2013 for testing. The testing facility was the Department of Dermatology at the Tokushima University Hospital, and the test was implemented by a resident dermatologist of the Department of Dermatology. Furthermore, study approval was received from the Ethics Committee of the hospital prior to the implementation of the test (Approval Number: 1656).

### 2.3. Test Samples

The product under study is a moisturizing lotion for the scalp developed by Tokiwa Pharmaceutical Co., Ltd., intended to improve dryness symptoms of the scalp. The product contains moisturizing components such as hyaluronic acid and antioxidative components such as tocophenol. Furthermore, the moisturizing lotion contained no fragrances or synthetic coloring and was prepared to ensure that the induction of primary irritation of the skin or allergic reaction would be low. Furthermore, the hair shampoo and conditioner, which were used in combination, were also devised to ensure that skin irritation would be low, with no disinfectant agents or cooling ingredients included in the product. The scalp moisturizing lotion (NOV® Scalp Lotion, Noevir Co., Ltd., Hyogo, Japan) is a product made by partially improving a formula for the purpose of increasing moisturizing effects of a product that is already available on the market in Japan. The hair shampoo (NOV® Hair Shampoo D, NOV® Hair Shampoo DS, Noevir Co., Ltd.) and hair conditioner (NOV® Hair Conditioner, Noevir Co., Ltd.) are all currently available on the market. In terms of the Pharmaceutical Affairs Law in Japan, the scalp moisturizing lotion is classified as a quasi-drug, while the hair shampoo and conditioner are categorized as cosmetic products. In the 48-hour closed patch tests, there was no difference in the degree of stimulation when compared to the simultaneously tested petrolatum (Kenei Pharmaceutical Co. Ltd., Osaka, Japan) and purified water (Kenei Pharmaceutical Co. Ltd., Osaka, Japan) and therefore, the shampoo and conditioner were confirmed to be highly safe. The hair shampoo is available as a refreshing type (NOV® Hair Shampoo D) and moisturizing type (NOV® Hair Shampoo DS), and were selected by the subjects according to the length of their hair and preference. The hair conditioner was used according to the preference of the subjects and was used, for instance, by women with longer hair.

## 2.4. Usage

The treatment (orally taken or externally applied) of the patients' underlying ailments prior to the commencement of the test, as well as treatment for any complication, was continued throughout the study, with no change in the type, usage, or dosage. However, if changes in the previously established treatment were necessary, and the physician-in-charge considered that such changes would affect the test, the patient was treated as an exception. The subjects washed their scalp and hair using the shampoo, as well as hair conditioner if preferred, once a day when they bathed, according to the scalp skin care method instructed by the physician-in-charge. After washing their hair, the subjects applied approximately 2 mL of moisturizing lotion over the entire scalp, while the amount of hair shampoo and hair conditioner used for shoulder-length hair was approximately 5 mL. Hair washing was to be performed once a day; however, if the subjects customarily washed their hair once every 2 days, then they were instructed to continue washing their hair at that frequency throughout the study. Any other skin care products being used prior to the study, such as hairdressing products or coloring agents, were allowed if they had been determined not to irritate the scalp.

## 2.5. Instructions on Hair Washing Method

The physician-in-charge provided each subject instructions on how to wash their hair, according to the contents in **Table 1**.

## 2.6. Observation and Evaluation Methods

The physician-in-charge entered the identification number, age, sex, complications, combined medications for use during the test period (medication name, usage, and dosage) of each anonymous subject (linkable anonymity) on the case card of each subject and observed the skin symptoms of the scalp.

    1) Skin observations

    a) The extent of dryness, itchiness, scratch marks, and erythema were judged according to the following criteria and rated in scores as follows:

**Table 1.** Washing method.

| 1) Shampoo |
|---|
| Place some shampoo on the palm of the hand and spread it on both hands softly, and then apply it to the back of the head and foam it towards the side of the head. Shampoo the hair from the back of the head and the top of the head to the front of the head gently, using the balls of the fingers, not the nails. |
| 2) Rinsing |
| Warm water does not reach the scalp only by pouring it from the top, which leaves shampoo ingredients on the scalp. Raise the roots using the finger comb to allow warm water to reach the roots. |
| 3) Moisturizing |
| Apply approximately 2 mL of scalp moisturizing lotion directly to the dry area of the scalp. Spread it gently using the balls of the fingers. |

4. Severe: Significant symptoms visible.

3. Intermediate: Symptoms are clearly visible.

2. Slight: Symptoms are somewhat visible.

1. Minute: Very little symptoms are visible.

0. None: No symptoms are visible.

b) The desquamation and scales observed to be falling off the scalp when the hair on the top of the head is parted, was judged according to the following criteria and rated in scores as follows:

3. Advanced: Considerable amount confirmed.

2. Intermediate: Easily confirmed.

1. Slight: Little amount confirmed.

0. None: None confirmed or very little confirmed with none attaching to the hair.

2) Collection of fungus from the scalp and quantitative analysis of *Malassezia* and bacterial DNA

a) Collection

The swab portion of an aseptic cotton swab with a test tube (JCB Industry Ltd., Tokyo, Japan) was immersed in distilled water (Otsuka Pharmaceutical Co., Ltd., Tokyo, Japan) and the swab portion was rubbed against the scalp within a specific area (3 cm × 3 cm) by making 15 roundtrips in the X-axis direction and 15 roundtrips in the Y-axis direction, while rotating the swab to collect fungus from the scalp. The swab was then stored in a refrigerator at 4°C.

b) Quantitative analysis of *Malassezia* and bacteria by qPCR

Fungal and bacterial DNA was extracted directly from the swab portion. The amounts of *Malassezia* and bacterial DNA were quantified using real-time PCR (Applied Biosystems, CA, USA) with a TaqMan probe [3] [4].

3) Safety

Details of adverse effects (symptoms, extent, whether or not the subject should stop participating in the test, treatments, and outcomes) were entered on the case card. When a causal relationship with the product under the study was confirmed, such reactions were considered adverse reactions.

4) QOL evaluation

The Skindex-16, a measure of specific skin ailments, was used to investigate the QOL of test subjects at the start and end of the test [5]. Furthermore, Skindex-16 was used to investigate the scalp condition.

5) Survey

The extent of "dryness" and "itchiness" of the scalp as felt by the subjects were investigated with a set of multiple choice questions at the start and end of the test.

a) Dryness
- Dry;
- Slightly dry;
- Not dry;
- Do not know.

b) Itchiness
- Itchy to the point it is not possible to refrain from scratching;
- Notice scratching unconsciously;
- Scratch slightly here and there;
- Scratch slightly but can refrain from scratching;
- Feel no itch.

## 2.7. Statistical Analysis

Correlations between the scalp condition scores at the start of the test, scores for the respective observation items, the levels of colonization by *Malassezia* and bacteria, Skindex-16 measures, and correlations between quantitative changes in the scores for the respective observation items before and after the test were examined using Spearman's rank-order correlation coefficient. Furthermore, whether any significance existed between the scores of respective observation items for scalp condition before and after the test, the levels of colonization by *Malassezia* and bacteria, and changes in the Skindex-16 measures, were analyzed using a paired t-test or Wilcoxon signed-rank test. A chi-square analysis of the survey response items was performed. A p-value < 0.05 was considered statistically significant.

## 3. Results

### 3.1. Cases and Test Subject Background

A total of 30 subjects (average age: 47 ± 14 years) consisting of 15 men (average age: 49 ± 15 years) and 15 women (average age: 46 ± 14 years) were included in the present study. Diagnostic descriptions included atopic dermatitis, seborrheic dermatitis, psoriasis vulgaris, and eczema capitis, among others.The following complications were observed: hypertension in 2 patients, and prostatic hypertrophy, pollinosis, asthma, Kimura's disease, depression, hyperthyroidism, follicular mucinosis, and reflux esophagitis in one patient each. Concomitant drugs included both topical agents and oral agents. The topical agents consisted of steroids, immunosuppressants, and others, which were used by 22, 2, and 12 patients, respectively. The oral agents consisted of anti-allergic agents, steroids, immunosuppressants, and others, which were used by 18, 5, 3, and 16 patients, respectively. During the trial period, there were no changes in the agents used (**Table 2**).

### 3.2. Safety

Out of the 30 cases, one was excluded because the subject with seborrheic dermatitis did not come in for an examination at the end of the test, and another case was considered to have deviated because the subject with psoriasis vulgaris suspended the use of Antebate lotion, which resulted in the occurrence of itchiness. The use of the product under study was suspended 8 days after the start of the test in one subject with seborrheic dermatitis, as papular eruption and itchiness occurred. No treatment was provided for this condition, but the symptom disappeared naturally 1 week later so the use of the product was restarted, with no problem occurring during the

**Table 2.** Characteristics of subjects.

|  |  | Men | Women |
|---|---|---|---|
| Age, years | 21 - 30 | 1 | 2 |
|  | 31 - 40 | 4 | 5 |
|  | 41 - 50 | 3 | 4 |
|  | 51 - 60 | 3 | 1 |
|  | ≥61 | 4 | 3 |
|  | Total, n | 15 | 15 |
|  | Mean ± SD | 49 ± 15 | 46 ± 14 |
|  | Mean ± SD | 47 ± 14 | |
| Diagnostic name (some overlapping) | Atopic dermatitis | 9 | |
|  | Seborrheic dermatitis | 3 | |
|  | Psoriasis (psoriasis vulgaris, pustular psoriasis) | 5 | |
|  | Eczema | 5 | |
|  | Prurigo | 4 | |
|  | Alopecia areata | 4 | |
|  | Contact dermatitis | 1 | |
|  | Scleroderma | 1 | |
| Complication (some overlapping) | Hypertension | 2 | |
|  | Prostatic hypertrophy, pollinosis, asthma, Kimura's disease, depression, hyperthyroidism, follicular mucinosis, reflux esophagitis | 1 each | |
| Concomitant drug External | Steroid | 22 | |
|  | Immunosuppressant | 2 | |
|  | Other than the above | 12 | |
| Concomitant drug Internal | Anti-allergic agent | 18 | |
|  | Steroid | 5 | |
|  | Immunosuppressant | 3 | |
|  | Other than the above | 16 | |

remaining 6 weeks. This instance was determined to have had "no" causal relationship with the product under study.

Itchiness in the head region occurred in 2 subjects with atopic dermatitis at 15 days and 27 days after starting the use of the product; the use of the product under study was suspended in these subjects. In one of these subjects, the symptom did not improve after the use of the product was suspended; however, this subject also presented a rash in regions other than the head. For this reason, the symptom was determined to have had no relationship with the product under study. No symptom improvement occurred in the other case, and while seasonal deterioration of the skin symptom was considered possible, since the causal relationship could not be ruled out, the determination was a "yes" for the existence of adverse effects. Twenty-six cases except for the 4 above-mentioned cases were aggregated.

### 3.3. Skin Observations

The scores at the start and end of the test for the respective observation items of scalp symptoms were: Dryness ($1.3 \pm 0.2$ and $0.4 \pm 0.1$); scale and desquamation ($0.9 \pm 0.2$ and $0.5 \pm 0.2$); itchiness ($2.2 \pm 0.2$ and $1.1 \pm 0.2$); scratches ($1.4 \pm 0.2$ and $0.7 \pm 0.2$); and erythema ($2.0 \pm 0.1$ and $1.2 \pm 0.2$), with all item scores showing a significant decline (**Figure 1**).

### 3.4. Colonization by Malassezia and Bacteria

The levels of colonization by *Malassezia* and bacteria decreased significantly from the start to the end of the 8-week testing period (**Figure 2**).

### 3.5. QOL

Of the measures of Skindex-16, which are "Symptoms", "Emotions", "Functioning", and "Global", the item scores of "Symptoms", "Emotions", and "Global" significantly decreased from the start to the end of the 8-week testing period (**Figure 3**).

### 3.6. Survey

The evaluations of dryness at the start and the end of the test were "dry" (5/1), "slightly dry" (8/3), and "not dry" (7/13); changes in the shape of dry-skin patches were considered to indicate improvement. The evaluations of itchiness at the start and the end of the test were "Itchy to the point it is not possible to refrain from scratching" (5/1), "Notice scratching unconsciously" (10/4), "Scratch slightly here and there" (5/10), "Scratch slightly but can refrain from scratching" (5/5), and "Feel no itch" (1/6), with significant changes (**Table 3**).

### 3.7. Statistical Analysis (Correlation)

The correlations between the scalp condition scores at the start of the test, scores for the respective observation items, the levels of colonization by *Malassezia* and bacteria, and the Skindex-16 measures are shown in **Table 4**. The correlations of quantitative changes in the scores for the respective observation items relating to the condition of the scalp before and after the test are shown in **Table 5**.

"Dryness" at the start of the test was found to be positively correlated with the observation items of the scalp and Skindex-16 measures "symptoms" and "global", while the level of *Malassezia* colonization was found to be negatively correlated. "Scales and desquamation" was found to be negatively correlated with the levels of colonization by *Malassezia* and bacteria; however, the correlation was only statistically significant between "scales and desquamation" and the level of *Malassezia* colonization.

Furthermore, with respect to the change in scores of respective observation items relating to the condition of the scalp ($\Delta$ at the end—at the beginning), "$\Delta$dryness" was positively correlated with all observation items.

## 4. Discussion

In 26 cases, the scalp symptoms before the test showed significant improvements by the end of the testing period, indicating that scalp skin care as performed in this study (moisturizing, use of hair shampoo and hair conditioners that present low levels of irritation, as well as the hair washing method that presents low levels of irritation)

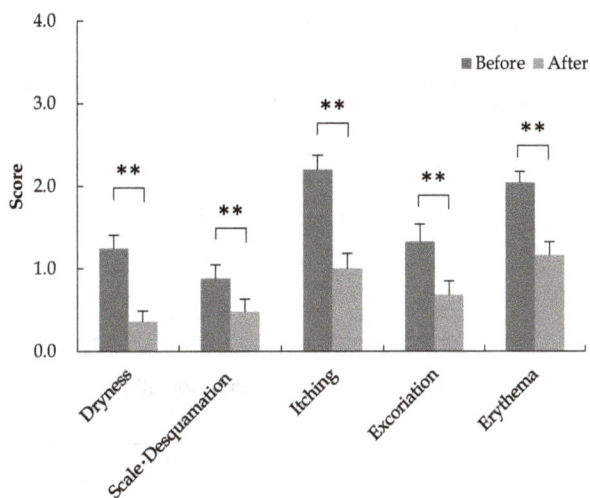

**Figure 1.** Skin findings.

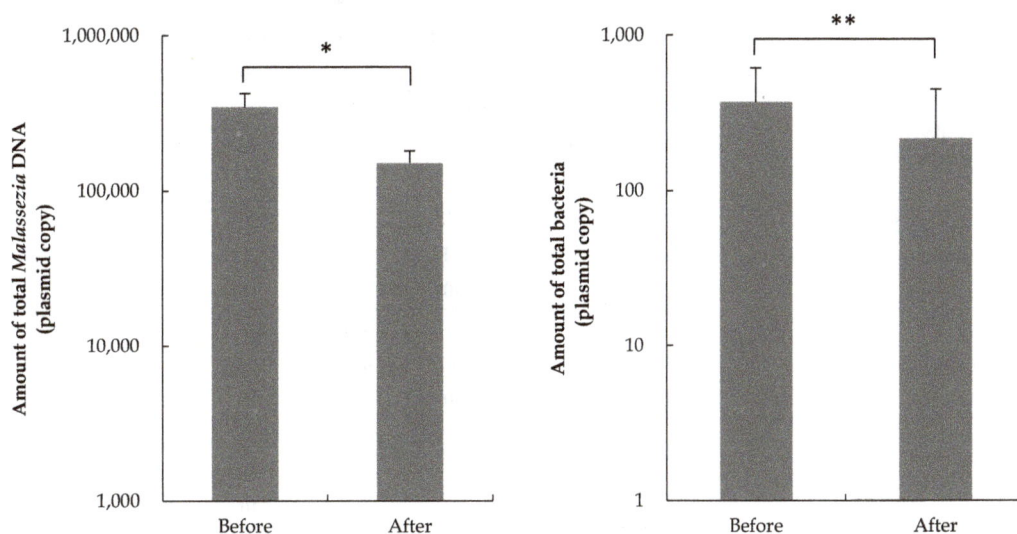

**Figure 2.** Evaluation of the levels of colonization by *Malassezia* and bacteria.

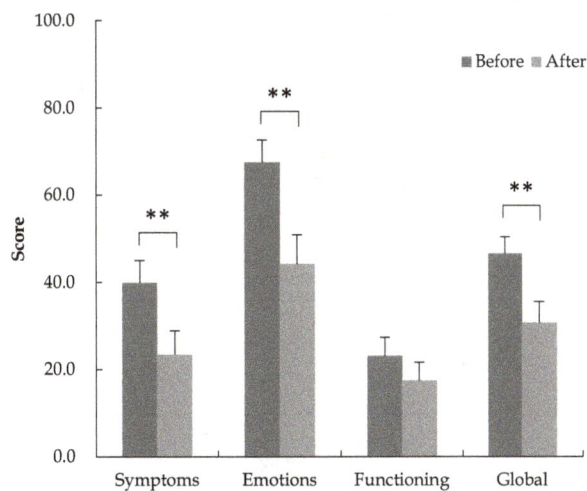

**Figure 3.** Evaluation of QOL score.

**Table 3.** Evaluation of severity of dryness and itchiness.

| Dryness n = 25 | Dry | | Slightly dry | | Not dry | | Do not know | | | | p-value $\chi^2$-test |
|---|---|---|---|---|---|---|---|---|---|---|---|
| Before | 5 | 20% | 8 | 32% | 7 | 28% | 5 | 20% | | | 0.059 |
| After | 1 | 4% | 3 | 12% | 13 | 52% | 8 | 32% | | | |

| Itchiness n = 26 | Itchy to the point it is not possible to refrain from scratching | | Notice scratching unconsciously | | Scratch slightly here and there | | Scratch slightly but can refrain from scratching | | Feel no itch | | p-value $\chi^2$-test |
|---|---|---|---|---|---|---|---|---|---|---|---|
| Before | 5 | 19% | 10 | 38% | 5 | 19% | 5 | 19% | 1 | 4% | 0.033 |
| After | 1 | 4% | 4 | 15% | 10 | 38% | 5 | 19% | 6 | 23% | |

**Table 4.** Correlation between skin findings, amount of colonization of the total *Malassezia* and total bacteria, and quality of life score.

| | | Skin findings | | | | Level of colonization | | Quality of life score | | | |
|---|---|---|---|---|---|---|---|---|---|---|---|
| | | Scale-Desquamation | Itching | Excoriation | Erythema | Total Malassezia | Total Bacteria | Symptoms | Emotions | Functioning | Global |
| Dryness | r | 0.55 | 0.48 | 0.48 | 0.42 | −0.44 | 0.03 | 0.57 | 0.20 | 0.19 | 0.40 |
| | p | 0.002 | 0.008 | 0.007 | 0.020 | 0.015 | 0.859 | 0.001 | 0.307 | 0.336 | 0.030 |
| | n | 30 | 30 | 30 | 30 | 30 | 30 | 29 | 29 | 29 | 29 |
| Scale-Desquamation | r | — | 0.02 | 0.16 | 0.18 | −0.58 | −0.15 | 0.34 | 0.34 | 0.26 | 0.38 |
| | p | — | 0.901 | 0.405 | 0.335 | 0.001 | 0.423 | 0.069 | 0.071 | 0.173 | 0.044 |
| | n | — | 30 | 30 | 30 | 30 | 30 | 29 | 29 | 29 | 29 |
| Itching | r | — | — | 0.83 | 0.45 | 0.15 | 0.19 | 0.36 | 0.09 | 0.12 | 0.24 |
| | p | — | — | 0.000 | 0.013 | 0.417 | 0.305 | 0.055 | 0.647 | 0.528 | 0.203 |
| | n | — | — | 30 | 30 | 30 | 30 | 29 | 29 | 29 | 29 |
| Excoriation | r | — | — | — | 0.47 | 0.17 | 0.40 | 0.29 | 0.06 | 0.18 | 0.24 |
| | p | — | — | — | 0.009 | 0.358 | 0.027 | 0.120 | 0.749 | 0.349 | 0.203 |
| | n | — | — | — | 30 | 30 | 30 | 29 | 29 | 29 | 29 |
| Erythema | r | — | — | — | — | −0.18 | 0.05 | 0.31 | −0.02 | −0.07 | 0.03 |
| | p | — | — | — | — | 0.341 | 0.803 | 0.100 | 0.904 | 0.706 | 0.861 |
| | n | — | — | — | — | 30 | 30 | 29 | 29 | 29 | 29 |

**Table 5.** Correlations between skin findings.

| | | Skin findings | | | |
|---|---|---|---|---|---|
| | | ΔScale-Desquamation | ΔItching | ΔExcoriation | ΔErythema |
| ΔDryness | r | 0.40 | 0.50 | 0.44 | 0.40 |
| | p | 0.045 | 0.009 | 0.026 | 0.045 |
| | n | 26 | 26 | 26 | 26 |
| ΔScale-Desquamation | r | — | 0.09 | 0.02 | 0.24 |
| | p | — | 0.662 | 0.915 | 0.239 |
| | n | — | 26 | 26 | 26 |
| ΔItching | r | — | — | 0.48 | 0.28 |
| | p | — | — | 0.013 | 0.164 |
| | n | — | — | 26 | 26 |
| ΔExcoriation | r | — | — | — | 0.21 |
| | p | — | — | — | 0.303 |
| | n | — | — | — | 26 |

is effective.

The "dryness" score of the scalp at the start of the testing period had a positive correlation with all other symptomatic scores, indicating that the level of dryness was associated with a variety of other symptoms; it can be surmised that dry symptom improvement is important for scalp care. This is also supported by the fact that the "Δdryness" had a positive correlation with the amount of change in all observation item scores from the start to the end of the testing period.

Seborrheic dermatitis has a negative effect on patients' QOL [6]. The fact that the "dryness" score was negatively correlated with the level of *Malassezia* colonization indicates that *Malassezia* prefers areas where the skin is moist and has a large quantity of sebum, and that it finds it difficult to multiply on a dry scalp. Although there was some concern that moisturizing a dry scalp may lead to bacterial multiplication, the quantities of *Malassezia* and bacteria decreased significantly at the end of the testing period. Moisturizing the dry scalp and washing the hair with a suitable shampoo resulted in a decrease in colonization by *Malassezia* and bacteria, which use sebum as their source of nutrition and produce decomposition products such as free fatty acids, possibly contributing to the improvement of symptoms such as erythema.

In conclusion, using a moisturizing lotion for dry scalp, washing hair with a shampoo and conditioner that cause low levels of irritation, and providing instructions on a hair washing method that avoids irritation led to the improvement of the scalp condition and to improved QOL and patient satisfaction. Adherence to the treatment of underlying ailments is therefore expected to improve by providing appropriate skin care to patients who have dry scalp symptoms.

## Declaration of Interest

All expenses, as well as documents required, were provided for by Tokiwa Pharmaceutical Co., Ltd.

## References

[1]    Ebling, F.J. (1965) The Sebaceous Glands. *Journal of the Society of Cosmetic Chemists*, **16**, 405-411.

[2]    Tajima, M., Sugita, T., Nishikawa, A. and Tsuboi, R. (2008) Molecular Analysis of *Malassezia microflora* in Seborrheic Dermatitis Patients: Comparison with Other Diseases and Healthy Subjects. *Journal of Investigative Dermatology*, **128**, 345-351.

[3]    Sugita, T., Tajima, M., Tsubuku, H., Tsuboi, R. and Nishikawa, A. (2006) Quantitative Analysis of Cutaneous Malassezia in Atopic Dermatitis Patients Using Real-Time PCR. *Microbiology and Immunology*, **50**, 549-552. http://dx.doi.org/10.1111/j.1348-0421.2006.tb03825.x

[4]    Gao, Z., Perez-Perez, G.I., Chen, Y. and Blaser, M.J. (2010) Quantitation of Major Human Cutaneous Bacterial and Fungal Populations. *Journal of Clinical Microbiology*, **48**, 3575-3581. http://dx.doi.org/10.1128/JCM.00597-10

[5]    Higaki, Y., Kawamoto, K., Kamo, T., Horikawa, N., Kawashima, M. and Chren, M.M. (2002) The Japanese Version of Skindex-16: A Brief Quality-of-Life Measure for Patients with Skin Diseases. *The Journal of Dermatology*, **29**, 693-698. http://dx.doi.org/10.1111/j.1346-8138.2002.tb00205.x

[6]    Szepietowski, J.C., Reich, A., Wesolowska-Szepietowska, E., Baran, E. and National Quality of Life in Dermatology Group (2009) Quality of Life in Patients Suffering from Seborrheic Dermatitis: Influence of Age, Gender and Education Level. *Mycoses*, **52**, 357-363. http://dx.doi.org/10.1111/j.1439-0507.2008.01624.x

# 23

# Assessing the Effects of a Health Belief Model-Based Educational Program on Knowledge Attitudes and Practice (KAP) among Patients with *Pemphigus vulgaris*

**Roya Sadeghi[1], Azar Tol[1], Masoud Baikpour[2], Azita Moradi[1], Mostafa Hossaini[3]***

[1]Deptartment of Education and promotion, School of Public Health, Tehran University of Medical Sciences, Tehran, Iran
[2]School of Medicine, Tehran University of Medical Sciences, Tehran, Iran
[3]Department of Epidemiology and Biostatistics, School of Public Health, Tehran University of Medical Sciences, Tehran, Iran
Email: *mhossein110@yahoo.com

## Abstract

**Introduction:** This study aimed to evaluate the effects of an educational program based on Health Belief Model on knowledge, attitudes and practice (KAP) in patients with *Pemphigus vulgaris* (PV) referred to Razi Hospital in Iran. **Materials and Methods:** This quasi-experimental study was conducted on 88 patients in 2013-2014. Subjects were divided into two intervention and control groups using block randomization. In addition to their usual care for both groups, the intervention group sat through a six-month self-care educational program in a specialized outpatient clinic. A self-designed questionnaire was used to gather information about demographic characteristics, PV related variables, and KAP-related questions. Data were analyzed using SPSS Software. p value of less than 0.05 was set as statistically significant. **Results:** mean scores of KAP increased significantly after intervention compared to control groups when adjusted for baseline differences of these scores and house ownership and employment status differences in two groups. **Conclusion:** study results show the effectiveness of an HBM based educational program on KAP in PV patients that can lead to adoption of self care behaviors and help them gain self efficacy in controlling their disease and assisting their treatment process, counting as a tertiary preventive measure.

## Keywords

KAP, HBM, Intervention, *Pemphigus vulgaris*

---

*Corresponding author.

# 1. Introduction

Categorized as one of the immunobullous diseases, pemphigus is characterized by widespread blistering and erosions affecting the skin and mucous membranes [1]. Of the six recognized variants of Pemphigus, *Pemphigus vulgaris* (PV) has the greatest prevalence [2]. The incidence of this disease varies from one to five cases per 1 million population per year but it is increased in patients of Ashkenazi Jewish descent and those of some Eastern countries including India, Malaysia, China, and Japan [1] [2]. As well as other parts of the world, PV is the most prevalent variant in Iran with prevalence rates of 0.64 - $1.5/10^5$ population/year, reported by some sporadic researches [3]-[5]. In a study conducted by Pemphigus Research Unit in Razi Hospital, a dermatology referral center in Tehran, Iran, its prevalence was reported to be approximately 1 per $10^5$ population per year [6]. Studies have shown differences in onset, occurrence and prognosis of the disease regarding age and gender in PV patients. Current evidence shows an earlier onset of the disease in Iran compared to other parts of the world [3]-[5]. As for the gender females are reported to be at greater risks of PV disease [3]-[7], strong evidence suggests that according to inadequate preventive measures for chronic diseases such as PV in routine clinical practice, patients could benefit from substitute measures such as self-care behaviour programs to limit the risk of recurrence. Adopting self care behaviours by the patients suffering from chronic conditions is very important since such diseases are basically managed by the patients themselves. Regarding the late onset of PV in the fourth decade of life along with other chronic diseases, the necessity of self-care behaviour is more prominent [8]. Therefore, the importance of employing self-care behaviours is emphasized by the guidelines of PV management, as well as other points such as the significance of medical regimen for symptomatic treatments, dealing with side effects of the medications and adherence to suggested dietary changes such as avoiding nuts and spicy foods containing garlic, onion or leek. Regarding the bulbous nature of PV, paying special attention to wound healing process, prevention and treatment of infection is of utmost importance [9]. Psychological stress is another important subject that should be considered in the management of this disease [10]. Health professionals are challenged to publicize the best of what is known in new conditions. Given a new condition or problem, health professionals are obligated to apply the best of what is known in their practice. The topic of implementing Health Behavior and Health Education in clinical practice is a dynamic argument among researchers trying to yield effective health education [11]. Health Belief Model (HBM), the theoretical framework applied in this study, is used to assess the patients' motivation to adapt to a health related behavior [11]. The impact of educational programs on self-care behaviour modifications in some chronic diseases is confirmed in existing literature [12]-[14]. This study aimed to evaluate the impact of an HBM based interventional program on the knowledge, attitudes and practice of the patients with pemphigus Vulgaris, referred to Razi Hospital in Tehran, Iran.

# 2. Patients and Methods

Approved by the Educational Deputy of Tehran University of Medical Sciences, the present study was a randomized educational intervention trial carried out in 2013-2014. The inclusion criteria for the study population included confirmed PV diagnosis through skin biopsy, being diagnosed with the disease for at least 6 months and tendency to participate in the study. The exclusion criteria were being unable to attend the educational program or missing one fourth of the planned sessions. 88 eligible patients with PV participated as intervention or control groups. The objectives of the study were clearly explained to them in their first visit to the dermatology center. Patients were invited to join group meetings in the center where they were asked queries about the study, gave verbal informed consent, provided baseline data and were divided randomly to two groups of intervention and control. The random allocation sort was performed using randomization block of size four. The subjects in intervention group were assigned to participate in a 6-month educational program including group discussions and problem solving strategies based on Health Belief Model to adopt self-care behaviors. The control group did not receive any further intervention more than that of the routine treatment plan of the center. At the start of study and three months after the last session of the self-care educational program, data were collected from patients in both groups.

The self-designed questionnaire comprised of two sections: First, demographic characteristics and PV related variables (14 items) including age, gender, level of education, family income, occupation, smoking, the time of disease incidence and recurrence, history of surgery and disease duration; Second, KAP including 22 items assessing knowledge, 10 items assessing attitudes based on 5-point Likert scale (completely disagree = 1 to completely agree = 5) and 10 items for practice whose score was based on a 4-point Likert scale (not at all = 1 to always = 4), ranging from 10 to 40. Higher score means higher tendency to adopt healthy practices. Cronbach's Alpha was computed for knowledge, attitude and practice and were 0.93, 0.93 and 0.91, respectively. The PV self-care educational program was instructed by one of the researchers aware of the health education models.

The educational program comprised of six group discussion and problem solving sessions focusing on self-care measures for the disease. The patient and the educator assessed the basic information in the initial session, to classify the patient's problems in order to find areas demanding more enforcement, and also to set goals. On the other five sessions materials based on HBM constructs were covered [11]. The program lasted 2 months. After intervention stage and filling the related questionnaire, patients had three months to get prepared for changing primary behaviors and trying to adopt self-care behaviors to promote their lifestyles. After three months, patients filled out the questionnaire again. This program aimed to help patients solve their self-care issues, to show the significance of self-care behaviors, to set up steps to reach the goals and also to enhance general knowledge about PV self-care measures. It should be mentioned that in this trial we did not change the medical treatment of the patients. Educational topics were set by the HBM constructs according to each session. Patients in both groups filled out the questionnaires based on study timetable. Data analysis was performed using SPSS software version 20 via descriptive and inferential statistical tests. Socio-demographic and disease related variables were compared at baseline between the two groups. Using independent samples T-test and Chi Square test, we compared the means and proportions in the study groups. Ordinal variables were compared by Mann-Whitney U test and ANCOVA was utilized to compare the mean score of KAP components after intervention, adjusting for possible differences in their baseline values and those demographic characteristics with different distributions compared to the study groups. A p value of less than 0.05 was considered as statistically significant.

## 3. Results

Demographic characteristics of the patients according to intervention are shown in **Table 1**. The mean age of patients in intervention and control group were $52.6 \pm 11.0$ and $56.5 \pm 8.8$ years, respectively (p = 0.06). In randomization of the patients, 28 female and 16 male were assigned to intervention and 34 female and 10 male to control group (p = 0.16). In intervention group, 8 (18.2%) patients were single and 36 (81.2%) married. In control group, these were 15 (34.1%) and 29 (65.9%), respectively (p = 0.09). Further analysis showed that the distribution education level, PV duration, history of chronic disease and other skin disease in two study group was not significantly different at the baseline (p > 0.05) although house ownership and employment status of subjects in two group was not the same (p < 0.05).

The mean scores of knowledge, attitudes and practice before intervention and three months after that are shown in **Table 2**. The mean score of the knowledge in the intervention group was $13.1 \pm 3.6$ before the intervention which increased to $21.8 \pm 0.4$, three months after the intervention. This rise was from $9.2 \pm 2.9$ to $11.2 \pm 3.4$ in the control group. The increase in knowledge score was significantly higher in intervention group compared with control group after adjusting for the significant difference of these scores at the baseline and also for the differences in house ownership and employment status in the two groups using ANCOVA (p < 0.0001).

Attitude's scores showed similar trends. The mean score of intervention group rose from $40.4 \pm 5.4$ to $44.0 \pm 3.8$ and in control group only from $34.5 \pm 4.8$ to $36.4 \pm 3.8$. Using ANCOVA and adjusting for the effect of baseline differences in attitude's scores, house ownership and employment the changes in intervention group was significant. As for the scores of the practice, it changed from $31.9 \pm 5.8$ to $37.8 \pm 2.6$ after intervention although the change in control group was from $25.9 \pm 4.6$ to $29.1 \pm 3.5$. The change in intervention group was significant after adjustment (ANCOVA; p < 0.0001).

## 4. Discussion

As shown scores of knowledge, attitude and practice showed promising changes after the intervention. The scores of knowledge and attitudes increased after the intervention in both groups of intervention and control, but the rise was greater in the intervention group. This indicates the positive effect of HBM based educational intervention on the patients' knowledge and attitudes regarding their disease. Namakin *et al.* investigated the impact of HBM based educational intervention on smoking habits of students in Birjand in 2005 [15]. Their results also showed the improvement of knowledge and attitude in these students, after this intervention. In another survey by Karimi *et al.* on the effect of HBM based educational intervention on adopting preventive behaviors to avoid

**Table 1.** Demographic characteristics of patients according to intervention.

| Demographic characteristics | | Intervention | | Controls | | p value |
|---|---|---|---|---|---|---|
| | | No | Percent (%) | No | Percent (%) | |
| Age | <50 yr | 19 | 43.2 | 13 | 29.5 | |
| | 50 - 59 yr | 16 | 36.4 | 13 | 27.3 | |
| | 60 - 69 yr | 6 | 13.6 | 17 | 38.6 | 0.06[*] |
| | ≥70 yr | 3 | 6.8 | 2 | 4.6 | |
| | Mean (±SD) | 52.6 ± 11.0 yr | | 56.5 ± 8.8 yr | | |
| Gender | Female | 28 | 63.6 | 24 | 72.3 | 0.16[**] |
| | Male | 16 | 36.4 | 10 | 22.7 | |
| Marital status | Single | 8 | 18.2 | 15 | 34.1 | 0.09[**] |
| | Married | 36 | 81.2 | 29 | 65.9 | |
| Education | Illiterate | 7 | 15.9 | 10 | 22.7 | |
| | Elementary | 9 | 20.4 | 18 | 40.9 | |
| | Guidance | 13 | 29.6 | 3 | 6.8 | 0.13[*] |
| | High school & diploma | 10 | 22.7 | 8 | 18.2 | |
| | University | 5 | 11.4 | 5 | 11.4 | |
| Employment status | Employed | 15 | 34.1 | 12 | 27.3 | |
| | Retired/Not-employed | 10 | 22.7 | 22 | 50.0 | 0.0.2[*] |
| | Housewife | 19 | 43.2 | 10 | 22.7 | |
| Family history of pamfigus | Yes | 3 | 6.8 | 3 | 6.8 | >0.99[***] |
| | No | 41 | 93.2 | 41 | 93.2 | |
| History of other skin diseases | Yes | 9 | 20.4 | 7 | 15.9 | 0.58[*] |
| | No | 35 | 79.6 | 37 | 84.1 | |
| House ownership | Owned | 32 | 72.7 | 40 | 90.9 | |
| | Rented | 9 | 20.5 | 0 | 0.0 | 0.003[***] |
| | Lives with a other | 3 | 6.8 | 4 | 9.1 | |
| Duration | <2 years | 17 | 38.6 | 8 | 18.2 | |
| | 2 - 4 years | 12 | 27.3 | 10 | 22.7 | |
| | 5 - 10 years | 10 | 22.7 | 26 | 59.1 | 0.566[****] |
| | >10 years | 5 | 11.4 | 0 | 0.0 | |
| | Mean (±SD) | 4.7 ± 4.2 yr | | 5.1 ± 2.6 yr | | |

[*]Mann-Whitney U test; [**]Chi squared test; [***]Fisher exact test; [****]Independent sample T-test.

**Table 2.** Mean (±SD) of knowledge, attitude and practice before and after intervention.

| Components | Group | Before intervention | p[*] | After intervention | p[**] |
|---|---|---|---|---|---|
| | | Mean ± SD | | Mean ± SD | |
| Knowledge | Intervention | 13.1 ± 3.6 | <0.0001 | 21.8 ± 0.4 | <0.0001 |
| | Control | 9.2 ± 2.9 | | 11.2 ± 3.4 | |
| Attitude | Intervention | 40.4 ± 5.4 | <0.0001 | 44.0 ± 3.8 | <0.0001 |
| | Control | 34.5 ± 4.8 | | 36.4 ± 3.8 | |
| Practice | Intervention | 31.9 ± 5.8 | <0.0001 | 37.8 ± 2.6 | <0.0001 |
| | Control | 25.9 ± 4.6 | | 29.1 ± 3.5 | |

[*]Independent sample T-test at baseline; [**]ANCOVA after educational intervention adjusting for house ownership and employment status duration and house ownership.

AIDS in 2009, the same results were obtained showing the positive influence of the intervention on knowledge and attitude of the subjects [16].

The intervention in our study also caused the patients to act as they learned. The practice score increased after the intervention. The study conducted by Rahnavard *et al.* on the changes in smoking habits in female adolescents after an HBM based educational intervention in 2011, also revealed the positive change in practice among the subjects [17].

Shakerinejad *et al.* evaluated the impact of an HBM based education on KAP variables in adolescent girls about dietary calcium in 2011. They also observed statistically significant improvements in the scores of these variables [18]. In another study investigating the effect of an HBM based educational program about gastric cancer on knowledge, attitude and practice of housewives in 2012 by Alidosti *et al.* the results showed patterns of improved KAP variables in subjects compatible with our results [19].

Effects of an HBM based education program on screening behavior in high risk women for breast cancer were assessed in a study conducted by Hajian *et al.* in 2011. After the educational sessions they found elevated rates of breast self examination and clinical examination due to increased scores of knowledge, attitude and practice of the patients [20].

Mahmoodi *et al.* also verified these findings by inspecting the changes in KAP scores after an HBM based educational program regarding osteoporosis prevention in women with low socioeconomic status in 2011 [21]. Knowledge, attitude and practice of the pharmaceutical industry employees in Tehran concerning breast cancer and the benefits of mammography were found to be improving after an educational program based on health belief model in a study conducted by Hatefnia *et al.* in 2010 [22].

In another survey, Goodarzi *et al.* assessed the impact of distance education via mobile phone text messaging on knowledge, attitude, practice and self efficacy of patients with type 2 diabetes mellitus in Iran. Their results also showed improvements in these variables confirming the effect of education via any means on improving knowledge, attitudes and practice of the patients [23]. As can be seen, all of the studies conducted to investigate the effects of education programs based on health belief model on knowledge, attitude and practice of the subjects, yield similar results, showing improvements in these variables after educating the patients. As discussed before, many studies have evaluated the effects of educational programs on promoting self care behaviors, but no similar study have investigated this effect in PV patients, so we used a unique study population for our survey. Regarding the low prevalence of PV in Iran, finding these many patients was a great challenge for our survey, so selecting Razi hospital as our research department was one of the strengths of this study, since it is a dermatology referral center. Applying more interactive educational methods such as group discussion and problem solving that are believed to be more effective than lecturing method, was another positive aspect in our survey. Not being able to directly observe the changes in the behaviors of our patients can be mentioned as an important limitation in our study, since our data are basically subjective and given to us by the subjects, so they might differ from the reality.

## 5. Conclusion

This study shows the effectiveness of an HBM based educational program on the patients' knowledge, attitudes and practice regarding their disease. This improvement can lead to adoption of self care behaviors and help them achieve self efficacy in controlling their disease and assisting their treatment process, counting as a tertiary preventive measure. As stated above according to inadequate preventive measures for chronic diseases such as PV in routine clinical practice, self-care behaviour programs are viable substitute choices for helping these patients. The management of chronic conditions is generally based on the patient adopting self care behaviors and based on the late onset of PV in the fourth decade of life and concurrence of other chronic diseases during this period, the necessity of self-care behavior is more eminent. So as shown in this article, educational interventions can be utilized to enhance the knowledge of these patients as well as their attitudes and their practice.

## Acknowledgements

The authors appreciatively thank all the personnel of Pemphigus Research Unit of Razi hospital, since this study could not have been carried out without their cooperation. Tehran University of Medical Sciences supported this survey as a part of MSPH thesis.

## References

[1]   Burns, T., Breathnach, S., Cox, N. and Griffiths, C. (2010) Rook's Textbook of Dermatology, 4 Volume Set. John Wiley & Sons, Hoboken.

[2]   Joly, P. and Litrowski, N. (2011) Pemphigus Group (Vulgaris, Vegetans, Foliaceus, Herpetiformis, Brasiliensis). *Clin-*

*ics in Dermatology*, **29**, 432-436. http://dx.doi.org/10.1016/j.clindermatol.2011.01.013

[3] Salmanpour, R., Shahkar, H., Namazi, M. and Rahman-Shenas, M. (2006) Epidemiology of Pemphigus in South-Western Iran: A 10-Year Retrospective Study (1991-2000). *International Journal of Dermatology*, **45**, 103-105. http://dx.doi.org/10.1111/j.1365-4632.2004.02374.x

[4] Ali, A., Ali Reza, Y. and Gita, F. (2006) *Pemphigus vulgaris* in Iran: Epidemiology and Clinical Profile. *SKINmed: Dermatology for the Clinician*, **5**, 69-71. http://dx.doi.org/10.1111/j.1540-9740.2006.03756.x

[5] Javidi, Z., Meibodi, N.T. and Nahidi, Y. (2007) Epidemiology of Pemphigus in Northeast Iran: A 10-Year Retrospective Study. *Indian Journal of Dermatology*, **52**, 188-191.

[6] Chams-Davatchi, C., Valikhani, M., Daneshpazhooh, M., Esmaili, N., Balighi, K., Hallaji, Z., *et al.* (2005) Pemphigus: Analysis of 1209 Cases. *International Journal of Dermatology*, **44**, 470-476. http://dx.doi.org/10.1111/j.1365-4632.2004.02501.x

[7] Chmurova, N. and Svecova, D. (2009) *Pemphigus vulgaris*: A 11-Year Review. *Bratisl Lek Listy*, **110**, 500-503.

[8] Ruocco, E., Wolf, R., Ruocco, V., Brunetti, G., Romano, F. and Lo Schiavo, A. (2013) Pemphigus: Associations and Management Guidelines: Facts and Controversies. *Clinics in Dermatology*, **31**, 382-390. http://dx.doi.org/10.1016/j.clindermatol.2013.01.005

[9] Pemphigus (2013) http://www.pemphigus.org/index.php

[10] Picardi, A. and Abeni, D. (2001) Stressful Life Events and Skin Diseases: Disentangling Evidence from Myth. *Psychotherapy and Psychosomatics*, **70**, 118-136. http://dx.doi.org/10.1159/000056237

[11] Glanz, K., Rimer, B.K. and Viswanath, K. (2008) Health Behavior and Health Education: Theory, Research, and Practice. John Wiley & Sons, Hoboken.

[12] Sharifirad, G., Entezari, M.H., Kamran, A. and Azadbakht, L. (2009) The Effectiveness of Nutritional Education on the Knowledge of Diabetic Patients Using the Health Belief Model. *Journal of Research in Medical Sciences: The Official Journal of Isfahan University of Medical Sciences*, **14**, 1-6.

[13] Sharifirad, G.R., Tol, A., Mohebi, S., Matlabi, M., Shahnazi, H. and Shahsiah, M. (2013) The Effectiveness of Nutrition Education Program Based on Health Belief Model Compared with Traditional Training. *Journal of Education and Health Promotion*, **2**, 15.

[14] Tol, A., Shojaeezadeh, D., Sharifirad, G., Alhani, F. and Tehrani, M.M. (2012) Determination of Empowerment Score in Type 2 Diabetes Patients and Its Related Factors. *JPMA-Journal of the Pakistan Medical Association*, **62**, 16-20.

[15] Namakin, K., Sharifzadeh, G. and Miri, M. (2008) Prevalence of Cigarette Smoking and Evaluation of Attitude and Knowledge in Its High School Boys in Birjand, 2005. *Journal of Birjand University of Medical Sciences*, **15**, 66-70.

[16] Karimi Mahmoud, G.F. and Heydarnia, A.R. (2009) The Effect of Health Education Based on Health Belief Model on Preventive Actions of Aids on Addict in Zarandieh. *Journal of Guilan University of Medical Sciences*, **18**, 64-73.

[17] Rahnavard, Z., Mohammadi, M., Rajabi, F. and Zolfaghari, M. (2011) An Educational Intervention Using Health Belief Model on Smoking Preventive Behavior among Female Teenagers. *Hayat*, **17**, 15-26.

[18] Shakerinejad, G. (Ed.) (2011) Impact of Nutrition Education on Knowledge, Attitude and Practice of Adolescent Girls about Dietary Calcium According to Health Belief Model (HBM). *The 1st International & 4th National Congress on Health Education & Promotion*, 2011, 21.

[19] Alidosti, M., Sharifirad, G.R., Golshiri, P., Azadbakht, L., Hasanzadeh, A. and Hemati, Z. (2012) An Investigation on the Effect of Gastric Cancer Education Based on Health Belief Model on Knowledge, Attitude and Nutritional Practice of Housewives. *Iranian Journal of Nursing and Midwifery Research*, **17**, 256-262.

[20] Hajian, S., Vakilian, K., Najabadi, K.M., Hosseini, J. and Mirzaei, H.R. (2011) Effects of Education Based on the Health Belief Model on Screening Behavior in High Risk Women for Breast Cancer, Tehran, Iran. *Asian Pacific Journal of Cancer Prevention*, **12**, 49-54.

[21] Mahmoodi, M. and Salehi, L. (2011) To Evaluate of Efficacy of Education Based on Health Belief Model on Knowledge, Attitude and Practice among Women with Low Socioeconomic Status Regarding Osteoporosis Prevention. *Iranian Journal of Epidemiology*, **7**, 30-37.

[22] Hatefnia, E., Niknami, S., Mahmoudi, M., Ghofranipour, F. and Lamyian, M. (2010) The Effects of Health Belief Model Education on Knowledge, Attitude and Behavior of Tehran Pharmaceutical Industry Employees Regarding Breast Cancer and Mammography. *Journal of Kermanshah University of Medical Sciences*, **14**, 42-53.

[23] Goodarzi, M., Ebrahimzadeh, I., Rabi, A., Saedipoor, B. and Jafarabadi, M.A. (2012) Impact of Distance Education via Mobile Phone Text Messaging on Knowledge, Attitude, Practice and Self Efficacy of Patients with Type 2 Diabetes Mellitus in Iran. *Journal of Diabetes & Metabolic Disorders*, **11**, 10.

# 24

# Product Containing "Skin Calm Complex" Improves Barrier Effect *in Vitro*

**María Matabuena-de Yzaguirre[1], Gabriela Bacchini[2], Eva Vila-Martínez[2], Ángeles Juarranz[1]**

[1]Department of Biology, Faculty of Sciences, Universidad Autónoma de Madrid, Madrid, Spain
[2]Medical Department, Ferrer Health Care, Barcelona, Spain
Email: maria.matabuena@uam.es

## Abstract

Epidermal Barrier integrity is deteriorated in many skin conditions, including Atopic Dermatitis, and could be responsible for many of the associated clinical symptoms. The aim of this study was to determine the effect of REPAVAR ATOPIC SKIN BODY CREAM EXTREME, product containing "SKIN CALM COMPLEX" on barrier epidermis structure. Morphologic and structural evaluations were conducted on reconstructed human epidermis, by qualitative (hematoxylin/eosin- and immune-staining) and quantitative (MTT assay) techniques. Immature (Age Day 10) and mature (Day 17) sample tissues were treated with the product for 24 hours or 7 days, respectively. Morphological and quantitative analysis revealed an increase in the thickness of the epidermis in both cases after the treatment. The study by immunostaining showed that Product-treated tissues presented excellent localization of: 1) E-cadherin in keratinocytes of the spinous layer; 2) Filaggrin and Loricrin, in the granular layer; and 3) increased expression of Involucrin and Keratin 10 in suprabasal layers and 4) elevated expression of Keratin 5 in the basal layer of the epidermis. The product REPAVAR ATOPIC SKIN BODY CREAM EXTREME increases the epithelial regeneration and differentiation determined by cell proliferation and the expression and localization of specific proteins, improving the epidermal barrier effect.

## Keywords

Atopic Dermatitis, Epidermal Barrier, Epithelial Regeneration and Differentiation

## 1. Introduction

Appropriate expression of proteins in epidermis is a basic condition for the formation of a competent epidermal barrier (EB). Keratinocytes undergo different molecular changes during the transition from the basal layer into the spinous layer, the granular and finally to the stratum corneum. This process includes the synthesis of basal (K5 and K14) and suprabasal keratins (K1 and K10).

Different proteins, such as filagrin, loricrin, trichohyalin, small proline-rich proteins, involucrine and keratines, are located in the cornified cell envelop and are cross-linked by the action of different transglutaminases [1]-[5]. In order to assure an optimal structure and function of epidermis, it is important that both differentiation and proliferation of keratinocytes are well balanced. Variations in these processes, as well as genetic abnormalities in the genes encoding proteins of the cornified cell envelop components can lead to an abnormal keratinization, which is typical from certain skin conditions, like Atopic Dermatitis [6]-[8].

Human skin models (*in vivo* studies) are the best way to analyze the main functions of skin, including the EB structure. However, the studies in human volunteers have major limitations to evaluate EB such as analysis by biopsy, because there is no ethic in humans. For this reason indirect parameters are evaluated (transepidermal water loss, skin capacitance, erythema, skyn surface analysis and/or SCORAD) [9]-[15] instead of localization and expression of proteins. Furthermore, other drawbacks including the genetic variation among individuals, can lean to different effects of environmental factors on individuals from the same population [2] [16]-[20], and of course the number of volunteers needed to obtain significant results [21].

There is a considerable amount of new topical products on the market aimed to improve or to relieve certain symptoms associated to skin diseases like the EB in Atopic Dermatitis [9] [11]-[15] [18] [22]-[25]. Many of them are formulated with different active substances which have been analyzed by *in vitro* approaches or in animal models [22] [25]-[32], but not in the pool of ingredients of the final product. This is important because of the complexity of the formulas, where ingredients of different mechanism of action can overlap and do not give significant results [22].

Nowadays, *in vitro* models are important tools for the evaluation of safety and efficacy of topical or dermatological products [33]. A reconstructed skin model should show protective barrier function and the same behavior to environmental contaminants. In this context, validated models that show a structure similar to human skin, with proliferative basal layer, spinous, granular and cornified layer and also similar expression and distribution of structural proteins such as keratins, constitute an excellent tool for studying the effects on the structure and function of different agents, chemicals or physicals [34]. This fact allows quantification measures out of direct parameters, like localization and protein expression or regeneration levels.

The aim of this work was to demonstrate that the product REPAVAR ATOPIC SKIN BODY CREAM EXTREME, containing "SKIN CALM COMPLEX", mix of scientifically tested efficacy actives, improves EB at structural level.

## 2. Methods

### 2.1. *In Vitro* Model

*In vitro* Reconstructed Human Epidermis of 0.33 cm$^2$, Age Day 10 (12 samples) or Age Day 17 (12 samples), produced by Skin Ethic laboratories (Nice, France) were used. The tissues were cultured and kept in chemically defined medium, provided by the same laboratory, during the assays. Tissue cultures were performed in an incubator with 5% of $CO_2$ at 37°C. The tissue manipulation process was carried out in sterile conditions.

### 2.2. Treatments

4 samples per group were used, 1) negative control (Skin Ethic Maintenance Medium-Skin Ethic laboratories, Nice, France), 2) positive control of proliferation and differentiation treatment with 100 nM Vitamin D (1,25-dihidroxivitamina D3) (Sigma, St. Louis, MO) [35]-[37], diluted in maintenance medium for 24 hours or 7 days and 3) Product, REPAVAR ATOPIC SKIN BODY CREAM EXTREME, applied topically to the epithelium (enough to cover the tissue).

Immature tissues (Age Day 10) were treated for 7 days (7 days-treatment) and the mature tissues were treated for 24 hours (24 hours-treatment).

### 2.3. Histological Processing

Samples (3 negative controls, 3 positive controls and 3 treated tissues, for 24 hours or 7 days of treatment) were fixed by immersion in 3.7% formaldehyde (Panreac, Barcelona, Spain) in phosphate buffered saline (PBS) (HyClone Laboratories, Inc., South Logan, UT) for 12 hours at 4°C. Subsequently, they were washed and dried in increasing ethanol (Panreac, Barcelona, Spain) series before inclusion in paraffin. Finally, histological sections (4 μm thickness) were placed on electrostatically charged slides (Superfrost® Plus) (Menzel-Gläser, Braunschweig, Germany).

## 2.4. Hematoxylin-Eosin- and Inmuno-Staining

For morphological evaluation, sections were deparaffinized for 15 minutes in xylene (Panreac, Barcelona, Spain), and hydrated in decreasing ethanol series and washed with distilled water. All samples were stained with hematoxylin/eosin (H&E), according to standard protocols, and examined under the microscope (Olympus BX61 coupled to a digital camera Olympus DP50).

For inmunostaining, sections were deparaffinized, hydrated and washed with distilled water. Inhibition of endogenous peroxidase was carried out with hydrogen peroxide (Panreac, Barcelona, Spain) at 3% in methanol (Panreac, Barcelona, Spain). Afterwards, the sections were washed with PBS. Next, antigen retrieval was performed in citrate buffer at pH 6 (0.25% citric acid and 0.038% sodium citrate in water). Sections were blocked with non-immune serum and incubated with the primary antibody against the proteins under study, anti-E-cadherin (BD Transduction Laboratories, Franklin Lakes, NJ), anti-Involucin, anti-Loricrin and anti-Filagrin (Sigma, St. Louis, MO), anti-Keratin-10 (Dako, Glostrup, Denmark) and anti-Keratin-5 (Abcam, Cambridge, UK) overnight. For immnunohistochemistry (IHQ), the excess primary antibody was washed with PBS and sections were incubated with biotinylated antiserum for 25 minutes at room temperature with streptavidin-peroxidase, developed with diaminobenzidine and counterstained with Harris hematoxylin for nuclear contrast. The processing for immunofluorescence (IF), sections were incubated with corresponding secondary antibody, mounted with ProLong® Gold Natifade Reagent (Invitrogen, Frederick, MD) with DAPI for nuclear contrast and observed under the fluorescence microscope.

## 2.5. MTT Assay

Cellular proliferation was assessed by MTT (3-[4,5-dimethylthiazol-2-yl]-2,5-diphenyl-2H-tetrazolium bromide) assay (Sigma, St. Louis, MO), a method based on the activity of mitochondrial dehydrogenases [38]. Stock solution of MTT (5 mg/ml) in PBS, was diluted (1 mg/ml) in Skinethic culture medium, and then the samples were incubated at 37°C, 5% $CO_2$, 95% humidified atmosphere, for 3 hours. The resulting formazan crystals were dissolved by the addition of isopropanol (Sigma, St. Louis, MO), at room temperature, for 2 hours with gentle agitation. Optical Densities (OD) were measured at 570 nm wavelength.

## 2.6. Optical Microscopy

Microscopic observations were carried out using an Olympus BX61 epifluorescence microscope equipped with filter sets for fluorescence microscopy: ultraviolet (UV, 365 nm, exciting filter UG-1), blue (450 - 490 nm, exciting filter BP 490), and green (545 nm, exciting filter BP 545). Photographs were obtained with the digital camera Olympus CCD DP70 and processed using the Adobe PhotoShop CS5 extended version 12.0 software (Adobe Systems Inc., USA). The expression of some proteins was quantified using ImageJ 1.37v (http://rsb.info.nih.giv/ij). The relative fluorescence intensity was determined from, at least, 20 areas of 500 μm$^2$ for each treatment condition.

## 2.7. Statistical Analysis

The statistical analysis was performed using the SPSS 15.0, 1 software (SPSS Inc., Chicago, IL), using Student's t test and analysis of variance (ANOVA), and considering a $p < 0.05$ as statistically significant.

# 3. Results and Discussion

## 3.1. Morphological Analysis

**Figure 1** shows the morphological analysis, by hematoxylin-eosin staining, of the treated reconstructed epidermis (Vitamin D positive control group, product REPAVAR ATOPIC SKIN BODY CREAM EXTREME) and untreated epidermis (negative control) for 1 or 7 days.

Tissue samples, in all cases, showed a normal stratification, appreciating the different layers, basal (B), spinous

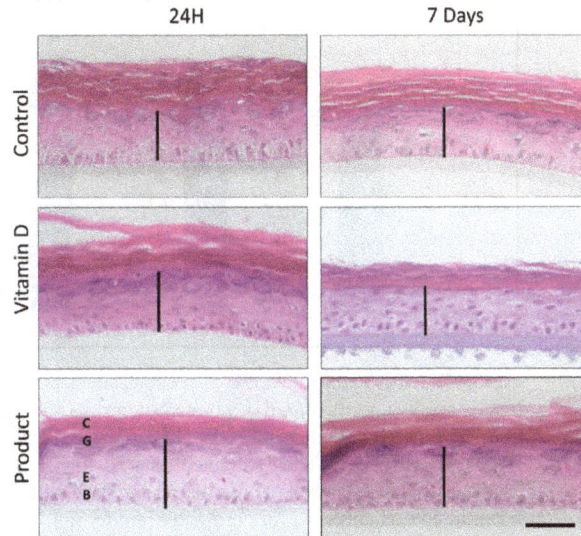

**Figure 1.** Histological sections of a representative reconstructed control (negative control), Vitamin D-treated (positive control) or REPAVAR ATOPIC SKIN BODY CREAM EXTREME-treated (product) epidermis for 24 hours (left panel) or 7 days (right panel), stained with H&E. All samples show a good arrangement of the layers: basal (B), spinous (S), granular (G) and cornified layer (C). Note the increased epidermal thickness in the treated group (Product). Scale bar: 50 μm.

(S), granular (G) and cornified (C). Similarly, in all cases, a good organization was observed in the different cell layers of the epidermis.

Interestingly, Vitamin D-treated epidermis as much as Product-treated tissues showed a thick increase compared to negative control, being greater in the case of Product treatments (24 hours and 7 days).

When assessing the epidermal thickness (cornified layer not included) by morphological evaluation, the results above described were confirmed. It is shown a statistically significant increase in the thickness of the epidermis treated for 24 hours ($p < 0.05$, Student t-test) (**Figure 2**).

All evaluations were carried out on immature (7 days-treatment) and mature tissues (24 hours-treatment) to confirm the effect of the product in both types of tissues but, because of thickness of cornified layer was smaller in all sections in immature epidermis, the analyses of this study were focused on mature epidermis treated for 24 hours (and non-treated).

All these results were confirmed by quantitative analysis. Product REPAVAR ATOPIC SKIN BODY CREAM EXTREME promotes an increase in epithelial proliferation of about 50% over the negative control (untreated tissue) and 30% more than Vitamin D, used as positive control (**Figure 3**).

## 3.2. Analysis of Protein Expression

The key proteins expression in organization and differentiation of epidermis was analyzed by IHC and immunofluorescence IF (**Figures 4-7**).

E-cadherin is a very important protein in epithelial cell organization, participating in cell-cell adhesion [5] [7]. The tissues treated for 24 h with Product show a good expression and localization of this protein on cell membrane, especially in the keratinocytes of the spinous layer and granulosum and lower in layer baseline (**Figure 4**). There were no differences in the amount of protein expression between the different sample groups, treated and controls.

An important protein which is frequently altered in Atopic Dermatitis and other skin conditions is Filaggrin [2] [39] [40]. This protein is produced from its precursor, the functionally inactive profilaggrin, which is proteolytically processed to Filaggrin during the transition from the granular layer of the cornified layer. Filaggrin is, therefore, an excellent marker of epidermal differentiation. **Figure 5** shows the high expression of this protein in

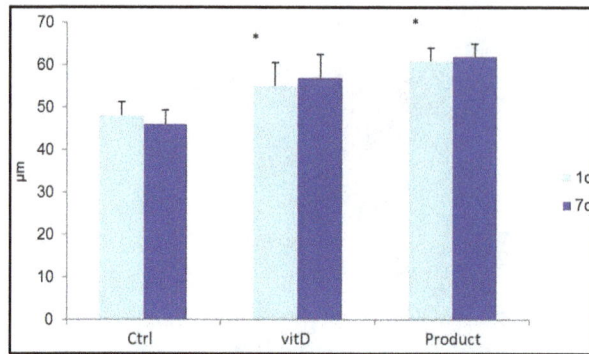

**Figure 2.** Measuring thickness of reconstructed epidermis: untreated tissues (control, Ctrl), positive control (Vitamin D, vit D-treated tissues, vit D) or Product (REPAVAR ATOPIC SKIN BODY CREAM EXTREME-treated tissues) for 24 hours (left) or 7 days (right). There is a significant increase of thickness in Vitamin D-treated and Product-treated epidermis for 24 hours ($p < 0.05$).

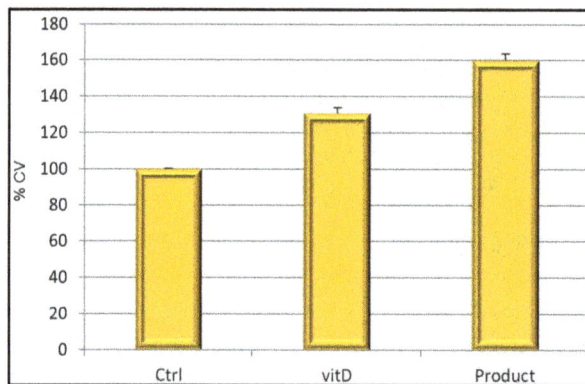

**Figure 3.** Cell viability (%) estimated by the MTT assay: untreated tissues (Ctrl), positive control (Vitamin D, vit D-treated tissues) or product (REPAVAR ATOPIC SKIN BODY CREAM EXTREME-treated tissues) for 24 hours. The Product-treated sample shows an increase in cell viability around 60%.

the keratinocytes located between the upper region of the granular layer, in contact with the keratin layer, in the reconstituted epidermis exposed to Vitamin D and Product, with a more precise localization, in both epidermis in relation to the untreated control, which is also located in spinous layer. This protein is not expressed in the *stratum corneum*. Greater thickness of Product-treated samples is noteworthy and good differentiation is shown by the marker Filaggrin.

Loricrin is the precursor protein of the *stratum corneum*, expressed mainly in the upper granular layer. Loricrin appears well defined and localized, with higher expression in Product-treated epidermis in relation to the Vitamin D-treated (positive control) for 24 hours and untreated (negative control) (**Figure 5**).

Involucrin expression was determinated by immunofluorescence, because no conclusions could be drawn by immunochemistry. A lower expression of the protein in the basal layer and a suitable location in suprabasal layers were detected in the case of Vitamin D-treated and Product-treated tissues (data not shown).

Finally the expression of two keratins, K10 and K5 were analyzed, by immunofluorescence. Keratin 10 (**Figure 6**) preferably located in the suprabasal layers. Meanwhile, keratin 5 (**Figure 7**) is preferentially expressed in the basal layer. The results show excellent labeling in all cases (treated and control samples) with Keratin 10, especially in Product-treated equivalents (**Figure 6(a)**). In this case, again, greater thickness is notable and good differentiation is shown by this new marker. Moreover, the measure of fluorescence intensity (**Figure 6(b)**) indicates a higher expression in suprabasal layers of treated epidermis compared to control

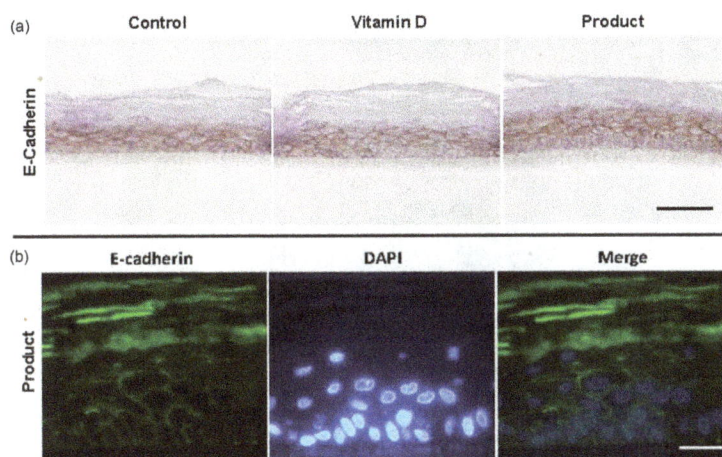

**Figure 4.** (a) Histological sections of representative reconstructed control (negative control), Vitamin D-treated (positive control) or REPAVAR ATOPIC SKIN BODY CREAM EXTREME-treated (Product) epidermis for 24 hours, and exposed to E-cadherin antibody for determination by immunohistochemistry. Scale bar: 50 μm; (b) Indirect immunofluorescence for the adhesion molecule E-cadherin in reconstituted REPAVAR ATOPIC SKIN BODY CREAM EXTREME-treated (Product) epidermis for 24 hours. Excellent membrane localization appreciated in spinous and cornified layers. In the basal layer is slightly lower. Scale bar: 25 μm.

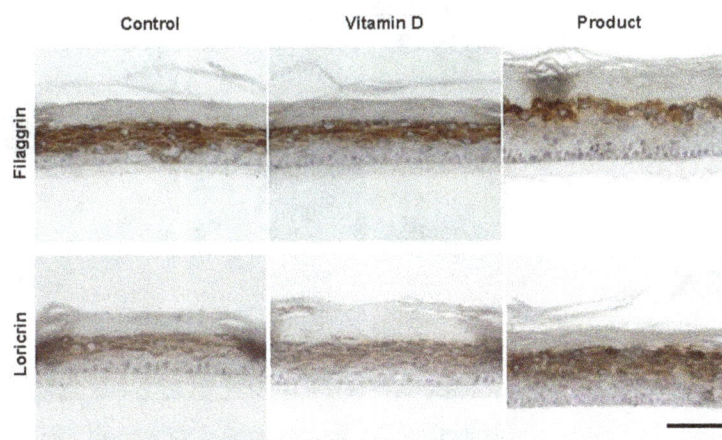

**Figure 5.** Immunohistochemistry for Filaggrin and Loricrin in representative reconstructed control (negative control), Vitamin D-treated (positive control) or REPAVAR ATOPIC SKIN BODY CREAM EXTREME-treated (Product) epidermis for 24 hours. An excellent location for all the proteins studied can be appreciated, both in positive control and Product-treated group. Scale bar: 50 μm.

samples. Keratin 5 (K5) analysis, by indirect immunofluorescence, revealed increased expression of this protein in the basal layer of both Vitamin D-treated and Product-treated epidermis. No striking differences were observed between Vitamin D and Product expression and localization.

All these results were confirmed after 7 days of treatment on immature (10 day aged) tissues.

Skincalm Complex® is a mix of scientifically tested efficacy actives that includes a skin-identicallipidic-complex (SK-influx®), γ linoleic acid (Railinol®), botanical hidrolized protein, pool of 7 botanical extracts, Di-hydroavenanthramide D and *Peumusboldus* extract. It restores EB [41] [42] and increases synthesis and functions of epidermal proteins [43].

Evaluating structural proteins involved in Atopic Dermatitis is not possible by human biopsy. For this reason

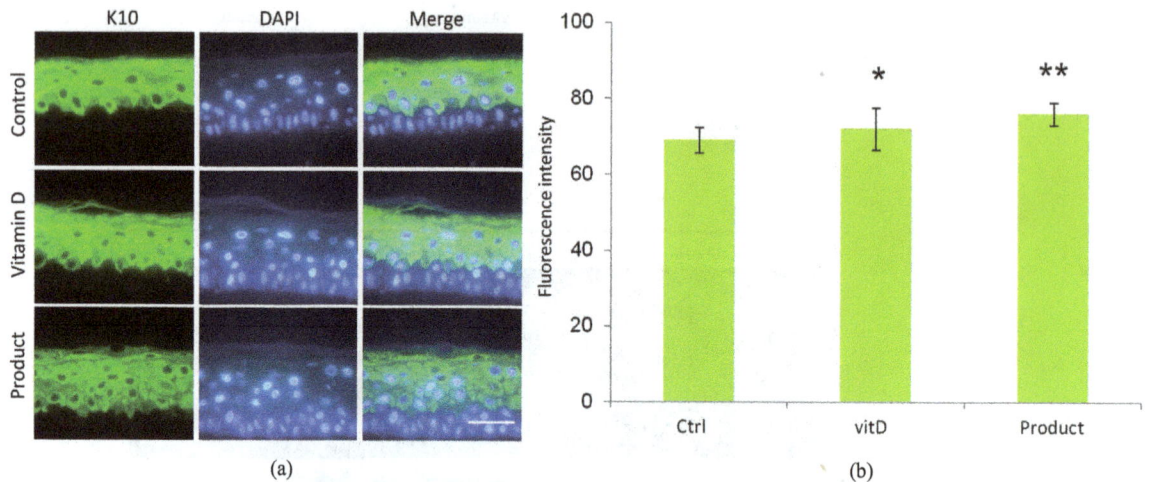

(a)                                                                    (b)

**Figure 6.** (a) K10 expression by indirect immunofluorescence in reconstructed normal, Vitamin D-treated (positive control) or REPAVAR ATOPIC SKIN BODY CREAM EXTREME-treated (Product) epidermis for 24 hours. It shows a greater thickening of the treated epidermis, especially the tissues exposure to product. Scale bar: 25 μm; (b) Quantification of K10 expression using imagenJ program. The differences are significant ($p < 0.05$), between Vitamin D-treated epidermis (positive control) and negative control, and between Product-treated epidermis and other groups.

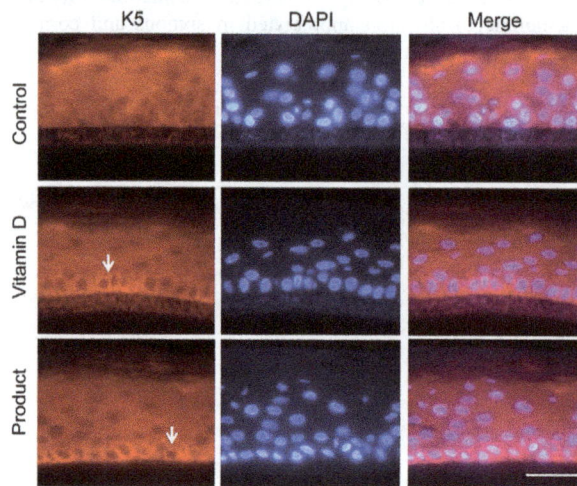

**Figure 7.** K5 expression by indirect immunofluorescence in reconstructed normal, Vitamin D-treated (positive control) or REPAVAR ATOPIC SKIN BODY CREAM EXTREME-treated (Product) epidermis for 24 hours. There is greater fluorescence intensity in the basal layer of the epidermis (white arrow) due to the increased expression of the protein in Vitamin D- (differentiation enhancer) or Product-treated epidermis, in relation to the untreated control. Scale bar 25 μm.

animal models are used. Nowadays, reconstructed human skin models allow this approach [34], representing a step forward in the evaluation of efficacy of human structural proteins involved in Atopic Dermatitis. The results obtained after treatment for 24 hours show that the product REPAVAR ATOPIC SKIN BODY CREAM EXTREME induces, compared to Vitamin D-treated and untreated tissues, 1) an excellent effect on the organization of the epidermal layers, showed in the histological sections stained with H/E; 2) enhances epidermal proliferation, showed in the increased thickness quantified by MTT assay; and, 3) promotes differentiation process, showed in the increased expression of the analyzed proteins Fillagrin, Loricrin and Keratins (10 and 5), and optimal distribution of all of them, as well as E-cadherin and Involucrin (by immunofluorescence or inmunochemistry analysis).

## 4. Conclusion

As a final conclusion, the study demonstrated that the product REPAVAR ATOPIC SKIN BODY CREAM

EXTREME is able to enhances skin regeneration, balancing both proliferation and differentiation of skin layers and thus, improving the epidermal barrier effect.

## References

[1] Alomar, A. (2008) Dermatitis atópica y alteración de proteínas estructurales. *Piel*, **23**, 159-161. http://dx.doi.org/10.1016/S0213-9251(08)71005-0

[2] Brown, S.J. and McLean, W.H. (2012) One Remarkable Molecule: Filaggrin. *Journal of Investigative Dermatology*, **132**, 751-762. http://dx.doi.org/10.1038/jid.2011.393

[3] Novak, N. and Leung, D.Y. (2011) Advances in Atopic Dermatitis. *Current Opinion in Immunology*, **3**, 778-783. http://dx.doi.org/10.1016/j.coi.2011.09.007

[4] Elias, P.M. (2010) Therapeutic Implications of a Barrier-Based Pathogenesis of Atopic Dermatitis. *Annals of Dermatology*, **22**, 245-254. http://dx.doi.org/10.5021/ad.2010.22.3.245

[5] Segre, J.A. (2006) Epidermal Barrier Formation and Recovery in Skin Disorders. *Journal of Clinical Investigation*, **116**, 1150-1158. http://dx.doi.org/10.1172/JCI28521

[6] Hara-Chikuma, M., Takahashi, K., Chikuma, S., Verkman, A.S. and Miyachi, Y. (2009) The Expression of Differentiation Markers in Aquaporin-3 Deficient Epidermis. *Archives of Dermatological Research*, **301**, 245-252. http://dx.doi.org/10.1007/s00403-009-0927-9

[7] Presland, R.B. and Dale, B.A. (2000) Epithelial Structural Proteins of the Skin and Oral Cavity: Function in Health and Disease. *Critical Reviews in Oral Biology Medicine*, **11**, 383-408. http://dx.doi.org/10.1177/10454411000110040101

[8] Rao, K.S., Babu, K.K. and Gupta, P.D. (1996) Keratins and Skin Disorders. *Cell Biology International*, **20**, 261-274. http://dx.doi.org/10.1006/cbir.1996.0030

[9] Breternitz, M., Kowatzki, D., Langenauer, M., Elsner, P. and Fluhr, J.W. (2008) Placebo-Controlled, Double-Blind, Randomized, Prospective Study of a Glycerol-Based Emollient on Eczematous Skin in Atopic Dermatitis: Biophysical and Clinical Evaluation. *Skin Pharmacology and Physiology*, **21**, 39-45. http://dx.doi.org/10.1159/000111134

[10] Solodkin, G., Chaudhari, U., Subramanyan, K., Johnson, A.W., Yan, X. and Gottlieb, A. (2006) Benefits of Mild Cleansing: Synthetic Surfactant Based (Syndet) Bars for Patients with Atopic Dermatitis. *Cutis*, **77**, 317-324.

[11] Lodén, M. (1995) Biophysical Properties of Dry Atopic and Normal Skin with Special Reference to Effects of Skin Care Products. *Acta Dermato-Venereologica. Supplementum*, **192**, 1-48.

[12] Draelos, Z.D. (2011) A Clinical Evaluation of the Comparable Efficacy of Hyaluronic Acid-Based Foam and Ceramide-Containing Emulsion Cream in the Treatment of Mild-to-Moderate Atopic Dermatitis. *Journal of Cosmetic Dermatology*, **10**, 185-188. http://dx.doi.org/10.1111/j.1473-2165.2011.00568.x

[13] Fontanini, C., Berti, I., Monasta, L. and Longo, G. (2013) Derma Silk in Long-Term Control of Infantile Atopic Dermatitis: A Double Blind Randomized Controlled Trial. *Giornale Italiano di Dermatologia e Venereologia*, **148**, 293-297.

[14] Bissonnette, R., Maari, C., Provost, N., Bolduc, C., Nigen, S., Rougier, A. and Seite, S. (2010) A Double-Blind Study of Tolerance and Efficacy of a New Urea-Containing Moisturizer in Patients with Atopic Dermatitis. *Journal of Cosmetic Dermatology*, **9**, 16-21. http://dx.doi.org/10.1111/j.1473-2165.2010.00476.x

[15] Tsuboi, H., Kouda, K., Takeuchi, H., Takigawa, M., Masamoto, Y., Takeuchi, M. and Ochi, H. (1998) 8-Hydroxy-deoxyguanosine in Urine as an Index of Oxidative Damage to DNA in the Evaluation of Atopic Dermatitis. *British Journal of Dermatology*, **138**, 1033-1035. http://dx.doi.org/10.1046/j.1365-2133.1998.02273.x

[16] Hall, J., Cruser D., Podawilt, A., Mummert, D.I., Jones, H. and Mummert, M.E. (2012) Psychological Stress and the Cutaneous Immune Response: Roles of the HPA Axis and the Sympathetic Nervous SysteminAtopic Dermatitis and Psoriasis (Review). *Dermatology Research and Practice*, **2012**, 1-11. http://dx.doi.org/10.1155/2012/403908

[17] Permatasari, F., Zhou, B. and Luo, D. (2013) Epidermal Barrier: Adverse and Beneficial Changes Induced by Ultraviolet B Irradiation Depending on the Exposure Dose and Time (Review). *Experimental and Therapeutic Medicine*, **6**, 287-292.

[18] Hong, J., Buddenkotte, J., Berger, T.G. and Steinhoff, M. (2011) Management of Itch in Atopic Dermatitis. *Seminars in Cutaneous Medicine and Surgery*, **30**, 71-86. http://dx.doi.org/10.1016/j.sder.2011.05.002

[19] Elias, P.M and Schmuth, M. (2009) Abnormal Skin Barrier in the Etiopathogenesis of Atopic Dermatitis. *Current Opinion in Allergy and Clinical Immunology*, **9**, 437-446. http://dx.doi.org/10.1097/ACI.0b013e32832e7d36

[20] Elias, P.M. (2008) Skin Barrier Function. *Current Allergy and Asthma Reports*, **8**, 299-305. http://dx.doi.org/10.1007/s11882-008-0048-0

[21] Van den Oord, R.A. and Sheikh, A. (2009) Filaggrin Gene Defects and Risk of Developing Allergic Sensitisation and

Allergic Disorders: Systematic Review and Meta-Analysis. *British Medical Journal*, **339**, 1-12. http://dx.doi.org/10.1136/bmj.b2433

[22] Reuter, J., Merfort, I. and Schempp, C.M. (2010) Botanicals in Dermatology: An Evidence-Based Review. *American Journal of Clinical Dermatology*, **11**, 247-67.

[23] Madaan, A. (2008) Epiceram for the Treatment of Atopic Dermatitis. *Drugs Today*, **44**, 751-755. http://dx.doi.org/10.1358/dot.2008.44.10.1276838

[24] Burkhart, C.N. and Burkhart, C.G. (2004) Pilot Study of Patient Satisfaction with Nonfluorinated Topical Steroids Compared with a Topical Immunomodulator in Atopiform Dermatitis. *International Journal of Dermatology*, **43**, 215-219. http://dx.doi.org/10.1111/j.1365-4632.2004.02118.x

[25] Gloor, M., Reichling, J., Wasik, B. and Holzgang, H.E. (2002) Antiseptic Effect of a Topical Dermatological Formulation That Contains Hamamelis Distillate and Urea. *Forsch Komplementarmed Klass Naturheilkd*, **9**, 153-159. http://dx.doi.org/10.1159/000064265

[26] Lee, Y.J., Kim, J.E., Kwak, M.H., Go, J., Kim, D.S., Son, H.J. and Hwang, D.Y. (2014) Quantitative Evaluation of the Therapeutic Effect of Fermented Soybean Products Containing a High Concentration of GABA on Phthalic Anhydride-Induced Atopic Dermatitis in IL-4/Luc/CNS-1 Tg Mice. *International Journal of Molecular Medicine*, **33**, 1185-1194.

[27] Dip, R., Carmichael, J., Letellier, I., Strehlau, G., Roberts, E., Bensignor, E. and Rosenkrantz W. (2013) Concurrent Short-Term Use of Prednisolone with Cyclosporine a Accelerates Pruritus Reduction and Improvement in Clinical Scoring in Dogs with Atopic Dermatitis. *BMC Veterinary Research*, **3**, 9, 173.

[28] Lee, T., Lee, S., Ho Kim, K., Oh, K.B., Shin, J. and Mar, W. (2013) Effects of Magnolialide Isolated from the Leaves of Laurusnobilis L. (Lauraceae) on Immunoglobulin E-Mediated Type I Hypersensitivity *in Vitro*. *Journal of Ethnopharmacology*, **149**, 550-556. http://dx.doi.org/10.1016/j.jep.2013.07.015

[29] Choi, S.E., Jeong, M.S., Kang, M.J., Lee do, I., Joo, S.S., Lee, C.S., Bang, H., Lee, M.K., Myung, S.C., Choi, Y.W., Lee, K.S., Seo, S.J. and Lee, M.W. (2010) Effect of Topical Application and Intraperitoneal Injection of Oregonin on Atopic Dermatitis in NC/Nga Mice. *Experimental Dermatology*, **19**, 37-43. http://dx.doi.org/10.1111/j.1600-0625.2009.00961.x

[30] Schlotter, Y.M., Veenhof, E.Z., Brinkhof, B., Rutten, V.P., Spee, B., Willemse, T. and Penning, L.C. (2009) A Genorm Algorithm-Based Selection of Reference Genes for Quantitative Real-Time PCR in Skin Biopsies of Healthy Dogs and Dogs with Atopic Dermatitis. *Veterinary Immunology and Immunopathology*, **129**, 115-118. http://dx.doi.org/10.1016/j.vetimm.2008.12.004

[31] Simonsen, L. and Fullerton, A. (2007) Development of an in Vitro Skin Permeation Model Simulating Atopic Dermatitis Skin for the Evaluation of Dermatological Products. *Skin Pharmacology and Physiology*, **20**, 230-236. http://dx.doi.org/10.1159/000104421

[32] Matsumoto, K., Mizukoshi, K., Oyobikawa, M., Ohshima, H., Sakai, Y. and Tagami, H. (2005) Objective Evaluation of the Efficacy of Daily Topical Applications of Cosmetics Bases Using the Hairless Mouse Model of Atopic Dermatitis. *Skin Research and Technology*, **11**, 209-217. http://dx.doi.org/10.1111/j.1600-0846.2005.00106.x

[33] Netzlaff, F., Lehr, C.M., Wertz, P.W. and Schaefer, U.F. (2005) The Human Epidermis Models EpiSkin®, SkinEthic® and EpiDerm®: An Evaluation of Morphology and Their Suitability for Testing Phototoxicity, Irritancy, Corrosivity, and Substance Transport. *European Journal of Pharmaceutics and Biopharmaceutics*, **60**, 167-178. http://dx.doi.org/10.1016/j.ejpb.2005.03.004

[34] http://www.skinethic.com/RHE.asp

[35] Bikle, D.D. (2010) Vitamin D and the Skin. *Journal of Bone and Mineral Metabolism*, **28**, 117-130. http://dx.doi.org/10.1007/s00774-009-0153-8

[36] Zbytek, B., Janjetovic, Z., Tuckey, R.C., Zmijewski, M.A., Sweatman, T.W., Jones, E., Nguyen, M.N. and Slominski, A.T. (2008) 20-HydroxyVitamin D3, a Product of Vitamin D3 Hydroxylation by Cytochrome P450scc, Stimulates Keratinocyte Differentiation. *Journal of Investigative Dermatology*, **128**, 2271-2280. http://dx.doi.org/10.1038/jid.2008.62

[37] Bikle, D.D. (2004) Vitamin D Regulated Keratinocyte Differentiation. *Journal of Cellular Biochemistry*, **92**, 436-444. http://dx.doi.org/10.1002/jcb.20095

[38] Merlin, J.L., Azzi, S., Lignon, D., Ramacci, C., Zeghari, N. and Guillemin, F. (1992) MTT Assays Allow Quick and Reliable Measurement of the Response of Human Tumour Cells to Photodynamic Therapy. *European Journal of Cancer*, **28**, 1452-1458. http://dx.doi.org/10.1016/0959-8049(92)90542-A

[39] Levin, J., Friedlander, S.F. and Del Rosso, J.Q. (2013) Atopic Dermatitis and the Stratum Corneum Part 1: The Role of Filaggrin in the Stratum Corneum Barrier and Atopic Skin. *The Journal of Clinical and Aesthetic Dermatology*, **6**, 16-22.

[40] Kubo, A., Nagao, K. and Amagai, M. (2012) Epidermal Barrier Dysfunction and Cutaneous Sensitization in Atopic

Diseases. *Journal of Clinical Investigation*, **122**, 440-447. http://dx.doi.org/10.1172/JCI57416

[41] Arikawa, J., Ishibashi, M., Kawashima, M., Takagi, Y., Ichikawa, Y. and Imokawa, G. (2002) Decreased Levels of Sphingosine, a Natural Antimicrobial Agent, May Be Associated with Vulnerability of the Stratum Corneum from Patients with Atopic Dermatitis to Colonization by *Staphylococcus aureus*. *Journal of Investigative Dermatology*, **119**, 433-439.

[42] Berardesca, E. (1998) Oral and Topical Supplementation of Linoleic Acid and Skin Disease. *Medecine Biologie Environnement*, **26**, 159-163.

[43] Kezic, S., O'Regan, G.M., Lutter, R., Jakasa, I., Koster, E.S., Saunders, S., Caspers, P., Kemperman, P.M., Puppels, G.J., Sandilands, A., Chen, H., Campbell, L.E., Kroboth, K., Watson, R., Fallon, P.G., McLean, W.H. and Irvine, A.D. (2012) Filaggrin Loss-of-Function Mutations Are Associated with Enhanced Expression of IL-1 Cytokines in the Stratum Corneum of Patients with Atopic Dermatitis and in a Murine Model of Filaggrin Deficiency. *Journal of Allergy and Clinical Immunology*, **129**, 1031-1039. http://dx.doi.org/10.1016/j.jaci.2011.12.989

# 25

# *In Vitro* Evaluations for a New Topical Anti-Aging Formulation

**Francesco Scarci, Federico Mailland**

Scientific Department, Polichem S.A., Lugano, Switzerland
Email: fscarci@polichem.com

## Abstract

The study aimed to evaluate the *in vitro* properties of a new gel formulation (P-3086) as anti-aging treatment. Two *in vitro* methods aimed to assess and compare the efficacy of the gel formulation in reducing oxidative damages, artificially induced by UVA on skin-derived keratinocytes and in promoting the synthesis of collagen, compared with other four formulations. P-3086 reduced reactive oxygen species production after UVA stress with the highest effect observed at 0.016 mg/ml and 0.031 mg/ml concentration. P-3086 also promoted the collagen synthesis faster when compared with other formulations. The new gel product, based on hyaluronic acid, Vitamin E and *Humulus lupulus*, showed a good efficacy as anti-aging effect reducing the oxidative damages derived by the action of ROS, moreover stimulating the synthesis of one of the components of the connective tissue, the collagen.

## Keywords

Skin, Wrinkles, Anti-Aging, Collagen Synthesis, Anti-Oxidant

## 1. Introduction

The desire for a long and healthy life is not an invention of modern times. In fact, the dream of eternal youth has accompanied humans since ancient time and in all cultures: from the Byzantine Empress Zoe Porphyrogenita, that tried to keep her youth appearance until a prolonged age, applying on herself cosmetic essences and fragrances made in her personal laboratory in the imperial palace [1] to Indian traditional medicine and the ayurvedic perspectives on theories and management of aging [2]. All of them tried to seek a remedy to rejuvenation. Even today, the demand for an anti-aging therapy is higher day by day. People want to look younger because a youthful appearance reflects also in a physical and mental health until very old age.

The skin aging is mainly genetically determined but also clinically associated with an increased fragility and loss of elasticity [3]; in addition, oxidative stress is an important contributor to the pathophysiology of various pathological conditions [4]. In fact, reactive oxygen species (ROS) are well-known as a cause of aging. Oxidative stress is one of the main causes of aging process as it is involved in the development of many serious human diseases. Intracellular formation of free radicals can occur by environmental sources, including ultraviolet light, ionizing radiation, and pollutants such as paraquat and ozone [5]; furthermore, diet, drugs intake or pathologies can increase the level of oxidant activity in the skin cells or decrease the effectiveness of endogenous antioxidant systems. Following exposure to oxidative stress, ROS damages the cells membrane and DNA, leading to cell transformation or even death [6].

The skin undergoes aging, genetic determinism and environmental factors, therefore it has to deal with uncounted changes on its structure. The outer layer of skin is the epidermis, made mainly by keratinocytes responsible for the formation of a barrier against environmental damages; the inner one, dermis, consists of connective tissue and structural components, such as collagen (responsible for the skin firmness), elastic fibres (responsible of the skin elasticity) and extracellular matrix (structural component). The skin ageing is characterized by an alteration of structural components of the connective tissue with the consequent formation of skin wrinkles, consisting in a disorganization or damage of these skin structures due to a lack of collagen or to its modification, thinning and/or fractioning and the stretching and repeated extension of some areas of the skin, especially the face [7]. Thus, at the level of epidermis, wrinkles appear as fold, deep lines, ridge or crease of the skin.

A lot of treatments are available for aging wrinkles: pharmaceutical, surgical and cosmetic solutions, which aim to change the nature of aging collagen, stretching the skin, filling in the depressions of the skin or paralyzing the muscles that cause the wrinkle. Retinoids, for example, decrease cohesiveness of follicular epithelial cells, stimulating mitotic activity and increasing the turnover of follicular epithelial cells [8], but they may produce redness, burning and general discomfort. Botulinum toxin treats wrinkles by immobilizing the muscles which cause wrinkles, but it is not indicated for all kind of wrinkles as it is indicated for the treatment of glabellar lines in adults; furthermore, it has high costs. In surgery, there are some techniques that could provide an excellent improvement acting as smoothers, but also produce significant side effects, including scarring and permanent changes in skin color. Or in other cases, the improvements last some months, but then they must be repeated. Moisturizers can make wrinkles look less prominent, keeping the skin hydrated, but their action is temporary. Hyaluronic acid promotes collagen synthesis, repairing and hydrating tissues, and preventing in this way the wrinkle formation. Antioxidants provide a sun protection, neutralizing the ROS. In this way, they could act preventing further worsening of wrinkle formation.

In this scenario, the best product to treat and prevent wrinkle formation should act in the sense of regenerating tissues, mostly collagen and opposing to oxidation. In front of these considerations, a new gel formulation, P-3086, based on hyaluronic acid, Vitamin E (for its antioxidant defence of the skin) and *Humulus lupulus*, has been developed for the treatment and prevention of wrinkle formation.

*Humulus lupulus* contains myrcene, humulene, xanthohumol, myrcenol, linalool, tannins, 8-prenylnaringenin and resin. Use of lupulus to relieve signs of skin ageing and to lead wrinkles be less evident or disappear has been disclosed in a paper where one of the flavonoids isolated from hop plant resulted efficacious in improving skin structure and firmness [9]. Lupulus is also employed mainly for its soothing, sedative, tonic and calming effect on the body and the mind [10].

P-3086 has been tested in the present study in order to evaluate its *in vitro* properties in the collagen synthesis and antioxidant activity, comparing our test product with other formulations of P-3086 where one or more of the elements have been deprived

## 2. Materials and Methods

### 2.1. Determination of Antioxidant Activity

*In vitro* method was used to evaluate anti-oxidant, regenerating and anti-age properties of cosmetic products. In the present study, we investigated the effectiveness of P-3086 to counteract oxidative damages, artificially induced by UVA on skin-derived keratinocytes, comparing the result with that of other formulations. The general compositions of the test products were as follows:

P-3086: *Humulus lupulus* (1%), hyaluronic acid (0.05%), ethanol (5%) and Vitamin E (0.02%);

Test Product 2: ethanol and Vitamin E;

Test Product 3: *Humuluslupulus*, ethanol and Vitamin E;

Test Product 4: hyaluronic acid, ethanol and Vitamin E;

Test Product 5: *Humuluslupulus*, hyaluronic acid and Vitamin E;

Reference standard (for ROS investigation): Vitamin C.

The concentration of the actives in the different test products reflects those of P-3086, taking into account that the excipients content is unchanged in the different test products.

The cells were exposed to a photo induced oxidative stress (UVA) with and without the tested products at different percentages, with the aim to evaluate their ability to neutralize the oxidative stress-induced damages.

We investigated ROS formation and their inhibition as a direct indicator of the anti-scavenger activity. Human primary keratinocytes come from paediatric foreskins, after ethic committee's permission, from pre-planned routine surgery. The epidermis was separated from dermis by incubation with dispase then trypsinized in order to generate a single cell suspension. Keratinocytes were cultivated in Dulbecco's modified Eagle's and Ham's F12 media (3:1) enriched with 10% foetal calf serum (v/v) and specific enrichments.

These cells multiply in culture until a cell monolayer is reached. In this study, the cells were seeded in 96-well plates and semi-confluency (30.000 cells/well) was reached in 24 hours. Once a confluence of 60% - 70% has been reached, fresh medium was added with scalar dilutions of the tested sample. Non-treated cells were used as negative controls. At this stage the cell cultures were treated with different dilutions of the test compound and of the controls to obtain final concentrations ranging from 0.5 to 0.016 mg/ml. For each dilution, three replicate tests were performed. The product was dissolved in the culture medium. 0.15 mg/ml Vitamin C were added separately as positive control. Part of the cells was checked for their vitality with the NRU assay (Neutral Red Uptake), based on the cell ability to incorporate and bind the Neutral Red (NR), a week cationic dye that penetrates the cell membrane through a mechanism of non-ionic diffusion and that is accumulated in the lysosomes, on matrix anionic sites. Cell and lysosome membrane alterations cause lysosomes fragility and gradual irreversible changes in the cells. These changes induced by xenobiotics determinate the decrease of NR uptake and of its linkage to lysosomes. This method is able to discriminate alive, damaged or dead cells. Cells were incubated with scalar concentrations of the products and with the Neutral Red solution (NR). If the membrane is damaged, it releases the dye in the medium. After incubation, the medium was replaced with fresh medium + NR medium and cells were incubated for 4 h at 37°C. Then cells were washed more times to eliminate exceeding dye wastes and read at the colorimeter.

The remaining cells were then exposed to 4' (1 J/cm$^2$), 8' (2 J/cm$^2$) and 12' (3 J/cm$^2$). At the end of the exposure period, the ROS formation was investigated in the cell supernatant. The cell vitality was determined after UVA exposure and without UV exposure.

After having exposed the cells to the tested sample, the cell culture medium was removed and the cells washed in PBS. The Dichlorofluorescein acetate (DCA) solution was added to each well. DCA reacts with free radicals in the medium, originating a fluorescent derivative, and the fluorimeter reading allows obtaining a quantitative data related to the ROS content in the cells. After suitable incubation, the DCA solution has been discharged and the cells have then been exposed for different times to UVA irradiation and soon after read in the fluorimeter [11].

The results are expressed in terms of viability:

% cell viability = Optical Density (OD) of treated cells × 100/OD untreated control cells.

## 2.2. Collagen Synthesis

We investigated the *in vitro* evaluation of the collagen synthesis in human skin fibroblasts (ATCC-CRL-2703) exposed to treatment with P-3086 at three different concentrations. The ex-novo synthesis of the extracellular matrix component collagen was measured by means of colorimetric assays, comparing the result with that of other formulations.

P-3086 was diluted in cell culture medium to achieve the final concentrations chosen for the tests. P-3086 was tested at 20%, 10%, 5%, 2.50%, 1.25%, 0.63% and 0.31% (w/v) for preliminary cytotoxicity test.

In accordance with toxicity data ($IC_{50}$ = 9.43%, non-cytotoxic), three different non-cytotoxic concentrations were chosen to continue the tests. The concentrations chosen for the efficacy test were 2.50%, 1.25% and 0.63% (w/v).

Cell exposure to P-3086 was prolonged for 24 and 48 hours. At the end of each experimental times cell proliferation and neo-synthesis of extracellular matrix elements were determined.

P-3086 was added to the wells containing cells in the $G_0$ phase of cell cycle (the cell number and the treatment to induce $G_0$ phase allow enough space for cell growing and avoid the contact inhibition phenomenon). Cells were exposed to P-3086 for 24 and 48 hours (medium was replaced every 24 h). At the end of incubation period, MTT test was performed in order to evaluate cell viability and the increasing proliferating rate compared to untreated control cell culture (CTR). For each determination 3 tests were carried out.

MTT assay [12]: MTT-medium was prepared by adding 15 mg of MTT to 30 ml of culture medium. After exposure of cells to the test items, they were washed with 200 μl of PBS. After removal of the washing solution, 200 μl of MTT-medium have been added to each culture well then incubated for 4 hours at 37°C and 5% $CO_2$. At the end of the incubation period, the MTT-medium was removed and 200 μl of MTT Solubilisation Solution (10% Triton X-100 plus 0.1 N HCl in anhydrous isopropanol) were added.

The plate was shaken on a rotatory plate for 20 - 30 minutes to ensure that all the crystals have been dissolved from the cells forming a homogeneous solution. The absorbance was measured at 570 nm on a microplate reader, with background reading at 690 nm. The results were expressed as % cell proliferation compared to an untreated control cell culture. Culture media with P-3086 was added to the wells containing cells in confluence (this feature allowed to maintain the cell number constant for the experiment duration time and avoids the influence of cell number in the observed trophism). Cells were exposed to each solution for 24 and 48 hours (medium was replaced every 24 h). At the end of incubation period, medium was collected in order to determine the concentration of collagen produced and released by the cells. For each determination 20 μl of medium was used. For each determination three tests were carried out.

The determination of collagen synthesis was carried out by quantitative dye-binding method. The chromogen agent used in the assay is Sirius Red (Direct red 80). Sirius red is an anionic dye with sulphonic acid side chain groups. These groups react with the side chain groups of the basic amino acids of collagen. The specific affinity of the dye for collagen, under the assay conditions, is due to the elongated dye molecules becoming aligned parallel to the long, rigid structure of native collagen that have intact triple helix organisation (dye affinity is much reduced when collagen is denatured).

Collagen concentration (μg in 20 μl of medium) was calculated by means of data interpolation on a standard curve obtained with known and increasing collagen concentrations.

## 2.3. Statistical Analysis

Data on ROS are presented with a descriptive statistics only providing the percentages of reduction for those experiments above the threshold (10%). Data on Collagen Synthesis were processed by a two-way ANOVA. Absolute collagen values (named ABS) recorded at 24 and 48 hours were pooled together and analyzed through an General Linear Model with Treatment (P-3086, test Product 2, test Product 3, test Product 4 and test Product 5), Dose (0.00625, 0.0125 and 0.025) and their interaction term (Treatment-by-Dose) as fixed effects (two-way ANOVA). Since the study objective consists in verifying whether the active compound P-3086 shows traits of superiority in comparison with other active compounds, the two-way ANOVA model was integrated with two sets of multiple comparisons. In the first set of comparisons, treatments (main effect regardless of dose) were compared with P-3086 used as control. In the second set of comparisons, treatments were compared with P-3086 used as control for each of the three doses. Statistical analyses were performed using NCSS 9 Software.

## 3. Results

### 3.1. Antioxidant Activity

In this test P-3086, at two out of three sub toxic tested concentrations, were able to reduce ROS production after UVA stress (at short time exposure). The results, summarized in **Table 1**, showed that P-3086 was able to reduce ROS production after UVA stress (at short time exposure) with the highest effect observed at 0.016 mg/ml and 0.031 mg/ml concentration showing therefore a superiority compared to the other formulations, without *Humuluslupulus*, hyaluronic acid and/or ethanol, having chosen preliminarily a threshold quote of <10% of ROS inhibition. P-3086 achieved a superiority even above the control (Vitamin C at 0.15 mg/ml, concentration 10- and 5-fold higher than P-3086).

**Table 1.** % reduction of UVA-induced ROS production after treatment (<under threshold)—a descriptive analysis.

| Composition | mg/ml | 4' UVA | 8' UVA | 12' UVA |
|---|---|---|---|---|
| P-3086 | 0.031 | 12.0 | 10.5 | 12.7 |
| | 0.016 | < | 14.0 | 19.4 |
| Test Product 2 | 0.031 | < | < | < |
| | 0.016 | < | < | < |
| Test Product 3 | 0.031 | < | < | < |
| | 0.016 | < | 13.6 | 11.7 |
| Test Product 4 | 0.031 | < | < | < |
| | 0.016 | 12.8 | 11.2 | < |
| Test Product 5 | 0.031 | < | < | < |
| | 0.016 | < | < | < |
| Vitamin C | 0.15 | 19.6 | 13.4 | 14.8 |

## 3.2. Collagen Synthesis

All the data are summarized in **Figure 1**. All treatments caused an increase of collagen synthesis at each tested dose. P-3086 was superior to all tested products.

The analysis on the pooled treatment effect significantly demonstrated the superiority of P-3086 on all the other tested formulations (**Table 2**).

The multiple comparisons among treatments at different dosages, demonstrated that the best dose of P-3086 was at 0.0125 which already reached the maximal effect and was superior on the same dose to all the other tested formulations at the same dose ($P < 0.05$). The lowest tested dose of P-3086 resulted inferior to the mid dose, but superior to almost all the other tested products. The highest dose of P-3086 had a similar effect of the mid dose, resulting to almost all the other test products, with the exception of test product 3 which demonstrated an evident dose effect relationship among the three tested dosages. Details of statistical analysis are displayed in **Table 3**.

## 4. Discussion

According to the data obtained in these *in vitro* studies, we could assess that the treatment of cell culture with P-3086 showed the efficacy of the test product against oxidative damages, artificially induced by UVA on skin-derived keratinocytes.

In fact, our results illustrated that at different time points (4', 8' and 12') of UVA exposure, P-3086 was able to reduce ROS production even at the lowest dose of those tested.

Moreover, comparing the result with that of the other formulations, P-3086 was able to increase collagen synthesis compared with untreated control cell culture, highlighting cell trophism enhancing properties. Hyaluronic acid showed modulate proliferation and collagen synthesis; this activity, combined with the antioxidant properties of hops extracts and their capabilities to soothe, to sedate and to provide a calming effect on the body, had been brought out by the presence of ethanol, which was able to synergise the interaction of hyaluronic acid, hops and Vitamin E, which on the contrary, taken on their own, did not show any relevant effect. Ethanol was therefore able to enhance the effect of these ingredients, boding excellent results in *in vivo* investigation of anti-aging capabilities of P-3086.

The above results account for the positive effect reported in humans [13] of this composition in terms of wrinkle profilometry, plastoelasticity and skin hydration. These results are consistent with other products that may serve as daily skin care to prevent UVA-induced skin damages by ROS-scavenging, promoting at the same time the collagen synthesis in dermis [14]. Moreover, P-3086 allows achieving comparable efficacious results without producing significant side effects or general discomfort in the subjects, acting in the way of tissue regeneration and not opposite to it, like chemical peels or cutaneous resurfacing [15]. Thanks to its antioxidant effects,

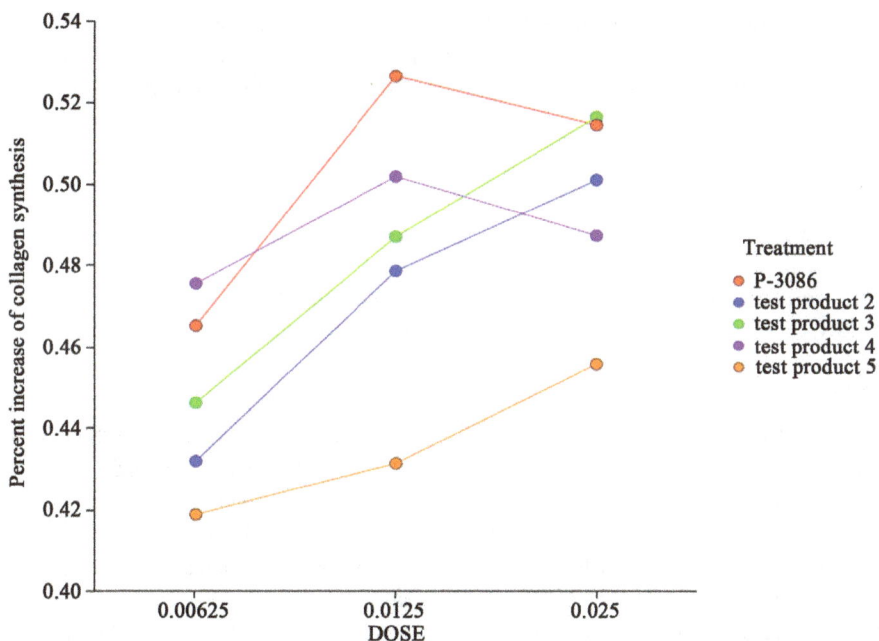

**Figure 1.** Percent increase of collagen synthesis versus untreated control by treatment and by dose (pooled data).

**Table 2.** Multiple comparisons of main treatment effects.

| Comparison | Significant |
|---|---|
| Test Product 2 vs. P-3086 | $P < 0.05$ |
| Test Product 3 vs. P-3086 | $P < 0.05$ |
| Test Product 4 vs. P-3086 | $P < 0.05$ |
| Test Product 5 vs. P-3086 | $P < 0.05$ |

**Table 3.** Multiple comparisons of treatment effects within dosages.

| Dose | Comparison | Significant |
|---|---|---|
| 0.00625 | Test Product 2 vs. P-3086 | $P < 0.05$ |
| | Test Product 3 vs. P-3086 | $P < 0.05$ |
| | Test Product 4 vs. P-3086 | N.S. |
| | Test Product 5 vs. P-3086 | $P < 0.05$ |
| 0.0125 | Test Product 2 vs. P-3086 | $P < 0.05$ |
| | Test Product 3 vs. P-3086 | $P < 0.05$ |
| | Test Product 4 vs. P-3086 | $P < 0.05$ |
| | Test Product 5 vs. P-3086 | $P < 0.05$ |
| 0.025 | Test Product 2 vs. P-3086 | $P < 0.05$ |
| | Test Product 3 vs. P-3086 | N.S. |
| | Test Product 4 vs. P-3086 | $P < 0.05$ |
| | Test Product 5 vs. P-3086 | $P < 0.05$ |

it can provide protection from the sun, neutralizing the free radicals responsible for the collagen breakdown. Finally, thanks to its moisturizing activity, P-3086 can make wrinkles look temporarily less prominent, keeping the skin hydrated. Due to all these properties, the product P-3086 can be definitely of benefit in skin rejuvenation practices.

## Acknowledgements

The authors would like to thank the following companies for their contribution in the conduction of the experiments described in this paper:

ABICH Srl, Verbania, Italy for the *in vitro* antioxidant evaluation;

FarcodermSrl, S. Martino Sicomario (PV), Italy for the *in vitro* evaluation of the collagen synthesis.

## References

[1]   Panas, M., *et al.* (2012) The Byzantine Empress Zoe Porphyrogenita and the Quest for Eternal Youth. *Journal of Cosmetic Dermatology*, **11**, 245-248. http://dx.doi.org/10.1111/j.1473-2165.2012.00629.x

[2]   Datta, H.S., *et al.* (2011) Theories and Management of Aging: Modern and Ayurveda Perspectives. *Evidence-Based Complementary and Alternative Medicine*, **2011**, Article ID 528527, 6 p. http://dx.doi.org/10.1093/ecam/nep005

[3]   Park, H.M., *et al.* (2012) Royal Jelly Increases Collagen Production in Rat Skin after Ovariectomy. *Journal of Medicinal Food*, **15**, 568-575. http://dx.doi.org/10.1089/jmf.2011.1888

[4]   Lee, N.J., *et al.* (2011) *In Vitro* Antioxidant Properties of a Ginseng Intestinal Metabolite IH-901. *Laboratory Animal Research*, **27**, 227-234. http://dx.doi.org/10.5625/lar.2011.27.3.227

[5]   Khansari, N., Shakiba, Y. and Mahmoudi, M. (2009) Chronic Inflammation and Oxidative Stress as a Major Cause of Age-Related Diseases and Cancer. *Recent Patents on Inflammation & Allergy Drug Discovery*, **3**, 73-80. http://dx.doi.org/10.2174/187221309787158371

[6]   Orrenius, S. (2007) Reactive Oxygen Species in Mitochondria-Mediated Cell Death. *Drug Metabolism Reviews*, **39**, 443-455. http://dx.doi.org/10.1080/03602530701468516

[7]   Fisher, G.J. (2005) The Pathophysiology of Photoaging of the Skin. *Cutis*, **75**, 5-9.

[8]   Stefanaki, C., *et al.* (2005) Topical Retinoids in the Treatment of Photoaging. *Journal of Cosmetic Dermatology*, **4**, 130-134. http://dx.doi.org/10.1111/j.1473-2165.2005.40215.x

[9]   Philips, N., *et al.* (2010) Direct Inhibition of Elastase and Matrixmetalloproteinases and Stimulation of Biosynthesis of Fibrillar Collagens, Elastin, and Fibrillins by Xanthohumol. *Journal of Cosmetic Science*, **61**, 125-132.

[10]  Chevallier, A. (1996) The Encyclopedia of Medicinal Plants: An Excellent Guide to over 500 of the More Well-Known Medicinal Herbs from around the World. Dorling Kindersley, London.

[11]  Kanthasamy, A., *et al.* (1997) Reactive Oxygen Species Generated by Cyanide Mediate Toxicity in Rat Pheochromocytoma Cells. *Toxicology Letters*, **93**, 47-54. http://dx.doi.org/10.1016/S0378-4274(97)00068-4

[12]  Mosmann, T. (1983) Rapid Colorimetric Assay for Cellular Growth and Survival: Application to Proliferation and Cytotoxicity Assays. *Journal of Immunological Methods*, **65**, 55-63.

[13]  Sparavigna, A., *et al.* (2014) An Innovative Concept Gel to Prevent Skin Aging. *Journal of Cosmetics, Dermatological Sciences and Applications*, **3**, 4.

[14]  Kato, S., *et al.* (2012) Hydrogen-Rich Electrolyzed Warm Water Represses Wrinkle Formation Against UVA Ray Together with Type-I Collagen Production and Oxidative-Stress Diminishment in Fibroblasts and Cell-Injury Prevention in Keratinocytes. *Journal of Photochemistry and Photobiology B: Biology*, **5**, 24-33. http://dx.doi.org/10.1016/j.jphotobiol.2011.09.006

[15]  Vedamurthy, M. (2006) Antiaging Therapies. *Indian Journal of Dermatology, Venereology and Leprology*, **72**, 183-186. http://dx.doi.org/10.4103/0378-6323.25776

# 26

# Grounding the Human Body Improves Facial Blood Flow Regulation: Results of a Randomized, Placebo Controlled Pilot Study

## Gaétan Chevalier

Developmental and Cell Biology Department, University of California at Irvine, Irvine, USA
Email: dlbogc@sbcglobal.net

## Abstract

Earthing (grounding) refers to bringing the human body in direct contact with the negative electric charge of the earth's surface by barefoot exposure outdoors or using special conductive indoor systems that are connected to the Earth. To determine if earthing improves facial blood circulation/flow, a double-blind study was designed with forty subjects either grounded or sham-grounded (27 grounded subjects and 13 sham-grounded subjects acting as controls) for at least one hour in a comfortable recliner chair equipped with conductive mat, pillow, and patches. The grounding systems were either grounded or sham-grounded via a wire to the ground port (third hole) of a power outlet. A Laser Speckle Contrast Imaging camera was used to continuously record changes in facial blood flow non-invasively. Facial blood flow regulation clearly improved among grounded—but not sham-grounded—subjects. The results demonstrate, for the first time, that even one-hour contact with the earth restores blood flow regulation to the face suggesting enhanced skin tissue repair and improved facial appearance with possible implications for overall health. Further studies, using larger comparison groups, longer monitoring times, and more measuring methods, are warranted in order to confirm the novel influence of the Earth as a protector of skin health and appearance.

## Keywords

Earthing, Grounding, Laser Speckle Contrast Imaging, Facial Blood Flow

## 1. Introduction

Earthing (or grounding, both words will be used interchangeably) is a practice whereby individuals are put in direct contact with the surface of the Earth. It includes walking barefoot outdoors, swimming in oceans and lakes, or sleeping, working and relaxing indoors with bare skin in contact with conductive mats, bed sheets, pillows, body bands and patches in order to maintain the body at Earth's electric potential. Unlike past cultures, most people today, particularly in industrial societies, rarely are in contact with the surface of the Earth. They wear shoes with synthetic soles that insulate them from the Earth's electric charge, and they no longer sleep on the ground. The Earth's negative electric surface charge is a virtually limitless reservoir of free electrons that is constantly replenished by the global atmospheric electric circuit [1] [2]. The Earthing hypothesis states that when direct skin contact is made with the Earth's surface or a grounded system indoors, the body's electric potential equalizes with the Earth's potential thereby maintaining the body's access to the Earth's negative surface charge (electrons). This contact with the Earth naturally prevents buildup of static electric charge on the body [3] and allows the body to store a supply of electrons [4] [5].

Published research indicates that Earthing yields a broad array of intriguing positive changes within the physiology and the bioelectrical construct of the body. Multiple reported benefits include improved sleep, decreased pain, a normalizing effect on cortisol, reduction of stress, diminished damage to muscles caused by delayed onset muscle soreness (DOMS), lessening of primary indicators of osteoporosis, and improved thyroid function, glucose regulation, immune response, and blood fluidity. A review of documented benefits of Earthing was published in 2012 [6].

Besides treatments such as plastic surgery (face lift), injections of botox, concentrated platelets and restylane, increasing blood flow to the face is seen as a major natural way to rejuvenate the skin of the face. There are a number of treatments to increase blood flow. Some use creams containing specific ingredients and others use direct skin stimulation (massages, ultrasound and lasers), chemical peel and dermabrasion [7]-[9]. While these treatments give results, they may have important short term or long term side effects; also some of these procedures require intensive post-treatment care and/or prolonged downtime. For example, many procedures designed to induce a controlled form of skin wound to promote dermal matrix remodeling and collagen synthesis require significant post-treatment care and may lead to complications, such as infection, pain, erythema, bleeding, oozing, burns and scaring [9]. Earthing, by comparison, is not a treatment per se. but a simple practice requiring little or no effort, which can be introduced easily into one's daily life.

The present double-blind study was designed to determine if Earthing for one hour produced measurable changes in facial blood flow (FBF). Based on previous studies, the hypothesis is that there will be a marked increase in FBF in grounded subjects vs. ungrounded subjects, as measured by the Laser Speckle Contrast method. Confirmation will suggest that Earthing is an effective and natural way to rejuvenate facial skin and appearance.

## 2. Materials and Methods

This pilot study was approved by BioMed IRB of San Diego, California (http://www.biomedirb.com/) and was conducted at a single center: Total Thermal Imaging, La Mesa, California.

### 2.1. Subjects

Forty (40) participants were recruited with an average age and standard deviation (SD) of 54.8 ± 9.8 (details in **Table 1**). Subjects were randomly assigned to 2 groups: Group A, with 27 grounded individuals; Group B, with 13 sham-grounded individuals (the control group). Subjects were scheduled in the order they signed up to participate.

Exclusion criteria were:
✧ Pregnancy;
✧ Below the age of 18 or above 70;
✧ Taking pain, anti-inflammatory medication, sedatives or prescription sleeping medication (less than 3 days prior to testing);
✧ Taking psychotropic drugs or diagnosed with mental disorder;
✧ Recent surgery (less than 3 months);
✧ Documented life threatening disease (such as cancer and AIDS);
✧ Consumption of alcohol within 48 hours of participation;
✧ Smoking;
✧ Use of recreational drugs;

**Table 1.** Age and gender distribution of subjects.

| | Grounded | | Controls | |
|---|---|---|---|---|
| | **Female** | **Male** | **Female** | **Male** |
| **No. of Subjects** | 20 | 7 | 9 | 4 |
| **Average Age** | 54.2 | 55.6 | 58.7 | 47.8 |
| **Age SD** | 10.2 | 12.1 | 6.48 | 8.73 |

◇ Previous utilization of Earthing products or similar grounding products;
◇ Going barefoot outside more than once a week and for more than half hour.

All potential subjects not fitting one or more of the exclusion criteria above were eligible to participate (*i.e.* there was no specific inclusion criterion).

## 2.2. Materials

Grounding equipment included conductive mats, pillows, and transcutaneous electrical nerve stimulation (TENS) patches (Earthing.com, Palm Springs, California, USA).

## 2.3. Earthing (Grounding) Method

Subjects were grounded with the use of a grounding mat, pillow and conductive patches connected, via conducting wires, into the ground port (third hole) of an electric power outlet. For sham-grounded subjects, conducting wires were similarly connected to the ground port, but modified into an open circuit to block conduction with the Earth's surface. The facility's grounding system was tested and found to be fully functional. All grounding wires contained a built-in 100 k$\Omega$ resistor for surge protection.

## 2.4. Measurements and Instrumentation

Changes in FBF were documented with the Laser Speckle Contrast Imaging (LSCI) technique, also called Laser Speckle Contrast Analysis (LASCA) [10] [11], that delivers real-time, high-resolution blood flow videos (MoorFLPI-2 Speckle Contrast Imager, Moor Instruments Ltd., Axminster, UK; website: http://us.moor.co.uk/ product/ moorflpi-2-speckle-contrast-imager/291).

The LSCI camera illuminates a selected area of tissue with low intensity laser light to produce a high contrast random interference effect known as a speckle pattern. The image processing software uses the fact that high perfusion produces rapid variation in the laser speckle pattern, which is integrated by the charge-coupled device (CCD) camera to produce an area of low contrast (seen as blurring of the speckle pattern in the video image). Conversely, low perfusion causes little variation in the speckle pattern and as a result a high contrast area of well-defined speckle is produced in the video image. Contrast is quantified and the resulting flux is color-coded to produce a perfusion image [10]-[12]. The LSCI camera measures to a maximum skin depth of approximately 1mm, thus covering mainly superficial skin blood flow [12].

The LSCI camera uses a near-infrared laser diode emitting at a wavelength of 785 nm and a 568 × 760 pixels CCD camera to capture blood flow over an area of up to 80 × 120 mm$^2$ (the working distance of the camera for providing reliable images is between 15 and 45 cm). Researchers and manufacturers generally agree that because of the nature of the flow in capillaries and connecting small blood vessels and the effect of varying skin color and structure, it is not appropriate to use absolute flow units such as ml/100 gm/minute. To justify the use of these units it is necessary to calibrate for the particular tissue type and site of the measurement, which is impractical except in special circumstances and not appropriate for normal day-to-day measurements. Consequently, arbitrary units are used for flux (blood flow) in common with most manufacturers' recommendation [12].

The LSCI camera has the capability of recording up to 25 images per second (called frames per second, or FPS) in standard resolution mode (152 × 113 pixels) and 1 FPS in high resolution mode (568 × 760 pixels) and to put them in a video file. In the present study, an intermediate frame rate of 10 FPS with an averaging period of 10 seconds was used. With this setup, each recorded image represents the average of 100 consecutive frames.

This setup has the advantage of eliminating very short-term (<1 sec) artifacts while at the same time enhancing durable blood flow features and real FBF changes over time. Blood flow analysis was conducted using appropriate computer software (MoorFLPI Review V4.0, Moor Instruments Ltd., Axminster, UK) installed on a standard desktop computer.

For each image recorded in the video, the analysis software averages the blood flow of the entire face to give a mean FBF value (or flux). The mean FBF values are then processed by the analysis software to generate a graph of mean FBF value over time (with a time increment of 10 seconds between recorded images).

## 2.5. Procedure

Each subject was tested in one individual session. Each grounding or sham-grounding session lasted approximately one hour, during which time the subject sat in a comfortable recliner chair. The reclining angle of the chair was adjusted to a comfortable 30 degrees in respect to the plane of the floor. The chair back and seat were covered with a grounding mat. A grounding pillow was placed at the head position, with a Styrofoam pad positioned under the pillow on each side to help stabilize the head and minimize movements. Patches were placed on both palms and soles (total of four patches). The connector ends of the wires from the patches, pillow, and mat were inserted into the jacks of a connector box placed next to the chair. The box, in turn, was connected by a single wire to the ground port of an adjacent power outlet. To allow or interrupt the conduction, a switch was installed in the middle of that single wire, between the connector box and the ground port. Once the subject was comfortably installed, the camera was positioned and turned on to record the subject's session.

The first ten minutes of each session was dedicated to collecting baseline measurements. After ten minutes, the switch was flipped allowing conduction in the single wire connecting to the ground port. However, the wires used to connect the mat, pillow and patches to the connector box did not permit grounding during the sham-grounding sessions. For both grounded and sham-grounded sessions, the grounding switch was turned off after at least one hour.

A double-blind procedure prevented researchers, study coordinators/technicians, and subjects from knowing whether an individual subject was actually grounded or sham-grounded. To accommodate the double blinded study design calling for about twice as many grounded subjects than sham-grounded subjects, three different colored-coded wires connecting the patches, pillow, and mat to the connector box were utilized. Wires with red and yellow tags permitted grounding; wires with the blue tag did not. The wires' color for a particular session was randomly selected by the study coordinators.

## 3. Results

Varying individual responses of the subjects dictated presenting only individual cases and space constrains to limit results presentation to three grounded subjects (A, B and C) and three sham-grounded (control) subjects (D, E and F). The results of these subjects were representative of the specific group results and are presented below according to age (youngest to oldest) for each group.

Linear regression analysis was applied to several graphs when appropriate. Curve smoothing was performed using the central moving average method with 5 points. Both regression analysis and curve smoothing were performed using Microsoft Office Excel 2003 SP2 software.

For each subject, two FBF images are presented first. The first image was extracted from the video just after an initial relaxation period or at 20 minutes after the start of the session when no clear relaxation period could be identified. The relaxation period is the time it takes for FBF to stabilize to a low value at the beginning of a session (corresponding to the time it takes for a subject to relax). The second image was extracted towards the end of the session for the sham-grounded session. After the relaxation period, peaks in blood flow were observed only among grounded subjects. For these subjects, the second image was taken at the highest point of the highest peak after the relaxation period.

Secondly, raw graphs of FBF values over time as calculated by the analysis software are presented. Each time a subject moved the head, a dip in mean FBF value (flux) can be seen, which is a movement artifact not related to the real mean FBF value. Blue arrows were added to these graphs to indicate when such movement artifact occurred.

Thirdly, the raw graphs were corrected for artifacts when needed and smoothed. Each dip in mean FBF value was replaced by the average of the mean FBF value immediately before and after the dip and then smoothed according to the procedure already described. Additionally, linear regression analysis was performed when a clear linear tendency could be found.

## 3.1. Grounded Subjects

### 3.1.1. Subject A—Female, Caucasian, 33

Subject A came with an overall body pain level at 3 (on a scale from 1 to 10). Most of the entire neck/back/arms/forearms/thighs/legs dropped to a 1 level after one hour of grounding. **Figure 1** shows two FBF images as recorded by the camera. The left image was taken at 11 minutes and 50 seconds (710 seconds, equivalent to frame 71, with each frame equal to 10 seconds) which corresponds to the end of the relaxation period. The right image was taken at 45 minutes and 10 seconds (2710 seconds, frame 271), corresponding to the highest mean FBF value of the highest peak after relaxation. Each time she moved her head, a dip in blood flow can be seen (movement artifact) in the top graph of **Figure 2**, which shows unprocessed mean FBF values (flux) over time. These dips are noted using blue arrows. The bottom graph of **Figure 2** shows the same graph but corrected for artifacts and smoothed. Each dip was replaced using the method previously described and then smoothed. From **Figure 2**, it can be seen that mean FBF decreased for about 12 minutes (corresponding to the relaxation period), remained more or less stable for another 28 minutes (with periodic peaks and troughs) and started to increase after that. The peaks and troughs produce a rhythmic fluctuation in mean FBF with a periodicity of 4 minutes and 20 seconds (260 seconds, corresponding to 26 periods of 10 seconds, as noted in the figure) that started after the relaxation period.

### 3.1.2. Subject B—Female, Caucasian, 49

**Figure 3** shows FBF images of Subject B at 20 minutes (left image), corresponding to the end of the relaxation period, and 39 minutes and 20 seconds (right image), corresponding to the high value of the highest peak after relaxation. **Figure 4** shows mean FBF values (flux) over time. In the top graph, which shows unprocessed mean FBF values, only one movement artifact was noted, indicating a very stable position for the entire session. The bottom graph shows mean FBF over time corrected for the artifact and smoothed. After the initial relaxation pe-

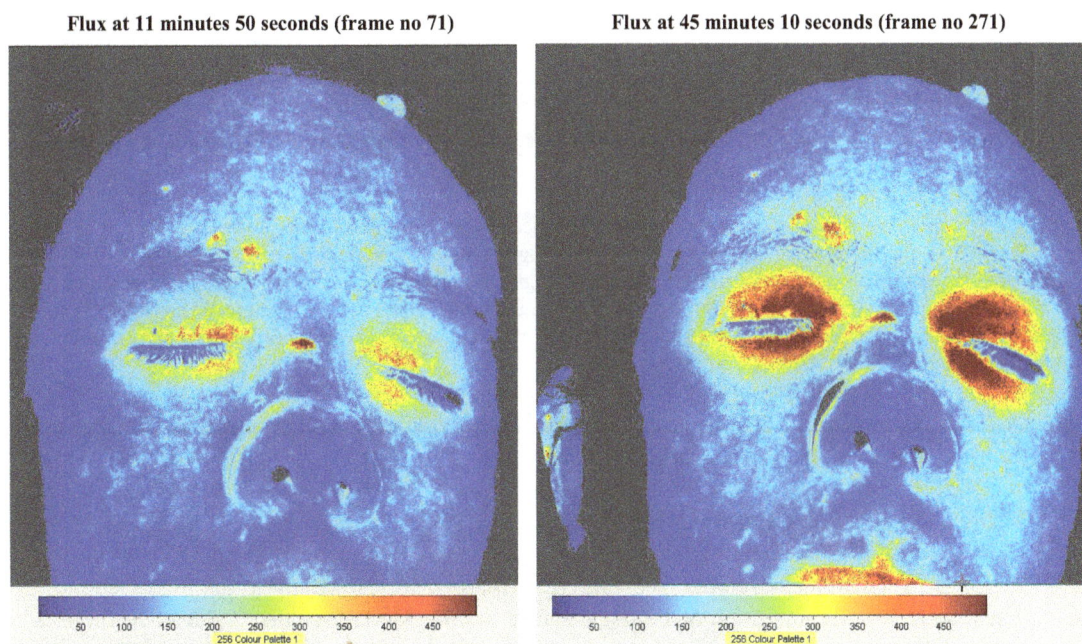

**Flux at 11 minutes 50 seconds (frame no 71)**          **Flux at 45 minutes 10 seconds (frame no 271)**

**Figure 1.** Subject A FBF images at 11 minutes and 50 seconds (left image) and 45 minutes and 10 seconds (right image). The flux intensity scale is shown below each image (dark blue = lowest flux; dark red = highest flux). There is a clear increase in FBF in the right image compared to the left image, especially around the eyes and the cheeks. Descriptive statistics for the left image: Mean Flux = 118.8; SD = 59.2; Flux min = 0; Flux max = 1129. Descriptive statistics for the right image: Mean Flux = 162.4; SD = 105.9; Flux min = 0; Flux max = 1053.

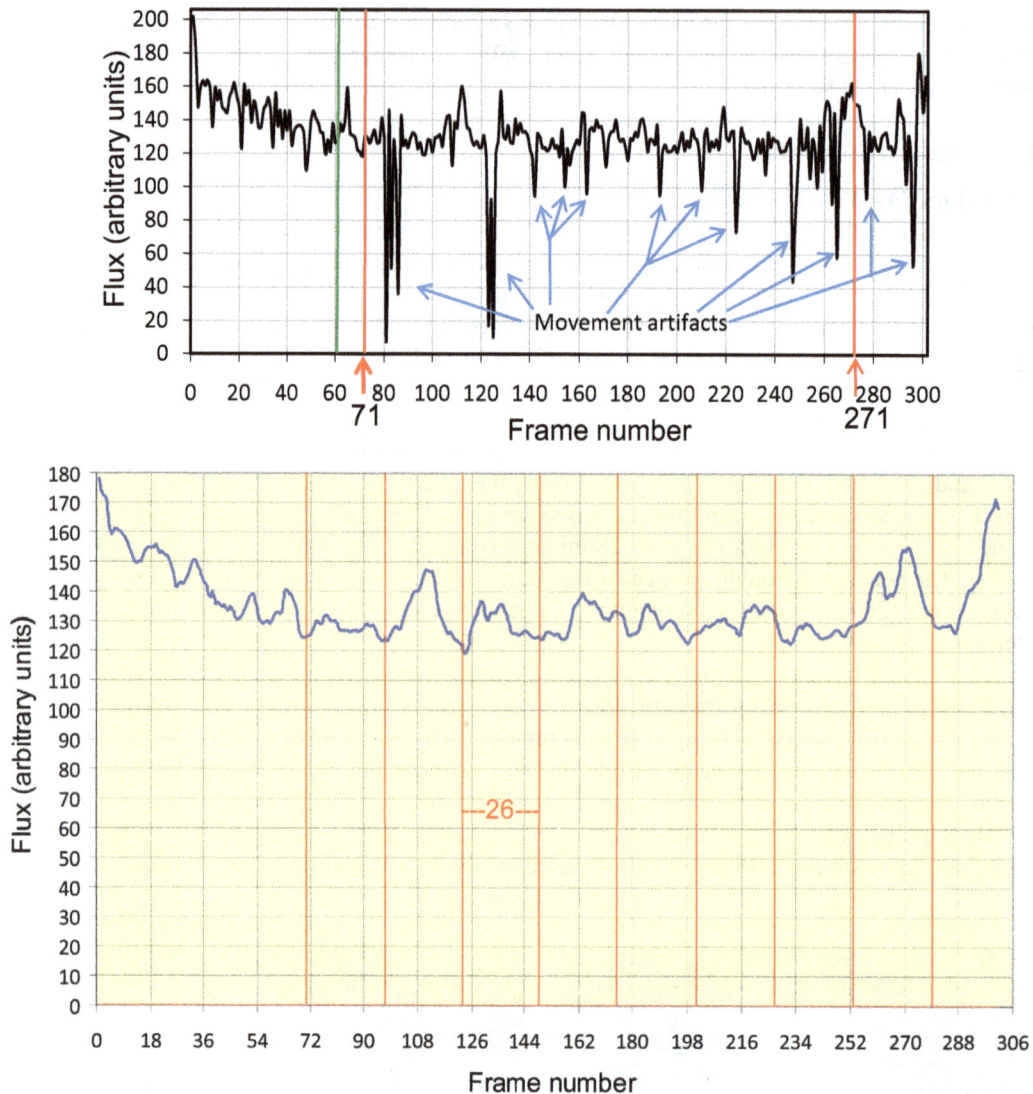

**Figure 2.** Top graph: Subject A unprocessed graph of mean FBF (in arbitrary units) over time. Red lines and numbers show the times at which the two images of **Figure 1** were extracted from the video. Blue arrows point to dips in flux caused by movement artifacts. The green line at 60 shows the time the grounding period started (10 minutes). Bottom graph: Same graph of mean FBF over time corrected for movement artifacts and smoothed. A rhythmic pattern of flux increases and decreases can be observed every 260 seconds (4 minutes and 20 seconds).

riod, no systematic increase in FBF is seen with time, only a rhythmic pattern of means FBF increases and decreases with a periodicity of 16 minutes (960 seconds).

### 3.1.3. Subject C—Female, Caucasian, 55

**Figure 5** shows FBF of Subject C at 28 minutes and 40 seconds (left image), corresponding to the end of the relaxation period) and 56 minutes and 40 seconds (right image), corresponding to the high value of the highest peak after relaxation. The top graph of **Figure 6** shows unprocessed mean FBF values over time, wherein no movement artifact was noted, indicating very stable head position. The bottom graph of **Figure 6** shows the same graph but smoothed (no artifact correction needed). Mean FBF started to increase about 40 minutes in the session. On top of that systematic increase, a rhythmic pattern of mean FBF fluctuations can be seen this time with a periodicity of 530 seconds (8 minutes and 50 seconds). It is interesting to note that the rhythmic fluctuations started before the relaxation period was completed.

**Flux at 20 minutes (frame no 120)**          **Flux at 39 minutes and 20 seconds (frame no 236)**

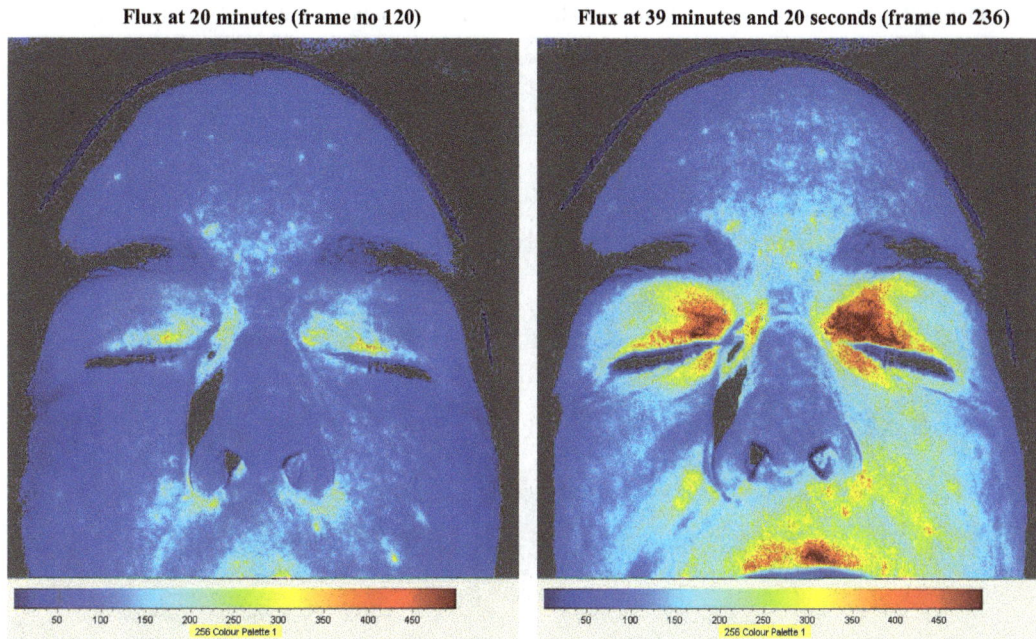

**Figure 3.** Subject B FBF images at 20 minutes (left image) and 39 minutes and 20 seconds (right image). There is a clear increase in FBF in the right image compared to the left image. Descriptive statistics for the left image: Mean Flux = 91.2; SD = 54.3; Flux min = 0; Flux max = 548. Descriptive statistics for the right image: Mean Flux = 150.8; SD = 93.9; Flux min = 0; Flux max = 810.

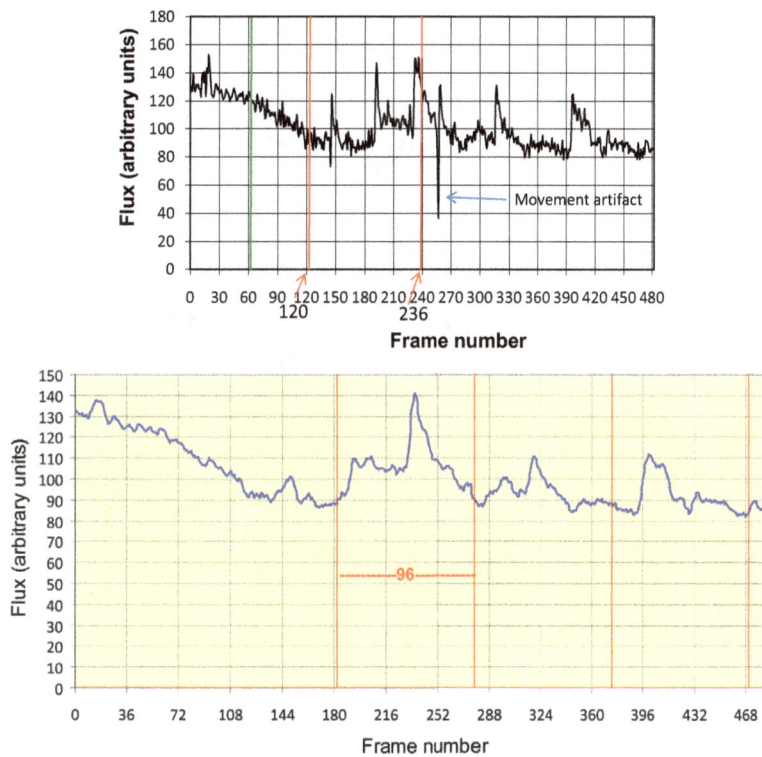

**Figure 4.** Top graph: Subject B unprocessed graph of mean FBF (in arbitrary units) over time. Red lines and numbers show the times at which the two images of **Figure 3** were extracted from the video. The blue arrow points to a dip in flux caused by movement artifacts. The green line at 60 shows the time the grounding period started. Bottom graph: same graph of mean FBF over time corrected for movement artifacts and smoothed. A rhythmic pattern of mean FBF increases and decreases can be observed every 960 seconds (16 minutes).

**Flux at 28 minutes and 40 seconds (frame no 172)**    **Flux at 56 minutes and 40 seconds (frame no 340)**

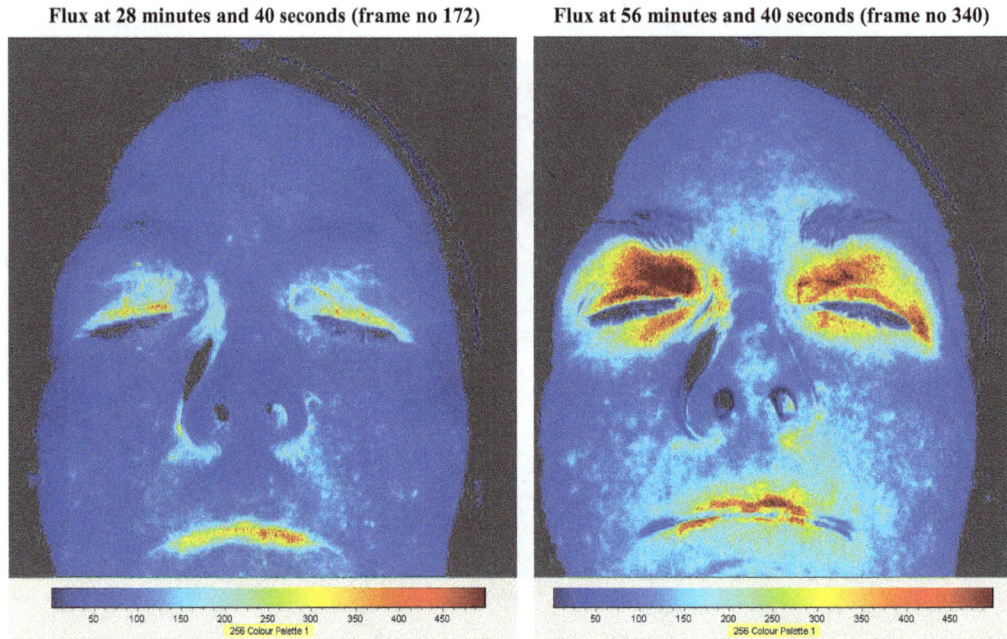

**Figure 5.** Subject C FBF images at 28 minutes and 40 seconds (left image) and 56 minutes and 40 seconds (right image). There is a clear increase in FBF in the right image compared to the left image. Descriptive statistics for the left image: Mean Flux = 78.5; SD = 47.6; Flux min = 0; Flux max = 517. Descriptive statistics for the right image: Mean Flux = 141.2; SD = 97.6; Flux min = 0; Flux max = 1050.

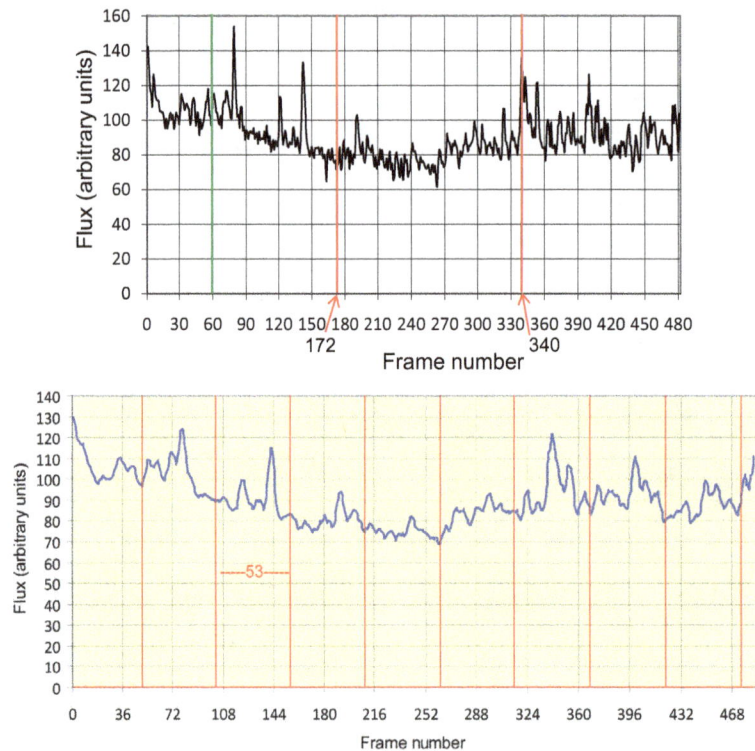

**Figure 6.** Top graph: Subject C unprocessed graph of mean FBF (in arbitrary units) over time. Red lines and numbers show the times at which the two images of **Figure 5** were extracted from the video. The green line at 60 shows the time the grounding period started. Bottom graph: same graph of mean FBF over time corrected for movement artifacts and smoothed. A rhythmic pattern of mean FBF increases and decreases can be observed every 530 seconds (8 minutes and 50 seconds).

## 3.2. Sham-Grounded (Control) Subjects

### 3.2.1. Subject D—Male, Caucasian, 42

**Figure 7** shows Subject D FBF images at 20 minutes (left image) and 54 minutes (right image). **Figure 8** shows change in mean FBF over time. In the top graph, which presents unprocessed mean FBF values, many movement artifacts are seen as noted. The bottom graph shows top graph data corrected and smoothed for movement artifacts. Linear regression analysis was performed on the bottom graph of **Figure 8** and shows that mean FBF decreased linearly with time (coefficient of determination $R^2 = 0.7171$), which explains the lower FBF observed in **Figure 7** at 54 minutes. No rhythmic pattern of fluctuations in mean FBF values can be observed.

### 3.2.2. Subject E—Female, Caucasian, 55

**Figure 9** shows FBF of subject E at 20 minutes (left image) and 79 minutes (right image). It is apparent that FBF in this sham-grounded subject is lower at 79 minutes. **Figure 10** shows variation of mean FBF values over time. Movement artifacts are identified by blue arrows in the top graph of **Figure 10** which presents unprocessed mean FBF values. The bottom graph of **Figure 10** shows the same graph corrected for artifacts and smoothed. Regression analysis shows that blood flow decreased linearly over time (coefficient of determination $R^2 = 0.9014$) which explains the lower FBF at 79 minutes in **Figure 9**. No rhythmic pattern of fluctuations in mean FBF values can be observed.

### 3.2.3. Subject F—Female, African-American, 68

**Figure 11** shows FBF of subject F after the relaxation period at 20 minutes (left image), and 43 minutes (right image). There is very little change in FBF between these 2 images. The time period shown in **Figure 12** is about 45 minutes because the subject was disturbed by someone inadvertently entering the room at that time. Only one movement artifact can be seen in the top graph of **Figure 12**, which presents change in unprocessed mean FBF values over time. Bottom graph of **Figure 12** shows change in mean FBF values over time corrected for that one artifact and smoothed. In her case, mean FBF fluctuated up and down for about 20 minutes (corresponding to the relaxation period) before settling down to a low stable value. This stable value after the initial relaxation period explains why the two images of **Figure 11** show about the same level of FBF. No rhythmic pattern in mean FBF value can be observed after the relaxation period.

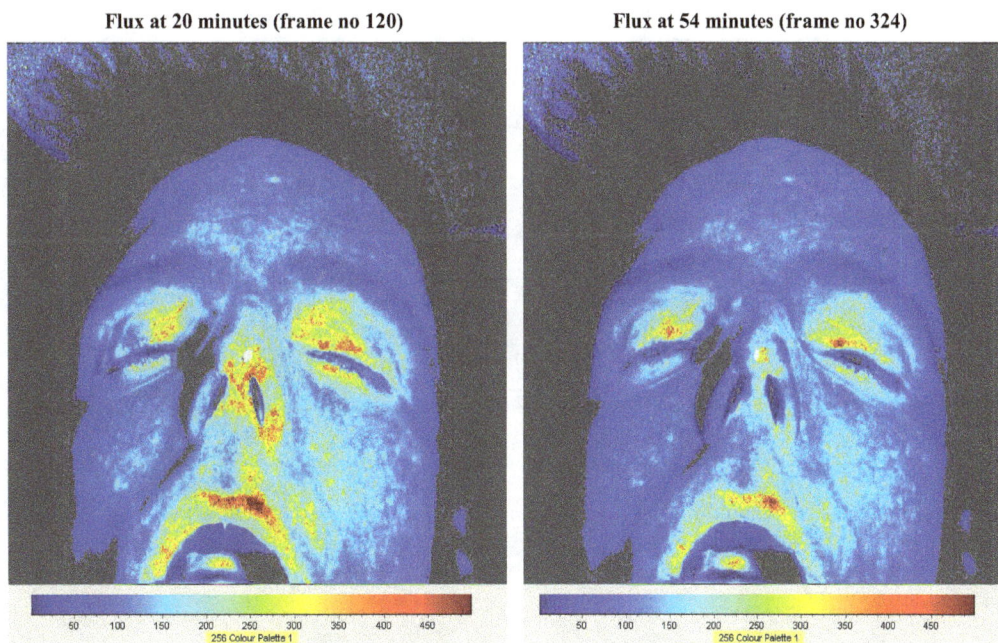

**Figure 7.** Subject D FBF images at 20 minutes (left image) and 54 minutes (right image). There is lower FBF in the right image compared to the left image. Descriptive statistics for the left image: Mean Flux = 127.9; SD = 80.1; Flux min = 0; Flux max = 784. Descriptive statistics for the right image: Mean Flux = 103.1; SD = 63.6; Flux min = 0; Flux max = 705.

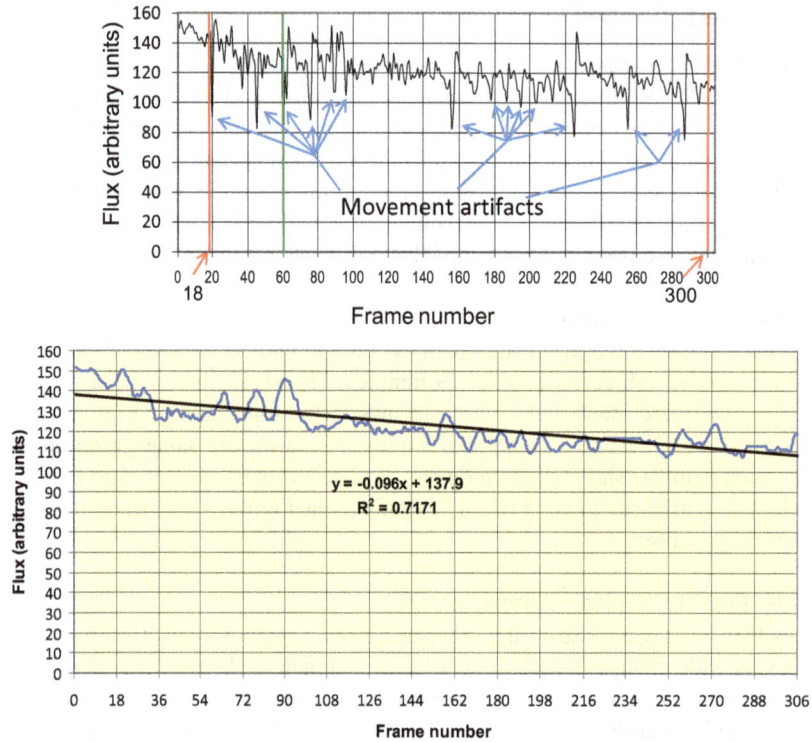

**Figure 8.** Top graph: Subject D unprocessed graph of mean FBF (in arbitrary units) over time. Red lines and numbers show the two frames at which the images of **Figure 7** were extracted from the video. Blue arrows point to dips in flux caused by movement artifacts. The green line at 60 shows the time when the switch was flipped (no grounding occurred). Bottom graph: Subject D graph of mean FBF (in arbitrary units) over time corrected for movement artifacts and smoothed with linear regression line, equation and $R^2$ value.

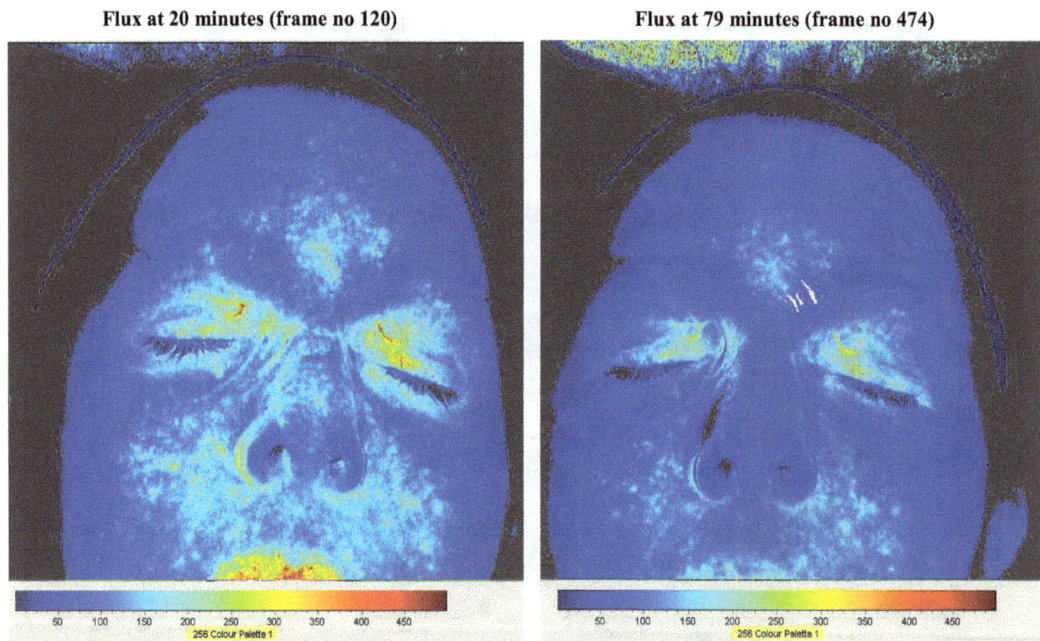

**Figure 9.** Subject E FBF images at 20 minutes (left image) and 79 minutes (right image). There is lower FBF in the right image compared to the left image. Descriptive statistics for the left image: Mean Flux = 103.7; SD = 55.9; Flux min = 0; Flux max = 606. Descriptive statistics for the right image: Mean Flux = 73.0; SD = 46.0; Flux min = 0; Flux max = 730.

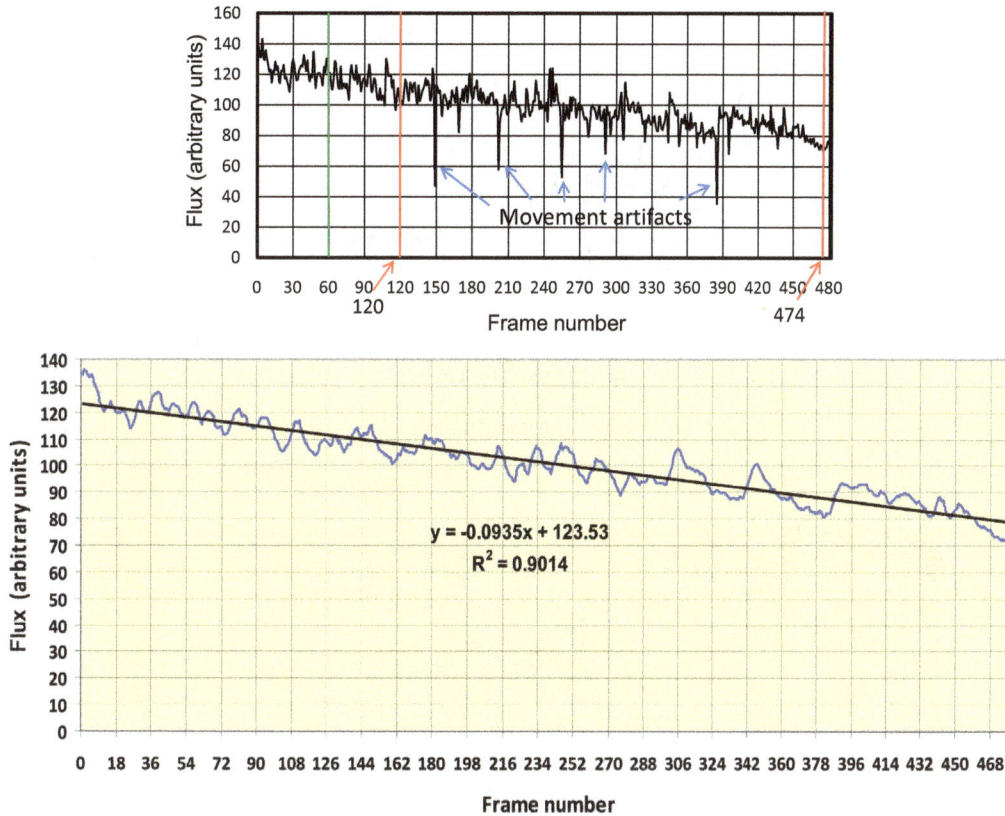

**Figure 10.** Top graph: Subject E unprocessed graph of mean FBF (in arbitrary units) over time. Red lines and numbers show the time at which the two images of **Figure 9** were extracted from the video. Blue arrows point to dips in flux caused by movement artifacts. The green line at 60 shows the time when the switch was flipped (no grounding occurred). Bottom graph: Subject E mean FBF graph (in arbitrary units) over time corrected for movement artifacts and smoothed with linear regression line, equation and $R^2$ value.

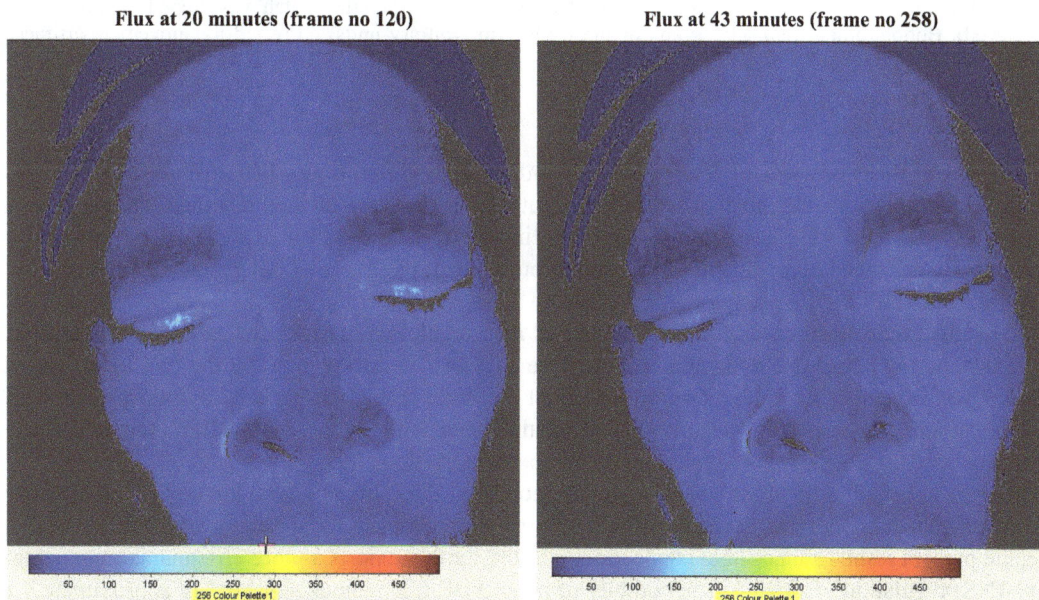

**Figure 11.** Subject F FBF images at 20 minutes (left image) and 43 minutes (right image). There is very little change in FBF. Descriptive statistics for the left image: Mean Flux = 33.4; SD = 19.1; Flux min = 0; Flux max = 248. Descriptive statistics for the right image: Mean Flux = 29.4; SD = 15.8; Flux min = 0; Flux max = 160.

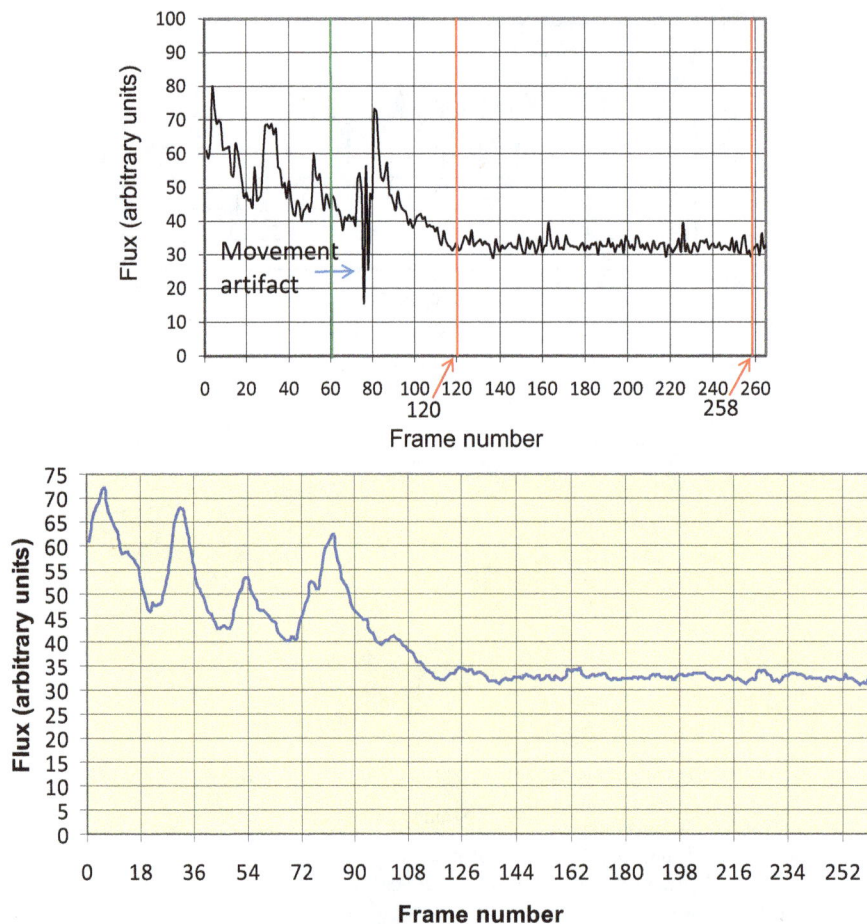

**Figure 12.** Top graph: Subject F unprocessed graph of mean FBF (in arbitrary units). Red lines and numbers show the time at which the two images of **Figure 11** were extracted. The blue arrow points to a dip in flux caused by movement artifacts. The green line at 60 shows the time when the switch was flipped (no grounding occurred). Bottom graph: Subject F graph of mean FBF (in arbitrary units) corrected for movement artifacts and smoothed.

## 4. Discussion

The purpose of this study was to determine if grounding the body promotes FBF. Improved facial microcirculation is a goal of various treatments used in the beauty industry. They include massage, the use of current emitting devices (DC and AC), lasers, ultrasound emitting devices, and acupuncture [8] [9]. Improved circulation may generate enhanced nourishment of the skin through greater delivery of oxygen and nutrients, as well as better resistance to the oxidative aging process [13].

The results of the present study showed improved FBF regulation in grounded subjects only. During the experimental period of about one hour, the FBF in these subjects, as documented by the LSCI camera, was seen to fluctuate with a regular rhythm and/or increase after an initial relaxation period varying from 12 to 29 minutes. By comparison, FBF decreased steadily and/or remained constant at a low value after a relaxation period during sham-grounded sessions of similar length with no apparent rhythmicity.

There are at least four neuronal mechanisms influencing FBF. Three of them are controlled by the sympathetic or parasympathetic nervous systems while the fourth one relates to local inflammatory responses [14]. Therefore, the present results suggest that connection with the Earth supports a more efficient autonomic nervous system (ANS) regulation of FBF. The periodicity of mean FBF fluctuations appeared in approximate 4 minute increments. While the reason for this incremental length in periodicity is not known, it is interesting to note that a rhythmic pattern of contraction/relaxation was seen for the first time in muscle tension after a grounding period of 28 minutes [15]. In relation to these observations, it is also interesting to mention that the baroreflex system, a mechanism by which the ANS control blood pressure, operates in a frequency range that overlaps our present observations [16]-[18].

The ANS regulation of FBF dynamics brings to mind an analogy of an efficient thermostat that activates or deactivates the heating or cooling system according to temperature fluctuations within the controlled environment. For the body, grounding may contribute to the restoration of regulation by the ANS of the distribution of blood, and therefore needed oxygen and nutrients, to the various organs and systems according to their needs.

Another explanation for improved FBF produced by grounding likely relates to the zeta potential (ZP) and aggregation of red blood cells (RBCs). RBC membranes naturally carry a negative electric charge that maintains cell spacing in the bloodstream by electrostatic repulsion. The potential difference between the RBC surface and the plasma produced by these charges is called zeta potential (ZP). ZP is an indicator of blood viscosity [19]-[21]. Elevated blood viscosity is associated with a number of clinical conditions, including hypertension, smoking, lipid disorders, advancing age, and diabetes mellitus. Research has found, for instance, a poor ZP among diabetics, and poorer yet among diabetics with cardiovascular disease [19]. The more negative the RBC surface charge is, the greater the repelling force between RBCs implying that the viscosity of the blood is lower which results in an improved blood flow [19]-[21]. In a previous study, grounding improved ZP and reduced RBC aggregation. Among the ten participants, the absolute value of the average ZP increased by a factor of 2.70—almost three-fold [21].

A third explanation for improved FBF is accumulated evidence that grounding improves overall physiology. If the body is healthier, it follows that the skin should be in better condition [8]. In support of this assertion, grounding has been shown to improve recovery from injury [22] [23], thyroid function and basic metabolism, calcium metabolism, glucose utilization by cells, the immune response [24], and oxygen consumption [25]. Some researchers consider that grounding may even be the primary factor regulating the endocrine and nervous systems [24].

It is instructive to raise the issue of stress. Numerous studies indicate that stress-induced sleep deficit can dramatically impair skin function and integrity [26]-[30]. Chronic insomnia, experienced by as much as a third of adults, can create damage to skin tissues ranging from premature aging [31] [32] to disorders like eczema, psoriasis, and dermatitis [33]-[36]. Previous grounding studies have produced results in which grounded participants subjectively reported better sleep and show lower stress levels [15] [25] [37]-[39].

According to the American Academy of Dermatology, stress can affect the skin in many ways [40]. Stress causes abnormalities in the level and oscillation of the central stress hormone cortisol that regulates a wide range of stress responses. Such disruption can trigger multiple neuroinflammatory conditions manifested in the skin, such as psoriasis, atopic dermatitis, acne, contact dermatitis alopecia areata, itch or pruritus, and erythema [41] [42]. Along with better sleep, grounding at night has been demonstrated to bring aberrant cortisol oscillations more in line with the natural cortisol pattern [37]. It should also be noted that grounding appears to promote balance in the sympathetic-parasympathetic function of the ANS, and thus exerts another stress reduction effect [15] [25] [39].

Through various measurements, grounding has also been documented to reduce inflammation [22] [43]. One mechanism of inflammation reduction is hypothesized to be the neutralization of oxidative free radical activity by added free electrons from contact with the Earth [4] [5]. Oxidative stress plays a central role in initiating and driving events that cause skin aging at the cellular level [44]. Oxidative stress breaks down protein (collagen), alters cellular renewal cycles, damages DNA, and promotes collagen glycation, cross-linking of proteins, and the release of pro-inflammatory mediators (cytokines), which trigger the generation of inflammatory skin diseases. It is also established that free radicals participate in the pathogenesis of allergic reactions in the skin [44]-[50]. The grounding effect may also be protective and/or therapeutic against UV radiation that produces oxidative stress in the cellular environment of the skin. Chronic free radical assault leads to aging skin, subverting the structural framework of the skin, and giving rise to wrinkles and sagging skin [46].

Another mechanism of inflammation reduction is the inflammatory reflex. Discovered about 15 years ago, this neural reflex mechanism controls inflammation and innate immune responses during tissue injury and pathogen invasion [51] [52]. A major constituent of the inflammatory reflex is the vagus nerve. Since grounding stimulates the parasympathetic branch of the ANS, it is reasonable to theorize that vagus nerve-mediated cholinergic signaling is also stimulated resulting in a decrease in inflammation.

Along with previous studies, the results of this study indicates that extended periods of grounding could be expected to produce further changes and benefits to facial skin. There's a saying that beauty comes from within.

It may also be appropriate to say that the beauty within comes from the ground.

## 5. Conclusion

The very Earth we live on possesses a form of easily accessible and beneficial natural electric energy that has been found to positively influence human physiology in various ways [6]. Previous studies have indicated improved cardiovascular and rheological (blood viscosity) dynamics, including autonomic nervous system regulation. In this study, the Laser Speckle Contrast Imaging camera further supports those findings by documenting a clear improvement in autonomic nervous system regulation of facial blood flow in grounded subjects but not in sham-grounded subjects. The results demonstrate, for the first time, that even one-hour contact with the Earth restores blood flow regulation to the face that may enhance skin tissue repair, health and vitality, and optimize facial appearance, which may also have broad implications for overall cardiovascular function and health. Further studies, using larger comparison groups, longer monitoring times and more measuring methods, are warranted in order to confirm the novel influence of the Earth as a protector of skin health and appearance.

## Acknowledgements

The author wishes to thank Earthing.com for providing the grounding equipment, Linda Hayes, C.C.T. and Theresa Williams, C.C.T., from Total Thermal Imaging, for recruiting study participants, collecting data and conducting all imaging activities, and Martin Zucker for reviewing the manuscript, for writing assistance, and for making useful suggestions. The study was funded by Earth FX, Inc.

## Conflict of Interests

The author is an independent contractor for Earth FX, Inc. and owns a very small number of shares in the company.

## References

[1] Williams, E. and Heckman, S. (1993) The Local Diurnal Variation of Cloud Electrification and the Global Diurnal Variation of Negative Charge on the Earth. *Journal of Geophysical Research*, **98**, 5221-5234. http://dx.doi.org/10.1029/92JD02642

[2] Anisimov, S., Mareev, E. and Bakastov, S. (1999) On the Generation and Evolution of Aeroelectric Structures in the Surface Layer. *Journal of Geophysical Research*, **104**, 14359-14367. http://dx.doi.org/10.1029/1999JD900117

[3] Applewhite, R. (2005) The Effectiveness of a Conductive Patch and a Conductive Bed Pad in Reducing Induced Human Body Voltage via the Application of Earth Ground. *European Biology and Bioelectromagnetics*, **1**, 23-40. http://www.earthingoz.com.au/pdf/Applewhite_earthing_body_voltage_2005.pdf

[4] Oschman, J.L. (2009) Charge Transfer in the Living Matrix. *Journal of Bodywork and Movement Therapies*, **13**, 215-228. http://dx.doi.org/10.1016/j.jbmt.2008.06.005

[5] Oschman, J.L. (2007) Can Electrons Act as Antioxidants? A Review and Commentary. *Journal of Alternative and Complementary Medicine*, **13**, 955-967. http://online.liebertpub.com/doi/pdfplus/10.1089/acm.2007.7048 http://dx.doi.org/10.1089/acm.2007.7048

[6] Chevalier, G., Sinatra, S.T., Oschman, J.L., Sokal, K. and Sokal, P. (2012) Earthing: Health Implications of Reconnecting the Human Body to the Earth's Surface Electrons. *Journal of Environmental and Public Health*, **2012**, Article ID 291541. http://dx.doi.org/10.1155/2012/291541

[7] Med-Health.net (2014) How to Tighten Face Skin. http://www.med-health.net/How-To-Tighten-Face-Skin.html

[8] Herman, J., Rost-Roszkowska, M. and Skotnicka-Graca, U. (2013) Skin Care during the Menopause Period: Noninvasive Procedures of Beauty Studies. *Postępy Dermatologii i Alergologii*, **30**, 388-395. http://www.ncbi.nlm.nih.gov/pmc/articles/PMC3907896/

[9] Avci, P., Gupta, A., Sadasivam, M., Vecchio, D., Pam, Z., Pam, N. and Hamblin, M.R. (2013) Low-Level Laser (Light) Therapy (LLLT) in Skin: Stimulating, Healing, Restoring. *Seminars in Cutaneous Medicine and Surgery*, **32**, 41-52. http://www.ncbi.nlm.nih.gov/pmc/articles/PMC4126803/

[10] Briers, J.D. and Webster, S. (1996) Laser Speckle Contrast Analysis (LASCA): A Nonscanning, Full-Field Technique for Monitoring Capillary Blood Flow. *Journal of Biomedical Optics*, **1**, 174-179. http://dx.doi.org/10.1117/12.231359

[11] Eriksson, S., Nilsson, J., Lindell, G. and Sturesson, C. (2014) Laser Speckle Contrast Imaging for Intraoperative Assessment of Liver Microcirculation: A Clinical Pilot Study. *Medical Devices: Evidence and Research*, **7**, 257-261.

http://dx.doi.org/10.2147/MDER.S63393

[12] Moor, F.L.P.I. (2012) User Manual, Issue 8.

[13] Schwartz, S.R. and Park, J. (2012) Ingestion of BioCell Collagen®, a Novel Hydrolyzed Chicken Sternal Cartilage Extract; Enhanced Blood Microcirculation and Reduced Facial Aging Signs. *Clinical Interventions in Aging*, **7**, 267-273. http://dx.doi.org/10.2147/CIA.S32836

[14] Drummond, P.D. (1994) Sweating and Vascular Responses in the Face: Normal Regulation and Dysfunction in Migraine, Cluster Headache and Harlequin Syndrome. *Clinical Autonomic Research*, **4**, 273-285. http://dx.doi.org/10.1007/BF01827433

[15] Chevalier, G., Mori, K. and Oschman, J.L. (2006) The Effect of Earthing (Grounding) on Human Physiology. *European Biology and Bioelectromagnetics*, **2**, 600-621. http://www.barefoothealth.com/science/physiology_study.pdf

[16] Task Force of the European Society of Cardiology and the North American Society of Pacing and Electrophysiology (1996) Heart Rate Variability: Standards of Measurement, Physiological Interpretation and Clinical Use. *Circulation*, **93**, 1043-1065. http://circ.ahajournals.org/content/93/5/1043.long
http://dx.doi.org/10.1161/01.CIR.93.5.1043

[17] Goldstein, D.S., Bentho, O., Park, M.Y. and Sharabi, Y. (2011) Low-Frequency Power of Heart Rate Variability Is Not a Measure of Cardiac Sympathetic Tone but May Be a Measure of Modulation of Cardiac Autonomic Outflows by Baroreflexes. *Experimental Physiology*, **96**, 1255-1261. http://ep.physoc.org/content/96/12/1255.long
http://dx.doi.org/10.1113/expphysiol.2010.056259

[18] Bonyhay, I., Risk, M. and Freeman, R. (2013) High-Pass Filter Characteristics of the Baroreflex: A Comparison of Frequency Domain and Pharmacological Methods. *PLoS ONE*, **8**, e79513.
http://dx.doi.org/10.1371/journal.pone.0079513

[19] Adak, S., Chowdhury, S. and Bhattacharyya, M. (2008) Dynamic and Electrokinetic Behavior of Erythrocyte Membrane in Diabetes Mellitus and Diabetic Cardiovascular Disease. *Biochimica et Biophysica Acta*, **1780**, 108-115.
http://dx.doi.org/10.1016/j.bbagen.2007.10.013

[20] Fontes, A., Fernandes, H.P., de Thomaz, A.A., Barjas-Castro, M.L. and Cesar, C.L. (2008) Measuring Electrical and Mechanical Properties of Red Blood Cells with Double Optical Tweezers. *Journal of Biomedical Optics*, **13**, Article ID: 014001. http://dx.doi.org/10.1117/1.2870108

[21] Chevalier, G., Sinatra, S.T., Oschman, J.L. and Delany, R.M. (2013) Earthing (Grounding) the Human Body Reduces Blood Viscosity: A Major Factor in Cardiovascular Disease. *Journal of Alternative and Complementary Medicine*, **19**, 102-110. http://dx.doi.org/10.1089/acm.2011.0820

[22] Brown, R., Chevalier, G. and Hill, M. (2010) Pilot Study on the Effect of Grounding on Delayed-Onset Muscle Soreness. *Journal of Alternative and Complementary Medicine*, **16**, 265-273. http://dx.doi.org/10.1089/acm.2009.0399

[23] Ober, C., Sinatra, S.T. and Zucker, M. (2010) Earthing: The Most Important Health Discovery Ever? Basic Health Publications, Laguna Beach, 193-205.

[24] Sokal, K. and Sokal, P. (2011) Earthing the Human Body Influences Physiologic Processes. *Journal of Alternative and Complementary Medicine*, **17**, 301-308. http://dx.doi.org/10.1089/acm.2010.0687

[25] Chevalier, G. (2010) Changes in Pulse Rate, Respiratory Rate, Blood Oxygenation, Perfusion Index, Skin Conductance and Their Variability Induced during and after Grounding Human Subjects for 40 Minutes. *Journal of Alternative and Complementary Medicine*, **16**, 81-87. http://dx.doi.org/10.1089/acm.2009.0278

[26] Kahan, V., Andersen, M.L., Tomimori, J. and Tufikm, S. (2010) Can Poor Sleep Affect Skin Integrity? *Medical Hypotheses*, **75**, 535-537. http://dx.doi.org/10.1016/j.mehy.2010.07.018

[27] Ghadially, R., Brown, B.E., Sequeira-Martin, S.M., Feingold, K.R. and Elias, P. (1995) The Aged Epidermal Permeability Barrier. Structural, Functional and Lipid Biochemical Abnormalities in Humans and a Senescent Murine Model. *The Journal of Clinical Investigation*, **95**, 2281-2290. http://dx.doi.org/10.1172/JCI117919

[28] Gupta, M.A. and Gupta, A.K. (1996) Psychodermatology: An Update. *Journal of the American Academy of Dermatology*, **34**, 1030-1046. http://dx.doi.org/10.1016/S0190-9622(96)90284-4

[29] Tausk, F.A. and Nousari, H. (2001) Stress and the Skin. *Archives of Dermatology*, **137**, 78-82.
http://dx.doi.org/10.1001/archderm.137.1.78

[30] Grice, K.A. (1980) Transepidermal Water Loss in Pathologic Skin. In: Jarrett, A., Ed., *The Physiology and Pathophysiology of the Skin*, Academic Press, London, 2147-2155.

[31] Rööst, M. and Nilsson, P. (2002) Sleep Disorders—A Public Health Problem. Potential Risk Factor in the Development of Type 2 Diabetes, Hypertension, Dyslipidemia and Premature Aging. *Läkartidningen*, **99**, 154-157.

[32] Edwards, B.A., O'Driscoll, D.M., Ali, A., Jordan, A.S., Trinder, J. and Malhotra, A. (2010) Aging and Sleep: Physiology and Pathophysiology. *Seminars in Respiratory and Critical Care Medicine*, **31**, 618-633.

http://dx.doi.org/10.1055/s-0030-1265902

[33] Altemus, M., Rao, B., Dhabhar, F.S., Ding, W. and Granstein, R.D. (2001) Stress-Induced Changes in Skin Barrier Function in Healthy Women. *The Journal of Investigative Dermatology*, **7**, 309-317. http://dx.doi.org/10.1046/j.1523-1747.2001.01373.x

[34] Kobayashi, S., Hayashi, K., Koyama, S., Tsubaki, H., Itano, T., Momomura, M., Koyama, T. and Yanagawa, Y. (2010) Actigraphy for the Assessment of Sleep Quality in Pediatric Atopic Dermatitis Patients. *Arerugi*, **59**, 706-715.

[35] Hanifin, J.M. and Reed, M.L., Eczema Prevalence and Impact Working Group (2007) A Population-Based Survey of Eczema Prevalence in the United States. *Dermatitis*, **18**, 82-91. http://dx.doi.org/10.2310/6620.2007.06034

[36] Choi, E.H., Brown, B.E., Crumrine, D., Chang, S., Man, M.-Q., Elias, P.M. and Feingold, K.R. (2005) Mechanisms by Which Psychologic Stress Alters Cutaneous Permeability Barrier Homeostasis and Stratum Corneum Integrity. *Journal of Investigative Dermatology*, **124**, 587-595. http://dx.doi.org/10.1111/j.0022-202X.2005.23589.x

[37] Ghaly, M. and Teplitz, D. (2004) The Biologic Effects of Grounding the Human Body during Sleep as Measured by Cortisol Levels and Subjective Reporting of Sleep, Pain and Stress. *Journal of Alternative and Complementary Medicine*, **10**, 767-776. http://74.63.154.231/here/wp-content/uploads/2013/06/Ghaly__Teplitz_cortisol_study_2004.pdf http://dx.doi.org/10.1089/acm.2004.10.767

[38] Ober, C. (2000) Grounding the Human Body to Neutralize Bioelectrical Stress from Static Electricity and EMFs. *ESD Journal*. www.esdjournal.com/articles/cober/ground.htm

[39] Chevalier, G. and Sinatra, S.T. (2011) Emotional Stress, Heart Rate Variability, Grounding and Improved Autonomic Tone: Clinical Applications. *Integrative Medicine: A Clinician's Journal*, **10**, 16-21. http://imjournal.com/pdfarticles/IMCJ10_3_p16_24chevalier.pdf

[40] American Academy of Dermatology (2014) Stress and Skin. http://www.aad.org/media-resources/stats-and-facts/prevention-and-care/stress-and-skin

[41] Senra, M.S. and Wollenberg, A. (2014) Psychodermatological Aspects of Atopic Dermatitis. *British Journal of Dermatology*, **170**, 38-43. http://dx.doi.org/10.1111/bjd.13084

[42] Chen, Y. and Lyga, J. (2014) Brain-Skin Connection: Stress, Inflammation and Skin Aging. *Inflammation & Allergy Drug Targets*, **13**, 177-190. http://www.ncbi.nlm.nih.gov/pmc/articles/PMC4082169/ http://dx.doi.org/10.2174/1871528113666140522104422

[43] Oschman, J.L., Chevalier, G. and Brown, D. (2014) The Effects of Grounding (Earthing) on Inflammation, the Immune Response, Wound Healing and Prevention and Treatment of Chronic Inflammatory and Auto-Immune Diseases. *Journal of Inflammation Research*, in Press.

[44] Masaki, H. (2010) Role of Antioxidants in the Skin: Anti-Aging Effects. *Journal of Dermatological Science*, **58**, 85-90. http://dx.doi.org/10.1016/j.jdermsci.2010.03.003

[45] Burke, K.E. and Wei, H. (2009) Synergistic Damage by UVA Radiation and Pollutants. *Toxicology and Industrial Health*, **25**, 219-224. http://tih.sagepub.com/content/25/4-5/219

[46] Fisher, G.J., Quan, T., Purohit, T., Shao, Y., Cho, M.K., He, T., Varani, J., Kamg, S. and Voorhees, J. (2009) Collagen Fragmentation Promotes Oxidative Stress and Elevates Matrix Metalloproteinase-1 in Fibroblasts in Aged Human Skin. *The American Journal of Pathology*, **174**, 101-114. http://dx.doi.org/10.2353/ajpath.2009.080599

[47] Pascucci, B., D'Errico, M., Parlanti, E., Giovannini, S. and Dogliotti, E. (2011) Role of Nucleotide Excision Repair Proteins in Oxidative DNA Damage Repair: An Updating. *Biochemistry (Moscow)*, **76**, 4-15. http://dx.doi.org/10.1134/S0006297911010032

[48] Röck, K., Grandoch, M., Majora, M., Krutmann, J. and Fisher, J.W. (2011) Collagen Fragments Inhibit Hyaluronan Synthesis in Skin Fibroblasts in Response to Ultraviolet B (UVB): New Insights into Mechanisms of Matrix Remodeling. *The Journal of Biological Chemistry*, **286**, 18268-18276. http://dx.doi.org/10.1074/jbc.M110.201665 Supplemental Material: http://www.jbc.org/content/suppl/2011/03/17/M110.201665.DC1.html

[49] Daniel, S., Reto, M. and Fred, Z. (2002) Collagen Glication and Skin Aging. *Cosmetics and Toiletries Manufacture Worldwide*. https://www.mibellebiochemistry.com/pdfs/Collagen_glycation_and_skin_aging_-_CT_2002.pdf

[50] Miwa, S., Beckman, K.B. and Muller, F., Eds. (2008) Oxidative Stress in Aging: From Model Systems to Human Diseases. Humana Press, New York.

[51] Borovikova, L.V., Ivanova, S., Zhang, M., Yang, H., Botchkina, G.I., Watkins, L.R., Wang, H., Abumrad, N., Eaton, J.W. and Tracey, K.J. (2000) Vagus Nerve Stimulation Attenuates the Systemic Inflammatory Response to Endotoxin. *Nature*, **405**, 458-462. http://dx.doi.org/10.1038/35013070

[52] Pavlov, V.A. and Tracey, K.J. (2012) The Vagus Nerve and the Inflammatory Reflex—Linking Immunity and Metabolism. *Nature Reviews Endocrinology*, **8**, 743-754. http://dx.doi.org/10.1038/nrendo.2012.189

# 27

# Development of Preparation Method for Microencapsulating Uycalyptus Oil Containing Fine Aqueous Droplets by Use of Interfacial Condensation Reaction between Hydroxy Propyl Methyl Cellulose and Tannic Acid

**Hiroyuki Sato, Yoshinari Taguchi, Masato Tanaka***

Graduate School of Science and Technology, Niigata University, Niigata, Japan
Email: *tanaka@eng.niigata-u.ac.jp

## Abstract

It was tried to develop the preparation method for microencapsulating the uycalyptus oil containing fine aqueous droplets by using the interfacial condensation reaction between hydroxyl propyl methyl cellulose and tannic acid. Uycalyptus oil containing fine aqueous droplets was dispersed in the continuous water phase to form the (W/O)/W emulsion. Tannic acid and hydroxyl propyl methyl cellulose were dissolved in the inner aqueous droplets and in the outer continuous water phase, respectively. Tannic acid transferred through the oil phase from the inner water droplets to the interface between the oil phase and the continuous water phase and then, reacted with hydroxyl propyl methyl cellulose. In the experiment, the concentrations of hydroxyl propyl methyl cellulose and tannic acid were mainly changed stepwise. The uycalyptus oil containing the fine water droplets could be microencapsulated satisfactorily. It was found that the microcapsules were composed of the gelated hydroxyl propyl methyl cellulose film as the shell, the fine aqueous droplets as the first core and the oil droplet as the second core.

## Keywords

Microcapsule, Uycalyptus Oil, Multiple Emulsion, Interfacial Condensation Reaction, Hydroxyl Propyl Methyl Cellulose, Tannic Acid

---

*Corresponding author.

## 1. Introduction

Many kinds of microcapsules have been developed and applied to the various fields such as cosmetics, paintings, catalyst, food industry, medicine, agriculture, and so on [1]-[3].

The purposes of microencapsulation are to optionally release the core material, to protect the core materials from environment, to modify the surface of core material, to mask the taste of core material and so on. These functions of microcapsules are strongly dependent on the physical properties of shell and core materials, the structure, size and morphology of microcapsules. Accordingly, in order to prepare the microcapsules with the desired functions, it is necessary to develop the preparation method which is suitable to the physical properties of the core and shell materials used.

Recently, many studies about the microencapsulation of essential oils have been reported [4]-[10]. These microcapsules have been applied to the textiles, fragrance, aromatherapy, insect repelling, stress reducing, antibiosis and so on.

Uycalyptus oil is known to have many physiological activities such as anti-aging effect, anti-inflammation effect, sterilization effect, anti-uilus and so on. If the microcapsules containing the uycalyptus oil could be prepared and the oil could be optionally released, the uycalyptus oil will be utilized extremely easily in the more fields. Furthermore, it will be expected that the microcapsules containing the uycalyptus oil have to develop the new fields and the applicable fields of oil will be dramatically increased. Until now, many kinds of oil species have been microencapsulated with the chemical methods such as interfacial gelling reaction method [11]-[13], the in-situ polymerization [14] [15], the interfacial polycondensation reaction [16] [17] and the physicochemical methods such as the coacervation method [18] [19], the spray-dried method [20]-[22], and the melting dispersion-cooling method [23]. In these preparation methods, a few harmful chemical species have been used and the complicated processes have been applied. However, if we are going to apply the microcapsules to the cosmetics, the food and the drug, the microcapsules have to be prepared with the materials suitable to the living body and the edible materials. Accordingly, it is necessary to newly develop the preparation method by using the designnated materials with the simple process. The purposes of this paper are to develop the microencapsulation procedure with the interfacial condensation reaction between hydroxyl propyl methyl cellulose and tannic acid, to investigate whether the microcapsules of uycalyptus oil containing the fine water droplets can be prepared or not, to characterize the microcapsules and to discuss the microencapsulation mechanism on the basis of the results obtained.

## 2. Experimental

### 2.1. Materials

Materials used to develop the preparation method for microencapsulating the uycalyptus oil containing the fine water droplets are as follows:

The first core material was Uycalyptus oil (UO) (Wako Junyaku Co., Ltd.). Span 80 (Wako Junyaku Co., Ltd.) and Soybean Lecithin (Wako Junyaku Co., Ltd.) were used as the oil soluble surfactant. Hydroxy propyl methyl cellulose (HPMC) (50SH-50: Shinetsu Chemical Ind Co., Ltd.) and Tannic acid (TA) were used as the reactants to form the microcapsule shell. These chemical species were used as received.

### 2.2. Pre-Microencapsulation

In order to investigate whether the microcapsules can be prepared by the microencapsulation mechanism presented in this study or not, the pre-microencapsulation experiment was tried as follows.

**Figure 1** shows the schematic diagram of pre-microencapsulation procedure. Namely, the HPMC aqueous solution and the UO were poured into the beaker as shown in **Figure 1**. The UO and the HPMC aqueous solution were separated to form the upper oil phase and the lower aqueous phase, respectively. Then, the TA aqueous solution was dropped into the oil phase through the nozzle by the syringe pump. If TA could transfer through the oil phase and react with HPMC on the interface between the oil phase and the HPMC aqueous solution, the gelated HPMC film should be formed on the interface. As a result, the TA aqueous droplet may be maintained on the formed film for a while.

According to this microcapsule shell formation mechanism, the pre-microencapsulation experiment was performed by changing the concentrations of HPMC and TA.

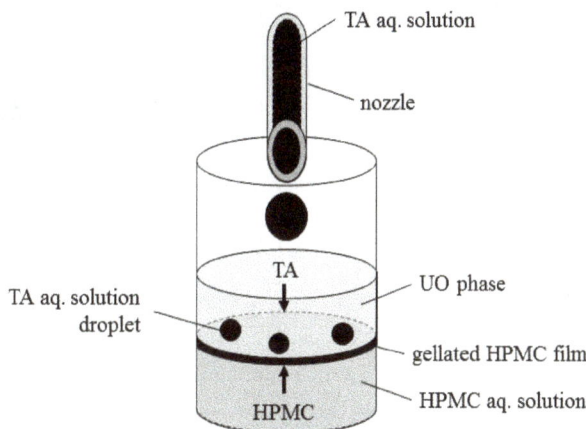

**Figure 1.** Pre-microencapsulation procedure.

## 2.3. Preparation of Microcapsules

**Figure 2** shows the schematic diagram of experimental apparatus used to prepare the microcapsules. The reactor was the separable flask with the effective volume of 500 cm$^3$. Four baffles made of aluminium plate were set on the wall of reactor. The six bladed disc turbine impeller with the diameter of 5 cm was used to stir the reaction mixture. The reactor was set in the thermos tatted water bath to keep temperature of reaction mixture constant. **Figure 3** shows the flow chart for microencapsulating the UO containing the fine water droplets by using the interfacial condensation reaction between HPMC and TA. The aqueous solution dissolving TA as a gelation agent was dispersed into the UO dissolving Soybean Lecithin (SL) of an oil soluble surfactant to form the (W/O) emulsion.

Then, the (W/O) emulsion was dispersed into the continuous water phase dissolving HPMC to form the (W/O)/W emulsion. The operation stated above was performed at room temperature.

After formation of the (W/O)/W emulsion, temperature of the (W/O)/W emulsion was raised to 30°C to perform the condensation reaction between TA and HPMC. When the reaction was continued for 1h, it was investigated whether the microcapsules of UO containing the fine water droplets could be prepared or not.

The formation of microcapsules was confirmed by observing the stability of the (W/O)/W emulsion after the microencapsulation process and by optical microscope. If the microcapsules were prepared well, the photographs of them were taken. Contrary to this, if the microcapsules were not prepared well, the emulsion should be broken rapidly.

In the fundamental experiment stated above, the concentrations of HPMC and TA were mainly changed. The experimental conditions in this experiment were shown in **Table 1**.

## 2.4. Characterization

### 2.4.1. Mean Diameter of Microcapsules
The microcapsules were observed by optical microscope and the photographs of them were taken. The diameter distributions and mean diameters of microcapsules were measured directly from these photographs.

### 2.4.2. Stability of Emulsion and Microcapsules
In order to investigate whether the microcapsules can be prepared or not, the (W/O)/W emulsion after microencapsulation process was set for 10 min. If the microcapsules could not be prepared well, the (W/O) droplets should be rapidly broken. The shape and inner structure of microcapsules were observed by taking the optical microscopic photographs.

### 2.4.3. Observation of Formation of Microcapsule Shell
The formation of microcapsule shell was observed to find the optimum concentrations of HPMC and TA.

Namely, the UO and the HPMC aqueous solution were poured into the beaker. The UO floated on the HPMC aqueous solution and the interface between the oil phase and the HPMC aqueous solution was formed as shown

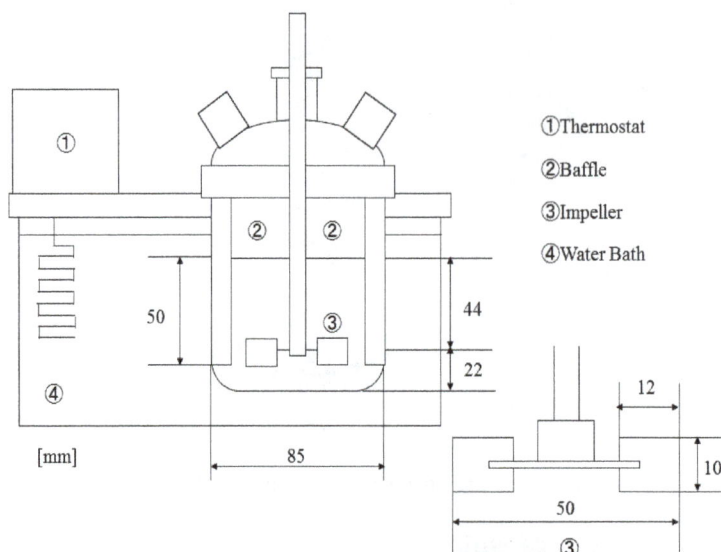

**Figure 2.** Schematic diagram of experimental apparatus.

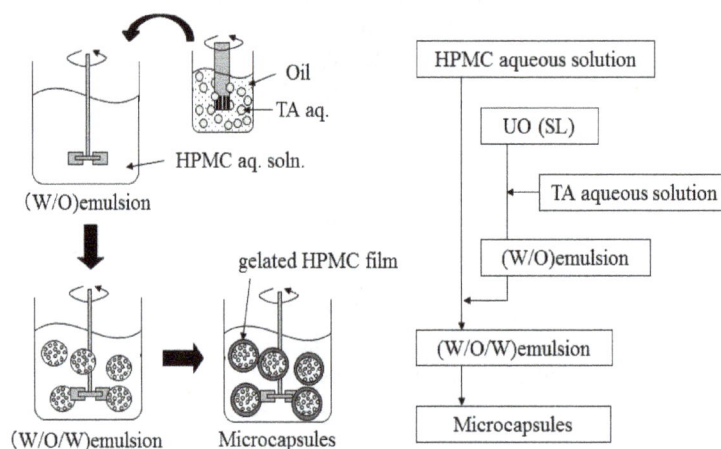

**Figure 3.** Flow chart for preparing microcapsules.

**Table 1.** Experimental conditions.

| | |
|---|---|
| • HPMC aq. soln. | 270 ml |
|    concent. of HPMC [$C_{HPMC}$] | 0.05 - 0.2 wt%-$H_2O$ |
| • Uycalyptus oil | 27 ml |
|    concent. of Lecithin [$C_{TA}$] | 0.1 wt%-Uycalyptus oil |
| • TA aq. soln. | 3 ml |
|    concent. of TA | 0 - 0.1 mol |
| • Revolution speed for formation of (W/O) emulsion | 1000 rpm |
|    Stirring time | 3 min |
| • Revolution speed for (W/O)/W emulsion [$N_r$] | 200 rpm |
|    Stirring time | 5 min |
|    Reaction Temp. | 30°C |
|    Reaction time | 1 h |

in **Figure 1**. The time elapsing from arrival of TA aqueous droplet at the interface to disappearance of droplet was measured. The concentrations of HPMC and TA required to form the gelated HPMC film could be estimated by observing the stability of a TA aqueous droplet on the interface.

# 3. Results and Discussion

## 3.1. Confirmation of Shell Formation and Microencapsulation Mechanism

**Figure 4** shows the photographs of the TA aqueous droplet and the interface on which the gelated HPMC film was formed according to the concentrations of HPMC and TA. When the concentrations of HPMC and TA were low ($C_{HPMC}$ = 0.05 wt%, $C_{TA}$ = 0.01 mol), the TA aqueous droplet was kept on the interface as shown in **Figure 4(a)**, but dissolved into the HPMC aqueous solution in a few min. The short life of TA aqueous droplet on the interface may be due to the formation of thinner film. On the other hand, when the concentrations of HPMC and TA were higher ($C_{HPMC}$ = 0.2 wt%, $C_{TA}$ = 0.06 mol), the TA aqueous droplet was kept on the interface for ca. 10 min as shown in **Figure 4(b)** due to the thicker film formation.

**Figure 5** shows the measured results of the time elapsing from arrival of a TA aqueous droplet at the interface to disappearance. From these results, it is found that the film was not formed at $C_{TA}$ = 0 in spite of elapsing of ca. 30 s and the gelated film was formed above the concentrations of $C_{HPMC}$ = 0.05 wt% and $C_{TA}$ = 0.01 mol. Here, ca. 8 min at $C_{HPMC}$ = 0.05 wt%, and ca. 10 min at $C_{HPMC}$ > 0.1 wt% don't mean that the TA aqueous droplet disappeared at these elapsing times, but mean that the measurement of elapsing time was finished at these times.

From these results, as the gelated HPMC film was found to be formed on the interface between the UO and the HPMC aqueous solution above $C_{HPMC}$ = 0.05 wt% and $C_{TA}$ = 0.01 mol. Taking these results into consideration, the formation mechanism of film may be stated as shown in **Figure 6**. TA should transfer from the TA aqueous droplet to the interface through the UO and react with HPMC on the interface to form the gelated HPMC film. If the concentrations of HPMC and TA are lower, the thinner shell film should be formed. Contrary to this, if the concentrations of HPMC and TA are higher, the thicker and stronger shell film should be formed.

Furthermore, it was investigated whether the microcapsules could be prepared or not by the preparation method presented in this study. Namely, the stability of the (W/O)/W emulsion was observed with and without the microencapsulation process.

**Figure 7** shows the photographs of the (W/O)/W emulsion just after the microencapsulation process (a) and after 10 min (b). The (W/O)/W emulsion without the microencapsulation process was separated rapidly into the oil phase and the water phase, but the observation result is not shown. Contrary to this, the (W/O)/W emulsion with the microencapsulation process, namely the (W/O) droplets microencapsulated floated on the water phase and was kept to stably disperse as shown in **Figure 7(b)**. From these results, the UO droplets containing the fine water droplets were estimated to be microencapsulated well by the gelated HPMC shell.

## 3.2. Observation of Microcapsules

**Figure 8** shows the optical microscopic photographs of microcapsules prepared by changing the concentration of HPMC at $C_{TA}$ = 0.06 mol. From these photographs, the following interesting results are obtained. The microcapsules could be prepared according to the formation mechanism presented in this study. The mean diameters of microcapsules changed from 780 μm to 1330 μm by changing the concentration of HPMC as shown in **Figure 8**. The fine water droplets were microencapsulated well, but become larger due to coalescence between the fine water droplets. In order to stably disperse the fine water droplets in the oil droplet and to utilize as the first core material, it must be necessary to select the optimum oil soluble surfactant species and the concentrations of them. The microcapsules become irregular with the concentration of HPMC. This result is considered to be due to the fact that the oil droplets containing the fine water droplets are hard to break by the stronger shell formed with the higher concentration and become irregular. These microcapsules could be stably dispersed in the continuous water phase under stirring of revolution speeds from 200 rpm to 500 rpm with the six bladed disc turbine impeller of 5 cm diameter.

## 3.3. Formation Mechanism of Microcapsules

From the results obtained above, the formation mechanism of microcapsules may be presented as shown in **Figure 9**. TA dissolved in the inner water droplets should transfer to the interface through the UO phase, react with HPMC on the interface and form the gelated HPMC film as the microcapsule shell.

In the case of the lower concentration of HPMC or TA, as the weak shell is formed, the (W/O) emulsion may be broken. As a result, the microcapsules cannot be prepared. Contrary to this, in the case of the higher concentration of HPMC and TA, as the stronger shell is formed, the microcapsules can be prepared well. The fine inner

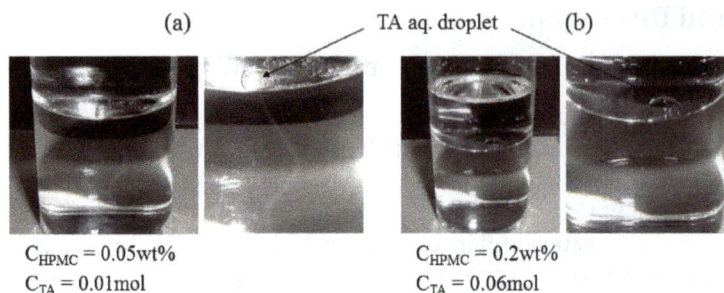

(a)                          TA aq. droplet      (b)

$C_{HPMC}$ = 0.05wt%                    $C_{HPMC}$ = 0.2wt%
$C_{TA}$ = 0.01mol                         $C_{TA}$ = 0.06mol

**Figure 4.** Confirmation of microcapsule shell formation.

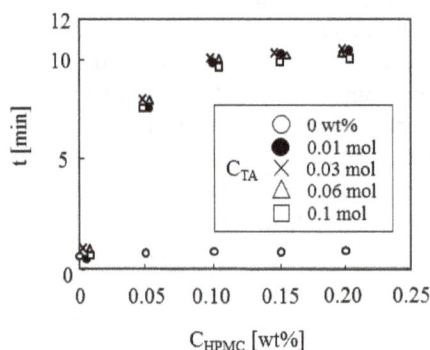

**Figure 5.** Effect of concentrations of HPMC and TA on film formations.

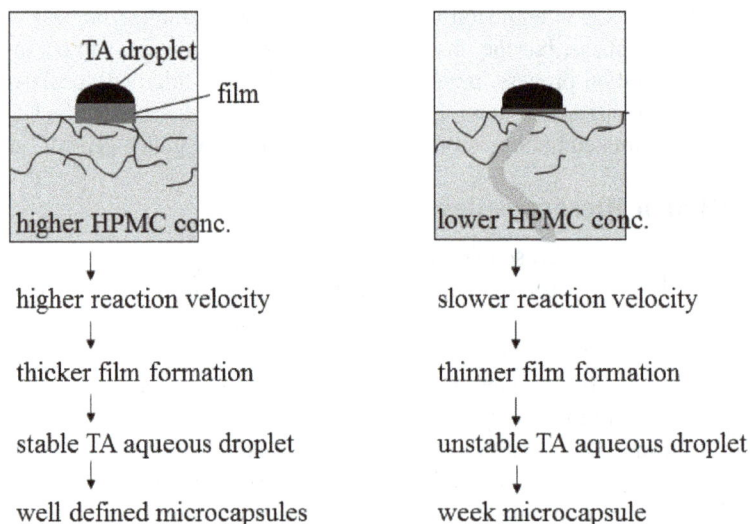

**Figure 6.** Formation mechanism of gelated HPMC film.

water droplets may coalesce each other to form the larger water droplets. If the fine water droplets could be dispersed stably, TA may transfer rapidly due to the larger interface area between the UO phase and the inner water phase. As a result, the shell may be formed rapidly and the microcapsules may be prepared more satisfactory. As many kinds of chemical species can be dissolved in the fine inner water droplets as the first core material and in the oil phase as the second core material at the same time, the microcapsules will be given the many kinds of functions. Namely, the microcapsules with the multiple functions can be prepared by using the microencapsulation method developed in this study.

However, it has to be investigated whether the microcapsules with the other oil species can be prepared by the microencapsulation mechanism presented here or not. Because, as it is necessary for TA to transfer through the

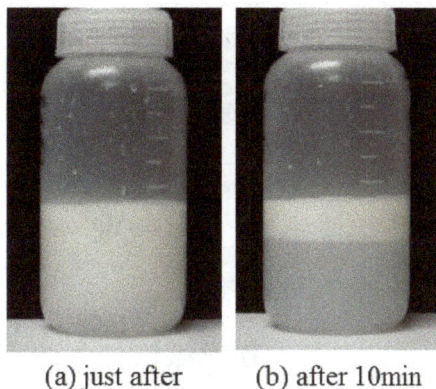

(a) just after          (b) after 10min

**Figure 7.** Photographs of (W/O)/W emulsion just after microencapsulation and after elepsing 10 min.

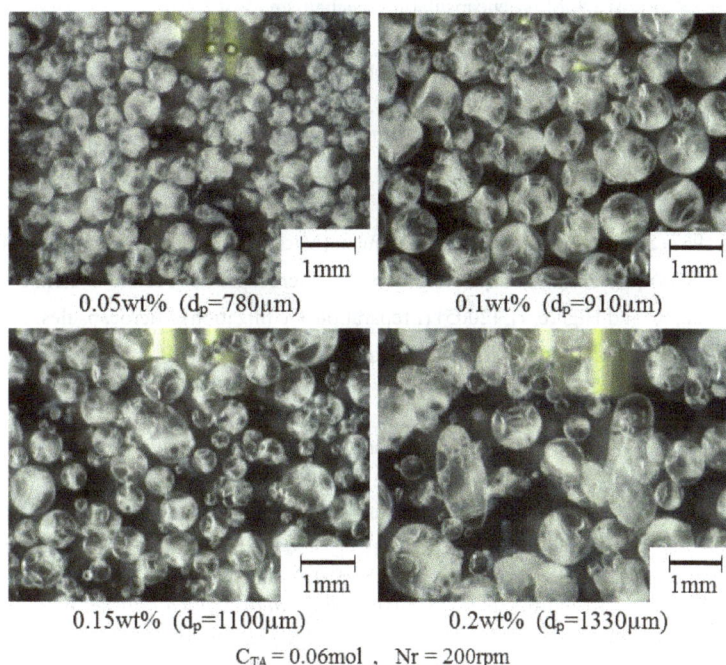

1mm
0.05wt%  ($d_p$=780μm)

1mm
0.1wt%  ($d_p$=910μm)

1mm
0.15wt%  ($d_p$=1100μm)

1mm
0.2wt%  ($d_p$=1330μm)

$C_{TA}$ = 0.06mol ,  Nr = 200rpm

**Figure 8.** Photographs of microcapsules prepared by changing concentrations of HPMC.

oil phase, the fundamental experiments with regard to mass transfer of TA in the other oil species have to be performed.

## 4. Conclusions

It was tried to microencapsulate the uycalyptus oil droplets containing the fine water droplets according to the microencapsulation mechanism presented. The following results were obtained.

1) TA transferred from the water droplets to the interface between the uycalyptus oil and the HPMC aqueous solution through the uycalyptus oil and reacted with HPMC.

2) The preparation method for microencapsulating the uycalyptus oil containing the fine water droplets could be developed.

3) There were the critical concentrations ($C_{HPMC}$ = 0.05 wt%, $C_{TA}$ = 0.01 mol) for HPMC and TA required to prepare the sound microcapsules.

4) The microcapsules become irregular with the concentrations of HPMC.

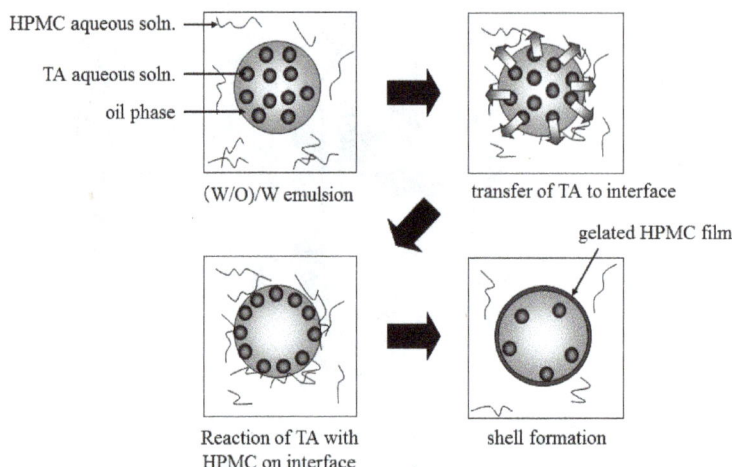

**Figure 9.** Microencapsulation mechanism.

5) The fine water droplets coalesced each other to form the larger water droplet.

6) As the microencapsulation method developed is the simple process with nontoxic materials, it may be expected that this method is going to be applied in many kinds of fields.

## References

[1]    Kondo, T. (1967) Saishin Maikurokapseruka Gijutsu (Microencapsulation Technique). TES, Tokyo.

[2]    Tanaka, M. (2008) Key Point of Preparation of Nano/Microcapsules. Techno System Publishing Co. Ltd., Tokyo.

[3]    Koishi, M., Eto, K. and Higure, H. (2005) (Preparation + Utilization) Microcapsules. Kogyo Chosakai, Tokyo.

[4]    Wang, J.M., Zheng, W., Song, Q.W., Zhu, H. and Zhou, Y. (2009) Preparation and Characterization of Natural Fragrant Microcapsules. *Journal of Fiber Bioengineering and Informatics*, **1**, 293-300.
http://dx.doi.org/10.3993/jfbi03200907

[5]    Lee, H., Jeong, C., Ghafoor, K., Cho, S. and Park, J. (2011) Oral Delivery of Insulin Using Chitosan Capsules Cross-Linked with Phytic Acid. *Bio-Medical Materials and Engineering*, **21**, 25-36.

[6]    Suthaphot, N., Chulakup, S., Chonsakorn, S. and Mongkholrattanasit, R. (2012) Application of Aroma Therapy on Cotton Fabric by Microcapsules. *International Conference*: *Textiles & Fashion* 2012, Bangkok, 3-4 July 2014.

[7]    Satapathy, D., Biswas, D., Behera, B., Sagiri, S.S., Pal, K. and Pramanik, K. (2013) Sunflower-Oil-Based Lecithin Organogels as Matrices for Controlled Drug Delivery. *Journal of Applied Polymer Science*, **129**, 585-594.
http://dx.doi.org/10.1002/app.38498

[8]    Hsieha, W.C., Changb, C.P. and Gaoc, Y.L. (2006) Controlled Release Properties of Chitosan Encapsulated Volatile Citronella Oil Microcapsules by Thermal Treatments. *Colloids and Surfaces B: Biointerfaces*, **53**, 209-214.
http://dx.doi.org/10.1016/j.colsurfb.2006.09.008

[9]    Iamrungraksa, T. and Charuchinda, S. (2010) Preparation and Characteristics of Galangal Essential Oil/Alginate Microcapsules. *Journal of Metals, Materials and Minerals*, **20**, 89-92.

[10]   Soliman, E.A., El-Moghazy, A.Y., Mohy El-Din, M.S. and Massoud, M.A. (2013) Microencapsulation of Essential Oils within Alginate: Formulation and *in Vitro* Evaluation of Antifungal Activity. *Journal of Encapsulation and Adsorption Sciences*, **3**, 48-55. http://dx.doi.org/10.4236/jeas.2013.31006

[11]   Paques, J.P., van der Linden, E., van Rijn, C.J. and Sagis, L.M. (2014) Preparation Methods of Alginate Nanoparticles. *Advances in Colloid and Interface Science*, **209**, 163-171. http://dx.doi.org/10.1016/j.cis.2014.03.009

[12]   Belyaeva, E., Valle, D.D., Neufeld, R.J. and Poncelet, D. (2004) New Approach to the Formulation of Hydrogel Beads Byemulsi & Cation/Thermal Gelation Using a Static Mixer. *Chemical Engineering Science*, **59**, 2913-2920.
http://dx.doi.org/10.1016/j.ces.2004.04.010

[13]   Wang, A., Tao, C., Cui, Y., Duan, L., Yang, Y. and Li, J. (2009) Assembly of Environmental Sensitive Microcapsules of PNIPAAm and Alginate Acidand Their Application in Drug Release. *Journal of Colloid and Interface Science*, **332**, 271-279. http://dx.doi.org/10.1016/j.jcis.2008.12.032

[14]   Katoh, K., Yoshimura, H. and Fujita, H. (2005) Preparation of Porous Matrices of Natural Polymer Using Microcapsules. *Aichiken Sangyou Gijutsu Kenkyuujo kenkyuu houkoku*, **4**, 200-203.

[15] Tian, K., Xie, C. and Xia, X. (2013) Chitosan/Alginate Multilayer film for Controlled Release of IDM on Cu/LDPE Composite Intrauterine Devices. *Colloids and Surfaces B: Biointerfaces*, **109**, 82-89. http://dx.doi.org/10.1016/j.colsurfb.2013.03.036

[16] Su, J.F., Wang, S.B., Zhang, Y.Y. and Huang, Z. (2011) Physicochemical Properties and Mechanical Characters of Methanol-Modified Melamine-Formaldehyde (MMF) Shell MicroPCMS Containing Paraffin. *Colloid and Polymer Science*, **289**, 111-119. http://dx.doi.org/10.1007/s00396-010-2328-1

[17] Yuan, Y., Zhang, N., Tao, W., Cao, X. and He, Y. (2014) Fatty Acids as Phase Change Materials: A Review. *Renewable and Sustainable Energy*, **29**, 482-498. http://dx.doi.org/10.1016/j.rser.2013.08.107

[18] Yang, Z., Peng, Z., Li, J., Li, S., Kong, L., Li, P. and Wang, Q. (2014) Development and Evaluation of Novel Flavour Microcapsules Containing Vanilla Oil Using Complex Coacervation Approach. *Food Chemistry*, **145**, 272-277. http://dx.doi.org/10.1016/j.foodchem.2013.08.074

[19] Chang, C.P., Leung, T.K., Lin, S.M. and Hsu, C.C. (2006) Release Properties on Gelatin-Gum Arabic Microcapsules Containing Camphor Oil with Added Polystyrene. *Colloids and Surfaces B: Biointerfaces*, **50**, 136-140. http://dx.doi.org/10.1016/j.colsurfb.2006.04.008

[20] Soottitantawat, A., Bigeard, F., Yoshii, H., Furuta, T., Ohkawara, M. and Linko, P. (2005) Influence of Emulsion and Powder Size on the Stability Ofencapsulated d-Limonene by Spray Drying. *Innovative Food Science and Emerging Technologies*, **6**, 107-114. http://dx.doi.org/10.1016/j.ifset.2004.09.003

[21] Polavarapu, S., Oliver, C.M., Ajlouni, S. and Augustin, M.A. (2012) Impact of Extra Virgin Olive Oil and Ethylenediaminetetraacetic Acid (EDTA) on the Oxidative Stability of Fish Oil Emulsions and Spray-Dried Microcapsules Stabilized by Sugar Beet Pectin. *Journal of Agricultural and Food Chemistry*, **60**, 444-450. http://dx.doi.org/10.1021/jf2034785

[22] Gharsallaoui, A., Saurel, R., Chambin, O., Cases, E., Voilley, A. and Cayot, P. (2010) Utilisation of Pectin Coating to Enhance Spray-Dry Stability of Pea Protein-Stabilised Oil-in-Water Emulsions. *Food Chemistry*, **122**, 447-454. http://dx.doi.org/10.1016/j.foodchem.2009.04.017

[23] Taguchi, Y., Ono, F. and Tanaka, M. (2013) Preparation of Microcapsules Containing $\beta$-Carotene with Thermo Sensitive Curdlan by Utilizing Reverse Dispersion. *Pharmaceutic*, **5**, 609-620. http://dx.doi.org/10.3390/pharmaceutics5040609

# 28

# Melanin Uptake Reduces Cell Proliferation of Human Epidermal Keratinocytes

Xianghong Yan[1], Ta-Min Wang[2*], Yung-Ching Ming[3*], Yuan-Ming Yeh[4], Tzu-Ya Chen[5], Jong-Hwei Su Pang[5#]

[1]P & G Innovation Godo Kaisha, Kobe, Japan
[2]Division of Urology, Department of Surgery, Chang Gung Memorial Hospital, Kwei-Shan, Taiwan
[3]Department of Pediatric Surgery, Chang Gung Children's Hospital, Chang Gung Memorial Hospital, Taiwan
[4]Molecular Medicine Research Center, Chang Gung University, Taiwan
[5]Graduate Institute of Clinical Medical Sciences, College of Medicine, Chang Gung University, Taiwan
Email: #jonghwei@mail.cgu.edu.tw

## Abstract

Melanin, synthesized by melanocyte, is transferred to neighboring keratinocyte and finally accumulates in perinuclear site. Except functioning as an internal sunscreen to protect from UV damage, the potential effect of melanin on modulating the bioactivity of keratinocyte has not yet been fully investigated. In this study, we added melanin directly to the culture of human epidermal keratinocytes and the uptake of melanin was found to be dose- and time-dependent as determined by spectrophotometric method. The uptaken melanin accumulated perinuclearly in keratinocytes that is similar to the pattern observed in human solar lentigo tissue by microscopic examination. Pretreatment of keratinocytes with either niacinamide or trypsin inhibitor reduced the uptake of melanin dose-dependently, indicating a PAR-2-dependent pathway involved. Melanin uptake by keratinocytes inhibited cell proliferation as demonstrated both by the decrease of cell number and nuclear Ki-67 expression. Inhibited Ki-67 expression in melanin-containing keratinocyte was also found in human lentigo tissue. The cell cycle arrested at G1 phase in melanin-uptaken keratinocytes was confirmed by flow cytometric method. The protein expressions of cyclin-dependent kinase 1 (CDK1), CDK2, cyclin E, cyclin A and cyclin B were significantly reduced by melanin treatment. Microarray analysis, RT/real-time PCR and western blot demonstrated the inhibited expression of DKK1, a protein known to reduce skin pigmentation, in melanin-uptaken keratinocytes. Together, the direct incubation of keratinocyte with melanin might serve as a useful model to study the potential mechanisms involved in melanin uptake and pigmentation process.

---

*Ta-Min Wang and Yung-Ching Ming contributed to this work equally.
#Corresponding author.

## Keywords

**Melanin, Epidermal Keratinocyte, Proliferation, Ki67, Cell Cycle, DKK1**

## 1. Introduction

Melanocytes produce specific organelles, termed melanosomes, in which melanin pigment is synthesized and deposited. Melanin is produced within melanosomes which later migrate into the melanocyte's dendrite tips using myosinV and dynein [1]. It is well known that tyrosinase is a rate limiting step in melanin production but melanosome transfer is also a decisive step responsible for melanogenesis [2] [3]. Therefore, instead of tyrosinase inhibitors that are mostly applied, a few hypopigmenting agents are now intended to inhibit the transfer of melanosomes [4]-[6].

Different mechanisms of melanosome transfer have been proposed including direct infusion of melanosomes into keratinocytes through nanotubular filopodia [7], uptake of released melanosomes by keratinocytes via phagocytosis [8], and partial cytophagocytosis of melanocyte dendrite tips containing melanosomes by keratinocytes [9]. A differernt mechanism for the transfer of melanosomes was reported in which pigment globules containing multiple melanosomes are released into the extracellular space from melanocytes and are then ingested by keratinocytes [10]. Recently, keratinocytes are found to predominantly induce a Rab11b-mediated exocytosis through remodeling of the melanosome membrane before subsequent endocytosis of melanin [11]. No matter which mechanism is acting, the result is the cellular uptake of melanin and finally forms perinuclear melanin caps [12].

Melanin, a natural pigment produced by stimulated melanocytes in the basal layer of skin epidermis, converts more than 99.9% of the absorbed UV light to heat and functions as an excellent photoprotectant that prevents cells from the DNA damage by UV [13]-[15]. Except functioning as an internal sunscreen, the potential effect of melanin on modulating the bioactivity of epidermal keratinocytes has not yet been fully investigated.

In this study, we attempted to investigate the biological effect of melanin in epidermal keratinocytes. Epidermal keratinocytes were incubated with melanin and the direct uptake of melanin was examined and compared with that in human lentigo tissues. Cell proliferation and the expressions of cell cycle-dependent genes were studied. Microarray analysis was carried out to further understand the effect of melanin uptake on the biological function of keratinocytes.

## 2. Materials and Methods

### 2.1. Cell Culture

Human epidermal keratinocytes were isolated from skin by enzymatic digestion method as described previously [16]. Skin samples were obtained from donors with informed consents, under the approval of the Institutional Review Board of Chang Gung Memorial Hospital in Tao-Yuan, Taiwan. Briefly, skin was rinsed in 10% iodine for 30 sec and cleaned with 1 × PBS, then incubated in dispase (type II, 2.5 mg/ml in 1 × PBS) for 2 h at 37°C to dissociate the epidermis from dermis. The epidermal layer was peeled off carefully and cut into small pieces and incubated in 0.25% trypsin for 30 min at 37°C to release single cell. Cells were centrifuged and the cell pellet was resuspended in keratinocyte serum-free medium (KSFM, GIBCO®) containing EGF and bovine pituitary extract and maintained at 37°C in a humidified atmosphere of 95% air and 5% $CO_2$. Keratinocytes between passages 3 and 5 were used for all the experiments. In the present study, epidermal keratinocytes at 70% - 80% confluence were treated with melanin (0 - 100 μg/ml) for 24 h or indicated time and used for the analysis. All experiments were performed in triplicate.

### 2.2. Measurement of Melanin Uptake

The content of melanin uptake in keratinocytes was determined by spectrophotometric method. Cells were washed thoroughly by 1 × PBS, homogenized with 1N NaOH and heated at 95°C for 30 min to dissolve intracellular melanin. The melanin content was determined by measuring the absorbance at 495 nm using a spectrophotometer.

## 2.3. Examination of Melanin Uptake in Cultured Keratinocytes and Solar Lentigo Tissue

Keratinocytes cultured on coverslips were fixed in 1 × PBS containing 4% paraformaldehyde for 15 min and stained with modified Wright-Giemsa stain (Sigma) for the microscopic examination of melanin uptake in cells. HE-stained tissue sections of solar lentigo was obtained from the tissue bank in Chang Gung Memorial Hospital (Tao-Yuan, Taiwan) and pathology was diagnosed and identified by Dr. Wen-Rou Wong who is a skin specialist. Solar lentigo is a small pigmented spot with a clearly defined edge on the skin associated with aging and exposure to ultraviolet radiation from the sun. Histologically, the hallmark of solar lentigo is an increase in basal melanin.

## 2.4. MTT Assay

Epidermal keratinocytes grown in 24-well culture plate with or without melanin treatment for 24 h were washed once with 1 × PBS, followed by addition of 0.5 ml KSFM containing 0.05 mg/ml 3-[4, 5-dimethylthiazol-2-yl]-2, 5-diphenyltetrazolium bromide (MTT). After incubation at 37°C for 1 h, the medium was removed and formazan crystals in the cells were dissolved in 1 ml DMSO for OD reading at 570 nm using a spectrophotometer.

## 2.5. Immunofluorescent Staining

Keratinocytes cultured on coverslips were fixed in 4% paraformaldehyde in 1 × PBS for 15 min and then in methanol at −20°C for 10 min. Cells were blocked in 1 × PBS containing 1% BSA and 1% goat serum for 30 min. Rabbit antibody against Ki67 (Lab Vision) was added to blocking solution in a ratio of 1:50 and incubated at 4°C overnight. After washing with 1 × PBS, FITC-conjugated goat anti-rabbit IgG (BioFX) was added (1:2000 in 1 × PBS) for 30 min. After washing with 1 × PBS, cell nuclei were counter-stained by propidium iodide for 10 min at 37°C. Coverslips were mounted with fluorescent specific medium for the examination under fluorescent microscope.

## 2.6. Immunohistochemistry

Rehydrated tissue section was pretreated in 10 mM citrate buffer, pH 6.0, at 95°C for 20 min followed by cooling at room temperature for 20 min. Tissue section was blocked in 1 × PBS containing 1% BSA and 1% goat serum for 30 min. Rabbit antibody against Ki67 (Lab Vision) was added to blocking solution in a ratio of 1:50 and incubated at 4°C overnight. After washing with 1 × PBS, section was incubated with biotinylated goat anti-rabbit IgG (Thermo Scientific) for 15 min. After washing with 1 × PBS, section was incubated with streptavidin-conjugated peroxidase (Thermo Scientific) for 10 min. In order to differentiate from the brown color of melanin in lentigo tissue, positive signals were developed by reacting peroxidase with ImmPACT™ SG substrate (VECTOR) for 15 min and Ki67 expression was developed into blue color. Cell nuclei were counterstained by nuclear fast red (VECTOR) for 10 min and mounted with VectaMount™ AQ mounting medium (VECTOR).

## 2.7. Flow Cytometry

Keratinocytes were harvested by trypsinization. After washing with 1 × PBS and centrifugation, the cell pellet was resuspended in 1 ml ice-cold 70% ethanol and incubated overnight on a rocker at 4°C. Cells were collected, washed and incubated in a solution of 0.5% Triton X-100 and 0.05% RNase at 37°C for 1 h. Cell nuclei were then stained by propidium iodide (PI) solution (50 mg/ml PI in 1 × PBS) and incubated at 4°C for 20 min. Cell cycle distribution was quantified with a FACS Calibur system (Becton-Dickinson). Percentages of cells in the $G_0/G_1$, S, and $G_2/M$ phases of the cell cycle were determined and analyzed using CellQuest Pro software (Becton Dickinson).

## 2.8. RNA Isolation and RT/Real-Time PCR

Total RNA was extracted from keratinocytes by acid guanidinium thiocyanate–phenol–chloroform extraction method, and complementary (c) DNA was synthesized using 1 μg total RNA in a 20 μl RT reaction mix containing 0.5 μg/μl of random primers, 0.1 mM dNTP, 0.1 M DTT and 5× first strand buffer. Real-time PCR was performed using an SYBR Green I technology and MxPro- Mx3000P QPCR machine (Stratagene), and a master mix was prepared with Smart Quant Green Master Mix with dUTP & ROX Kit (Protech). Relative gene expressions between experimental groups were determined using MxPro software (Stratagene) and GAPDH was used as an internal control. All real-time PCRs were performed in triplicate, and changes in gene expressions were reported as multiples of increases relative to the controls. The following primers were used: GAPDH: 5'-GAGGGGCCATCCACAGTCTT-3' (forward) and 5'-TTCATTGACCTCAACTACAT-3' (reverse). DKK1: 5'-CGTTGTTACTGTGGAGAA-3' (forward) and 5'-GTGTGAAGCCTAGAAGAAT-3' (reverse).

## 2.9. Western Blot Analysis

Epidermal keratinocytes were rinsed with cold $1 \times$ PBS, scraped and solubilized in lysis buffer (20 mM Tris-Cl, pH 7.5, 150 mM NaCl, 1 mM $Na_2EDTA$, 1 mM EGTA, 1% Triton, 2.5 mM sodium pyrophosphate, 1 mM β-glycerophosphate, 1 mM $Na_3VO_4$, 1 mM PMSF, 1 μg/ml aprotinin, and 1 μg/ml leupeptin), followed by sonication and centrifugation at 12,000 g for 20 min at 4°C. The protein concentration in the supernatant was determined by Bradford protein assay kit (Bio-Rad). Cell lysates containing equal amounts of protein were separated by 10% SDS-PAGE, and transferred onto PVDF membrane (Millipore). The membrane was incubated in blocking solution (1% BSA, 1% goat serum in $1 \times$ PBS) for 1 h, followed by incubation with primary antibody diluted in blocking solution. After washing, the membrane was incubated in $1 \times$ PBS containing secondary antibody conjugated with horseradish peroxidase for 1 h. The membrane was washed and the positive signals were developed with enhanced chemiluminescence reagent (Amershan Pharmacia Biotech). The following primary antibodies were used: anti-CDK1 antibody (MS-110-P1, Thermo), anti-CDK2 antibody (MS-459-P0, Thermo), anti-cyclin A antibody (ab38, Abcam), anti-cyclin B antibody (MS-338, Thermo), anti-cyclin E antibody (14-6714, eBioscience), anti-DKK1 (AF1096, R&D systems) and anti-tubulin-α antibody (MS-581-P, Thermo). Tubulin was used as the sample loading control.

## 3. Results

### 3.1. Direct Uptake of Melanin in Human Epidermal Keratinocytes

In order to study the direct effect of melanin on the cellular function of epidermal kerationcytes, we incubated keratinocytes with melanin in culture medium for 24 h and the uptake of melanin was measured by spectrophotometric method. The uptake of melanin by keratinocytes occurred soon after the addition of melanin for 1 h and the extent of uptake significantly increased in a dose- and time-dependent manner (**Figure 1(a)** and **Figure 1(b)**, respectively). The uptaken melanin was revealed to be accumulated surrounding the nucleus (**Figure 1(c)**) which was similarly observed in human lentigo tissue (**Figure 1(d)**) as indicated by yellow arrows.

### 3.2. Niacinamide and Trypsin Inhibitor Suppressed Melanin Uptake in Epidermal Keratinocytes

To understand the possible mechanism for epidermal keratinocytes to directly uptake melanin, we tested two well-known inhibitors for the transfer and uptake of melanosome into epidermal keratinocytes on this simplified cell model. Epidermal keratinocytes were pretreated with niacinamide or trypsin inhibitors for 3 h and then 50 μg/ml melanin was added for 24 h. The amount of melanin uptaken by epidermal keratinocytes was demonstrated to be dose-dependently suppressed by niacinamide or trypsin inhibitor (**Figure 2(a)** and **Figure 2(b)**, respectively).

### 3.3. Melanin Inhibited Cell Proliferation and Ki-67 Expression in Epidermal Keratinocytes

The uptake of melanin appeared to reduce the cell density of epidermal kertinocytes from microscopic observation. Epidermal keratinocytes with different concentration of melanin treatment for 24 h were analyzed by MTT assay. Results in **Figure 3(a)** demonstrated the dose-dependent effect of melanin on decreasing the cell number of epidermal keratinocytes. To further prove the inhibitory effect of melanin on the cell proliferation of epidermal keratinocytes, the expression of Ki-67, a cell proliferating marker, was fluorescently stained in epidermal keratinocytes. As clearly shown in **Figure 3(b)**, the number of cells with positively stained Ki-67 expression (green fluorescent signal) in the nucleus was significantly decreased after melanin treatment. The dose-dependent effect of melanin on suppressing the Ki-67 expression in keratinocytes was calculated and confirmed in

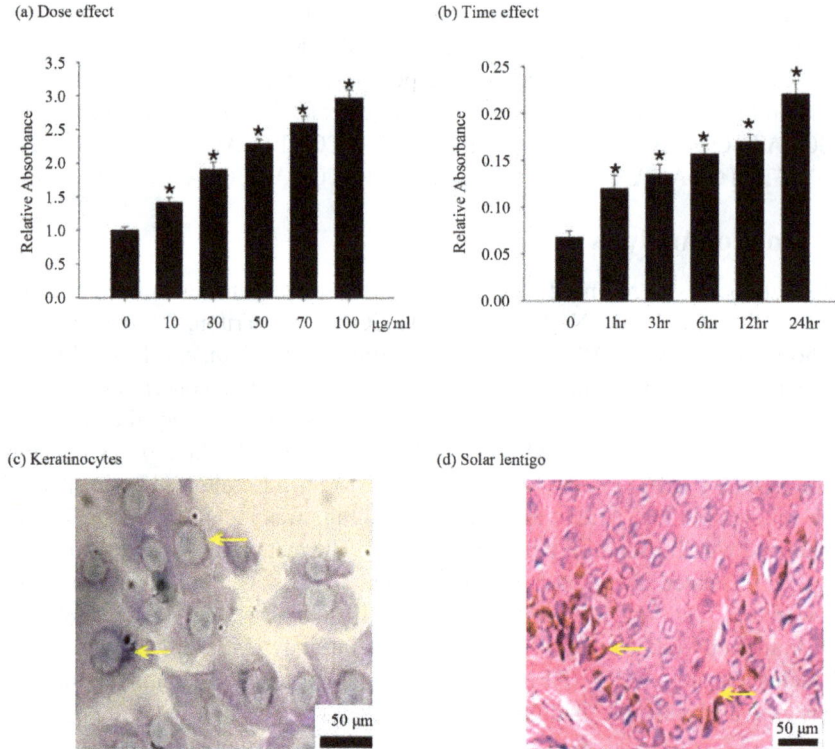

(a) Dose effect

(b) Time effect

(c) Keratinocytes

(d) Solar lentigo

50 µm

50 µm

**Figure 1.** Melanin uptake in human epidermal keratinocytes was dose- and time-dependent. (a) Melanin at the concentration from 0 to 100 µg/ml as indicated was added to 70% - 80% confluent human epidermal keratinocytes for 24 h and the melanin uptake was measured by spectrophotometric method. (b) Melanin at the concentration of 100 µg/ml was added to 70% - 80% confluent human epidermal keratinocytes and the melanin uptake was measured by spectrophotometric method at 0, 1, 3, 6, 12 and 24 h. The perinuclear accumulation of melanin was observed in (c) cultured human epidermal keratoinocytes and in (d) human lentigo tissue.

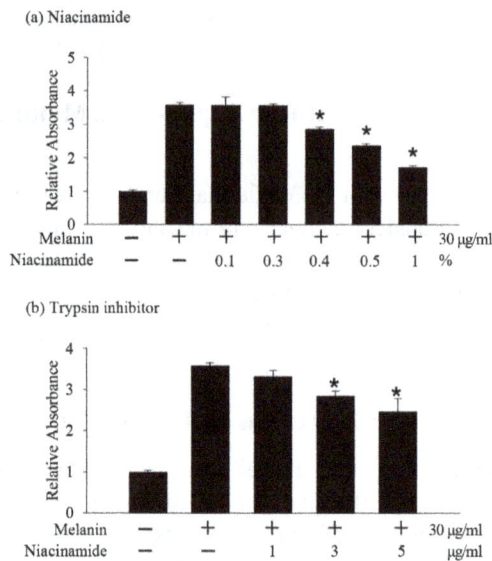

(a) Niacinamide

(b) Trypsin inhibitor

**Figure 2.** Niacinamide and trypsin inhibitor reduced the melanin uptake in epidermal keratinocytes. Human epidermal keratinocytes at 70% - 80% confluency were pretreated with (a) niacinamide (0% - 0.5% as indicated) and (b) trypsin inhibitor (0 - 10 µg/ml as indicated) for 3 h and then melanin at the concentration of 50 µg/ml was added for 24 h. Melanin uptake was measured by spectrophotometric method.

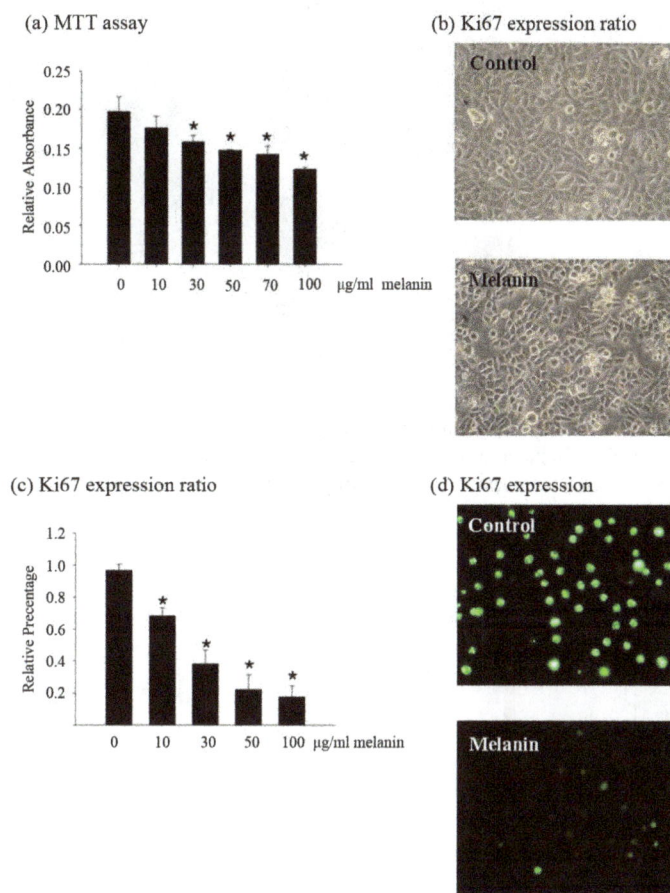

**Figure 3.** Melanin inhibited the proliferation of human epidermal keratinocytes. (a) Melanin at the concentration from 0 to 100 μg/ml as indicated was added to 70% - 80% confluent human epidermal keratinocytes for 24 h and MTT assay was performed. (b) Representative photo for the fluoresecently labeled Ki-67 expression in epidermal keratoinocytes without (upper panel) or with (lower panel) 50 μg/ml melanin treatment for 24 h. (c) The dose-dependent effect of melanin on the number of Ki-67 positive epidermal keratonicytes was quantified.

**Figure 3(c)**. Similar correlation was also found in human solar lentigo tissue as shown in **Figure 4**. Yellow arrow pointed out the cell with perinuclear accumulation of melanin (brown color) in which Ki67 expression was observed to be reduced. On the other hand, cell with positive Ki67 signal (blue color) as pointed out by red arrow was found to contain less melanin accumulation in the cells.

## 3.4. Melanin Arrested the Cell Cycle Progression of Epidermal Keratinocytes

The inhibitory effect of melanin on the proliferation of epidermal keratinocytes was further confirmed by the cell cycle distribution analysis using flow cytometry. Results in **Figure 5(a)** clearly revealed that the melanin treatment resulted in the increase of G1phase-cells from 41.84% to 57.57% and the decrease of S phase-cells from 45.52% to 30.09%. Clearly, the cell cycle progression of epidermal keratinocytes was delayed and partially arrested at G1 phase by melanin. The expressions of cell cycle-dependent genes including CDK1, CDK2, cyclin E, cyclin A and cyclin B were dose-dependently suppressed in epidermal keratinocytes by the treatment with melanin for 24 h (**Figure 5(b)**).

## 3.5. Microarray Study Revealed the Down-Regulation of DKK1 Gene Expression in Human Epidermal Kerationocytes by Melanin

To further explore the potential effect of melanin on the biological functions of epidermal keratinocytes, we

Solar lentigo (Ki67: blue color; melanin: brown color)

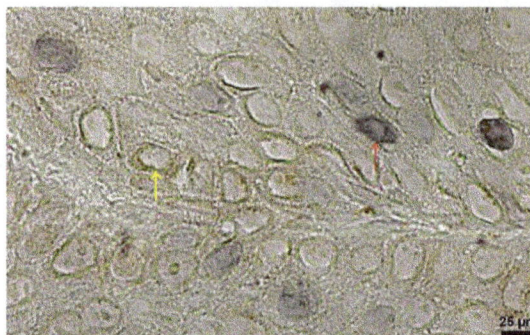

**Figure 4.** Melanin inhibited the in vivo Ki-67 expression in keratinocytes. The Ki-67 expression in human lentigo tissue was revealed by immunostaining the protein and developed into blue color. Yellow arrow indicated the cell with melanin uptake and red arrow indicated the cell without melanin uptake. Representative photo was shown from five different lentigo tissues with similar results.

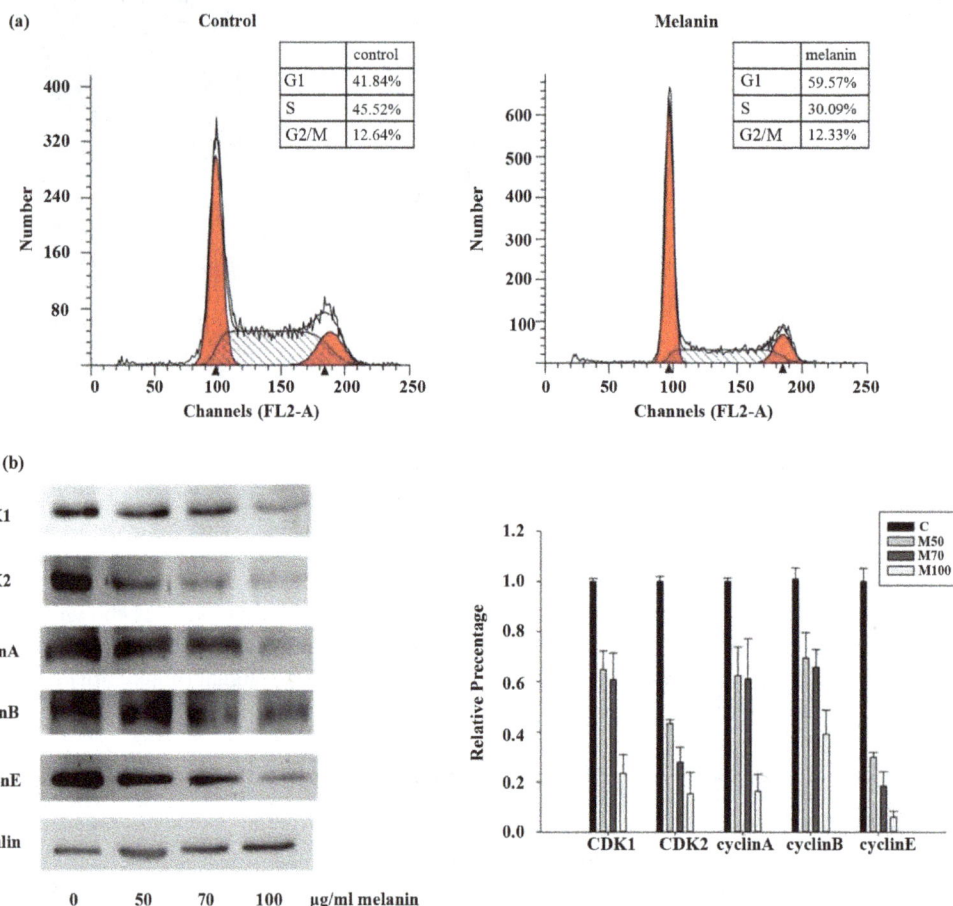

**Figure 5.** Melanin inhibited cell cycle progression and the gene expressions of cell cycle-dependent genes. (a) Epidermal keratinocytes were treated with 50 μg/ml melanin for 24 h and processed for the analysis of cell cycle distribution by flow cytometry. (b) Protein lysates were prepared from cells treated with different concentrations of melanin and western blot analysis was performed.

isolated RNA isolated from this simplified cell model and microarray analysis was performed by Phalanx Biotech Group (Hsinchu, Taiwan, R.O.C.) using The Human Whole Genome One Array® v6 containing 32,679 DNA oligonucleotide probes to reveal the gene expression profile changed by melanin. Results shown in **Figure 6(a)**

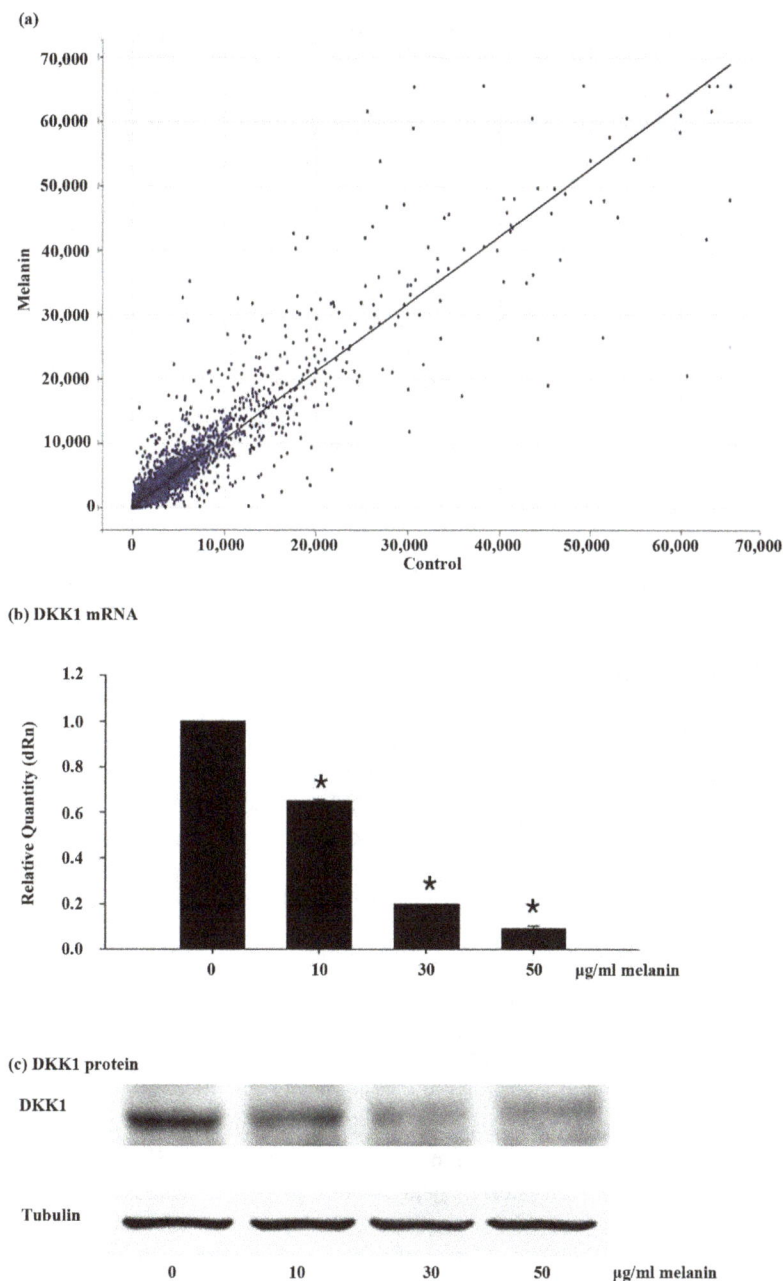

**Figure 6.** Microarray analysis revealed the inhibition of DKK1 gene expression in keratinocytes by melanin. (a) Full microarray data of expressed gene probes plotted as melanin-treated cells mean signal vs. control mean signal. Melanin at the concentration from 0 to 50 μg/ml as indicated was added to 70% - 80% confluent human epidermal keratinocytes for 24 h and the mRNA level was measured by (b) RT/real-time PCR and (c) western blot analysis, respectively.

revealed 800 genes with more than two-fold changes in melanin-treated keratinocytes. Among them, DKK1 was found to be remarkably suppressed in epidermal keratinocytes by melanin. In **Figure 6(b)** and **Figure 6(c)**, the mRNA and protein expression levels of DKK1 in epidermal keratinocytes were further confirmed to be decreased in a dose-dependent manner.

# 4. Discussion

The process of melanosome transfer has been investigated for decades either by co-culturing epidermal keratinocytes with melanocytes or incubating epidermal keratinocytes in the presence of isolated melanosomes mostly from melanoma cells. Although several mechanisms of melanosome transfer are likely to occur in the skin, recently, a new mechanism of melanosome transfer has been reported that involves the release of melanosome-containing globules and then uptake by keratinocytes [10]. However, it has been found that the removal of melanosomal membranes due to the detergent treatment during the purification process did not block the transfer into keratinocytes, suggesting that the melanosomal membrane is not critical for the ingestion by keratinocytes.

In the present study, we demonstrated that keratinocytes could uptake melanin directly into cytoplasm. Melanin alone in cytoplasm could also be accumulated to perinuclear site that did not require the components from melanosome. The direct uptake of melanin alone could also be inhibited by trypsin inhibitor and niacinamide, indicating the involvement of protease-activated receptor-2 (PAR-2) in this process, which was similar to previous studies using co-cultured cell model or incubation with isolated melanosomes.

Compared to the previous studies using co-cultured cell model or incubation with isolated melanosomes, this simplified cell model for direct uptake of melanin can be used to investigate the pure effect of melanin on the biological activity of epidermal keratinocyte without being interfered by some unknown factors in the melanosomes particularly those isolated from cancerous melanoma cells instead of normal cells. This cell model was apparently much easier and could avoid the experimental complication due to the different preparation of melanosomes and therefore data with higher reproducibility could be obtained.

Melanin plays an important role in protecting human skin from the UV irradiation. Nuclear accumulation forms a melanin cap above cell nuclei and functions to protect DNA from UV-induced damage. The uptake of melanin in keratinocytes resulted in the inhibition of cell proliferation not only in cultured epidermal keratinocytes, but also being observed in human solar lentigo tissue. The inhibition of cell proliferation is consistent to the result of delay of cell cycle, which may allow the cells to repair the potential damage of DNA and prevent the change of DNA sequence that could be fixed after the replication of DNA in keratinocytes. A recent study reported an inhibited cell proliferation of SV40T-transformed human epidermal keratinocytes (SV-HEKs) after the treatment with isolated melanosomes also in a PAR-2 dependent manner [17]. It is very likely that the inhibition of cell proliferation was caused by the melanin that got inside the cells through the uptake of melanosomes. In addition, based on the results of our microarray results, melanin was indeed found to down-regulate the expressions of many cell cycle-dependent genes in epidermal keratinocytes that contributed to the inhibition of cell proliferation.

Dickkopf 1 (DKK1), an inhibitor of Wnt signaling, not only functions during the embryonic development [18], but also regulates joint remodeling [19] and bone formation [20]. DKK1 is therefore believed to play a role in the pathogenesis of rheumatoid arthritis [21] and multiple myeloma [22]. Recently, the levels of DKK1 in palmoplantar dermal fibroblasts were found to be higher than those observed in non-palmoplantar dermal fibroblasts [23]. In a paracrine signaling way, DKK1 secreted from fibroblasts can suppress melanocyte function through the regulation of microphthalmia-associated transcription factor (MITF) and beta-catenin [24]. In addition, DKK1 can also induce the expression of keratin 9 and alpha-Kelch-like ECT2-interacting protein (alphaKLEIP) but decrease the expression of beta-catenin, glycogen synthase kinase 3beta, protein kinase C, and proteinase-activated receptor-2 (PAR-2) in epidermal keratinocytes which is consistent with the expression pattern in human palmoplantar skin [25]. More interestingly, treatment with exogeneous DKK1 could result in the hypopigmentation and thickening of a reconstructed skin model, elucidating why human palmoplantar skin is thicker and paler than non-palmoplantar skin [26]. Therefore, DKK1 can potentially be used to reduce skin pigmentation or to repair certain damaged skins. Our study, for the first time, demonstrated that keratinocytes can also produce DKK1 by themselves and the DKK1 gene expression in epidermal keratinocytes could be down-regulated by the uptake of melanin. Also, the decrease of DKK1 by melanin uptake was correlated well with the inhibited proliferation of epidermal keratinocytes. In other words, the uptake of melanin in epidermal keratinocytes might play a crucial role in the process of pigmentation that is likely mediated by the suppression of DKK1 gene expression. These interesting results warrant further extensive investigation.

## 5. Conclusion

In conclusion, our findings demonstrated a cell model that was potentially useful to study the effects of melanin uptake in epidermal keratinocytes; in addition, our findings demonstrated that after melanin uptake, keratinocyte cell cycle is delayed, which is consistent to the observation that in the solar lentigo area, the cell proliferation is inhibited. The discovery that DKK1 gene expression in this cell model was down-regulated by melanin uptake further confirmed the physiological meaning of this cell model which could be used to quickly screen drugs that might potentially result in hyper- or hypopigmentation. This simplified cell model could also be useful for exploring the molecular mechanism of melanin uptake and how melanin impacts keratinocyte biological activities, in addition, except DKK1, target proteins of skin pigmentation could be identified and help us to further understand the skin pigmentation issue.

## Acknowledgements

The authors would like to specially thank Dr. Wen-Rou Wong for providing tissue sections of lentigo obtained from the tissue bank in Chang Gung Memorial Hospital (Tao-Yuan, Taiwan). This study was supported by SCRPD190031 and SCRPD1A0061 from P & G Design Center Godo Kaisha, Procter & Gamble Japan K.K.

## Conflict of Interests

The authors declared no conflicts of interest.

## References

[1] Jordens, I., Westbroek, W., Marsman, M., *et al.* (2006) Rab7 and Rab27a Control Two Motor Protein Activities Involved in Melanosomal Transport. *Pigment Cell Research*, **19**, 412-423.
http://dx.doi.org/10.1111/j.1600-0749.2006.00329.x

[2] Park, H.Y., Kosmadaki, M., Yaar, M. and Gilchrest, B.A. (2009) Cellular Mechanisms Regulating Human Melanogenesis. *Cellular and Molecular Life Sciences*, **66**, 1493-1506. http://dx.doi.org/10.1007/s00018-009-8703-8

[3] Boissy, R.E. (2003) Melanosome Transfer to and Translocation in the Keratinocyte. *Experimental Dermatology*, **12**, 5-12. http://dx.doi.org/10.1034/j.1600-0625.12.s2.1.x

[4] Reish, O., Townsend, D., Berry, S.A., Tsai, M.Y. and King, R.A. (1995) Tyrosinase Inhibition Due to Interaction of Homocyst(e)ine with Copper: The Mechanism for Reversible Hypopigmentation in Homocystinuria Due to Cystathionine Beta-Synthase Deficiency. *The American Journal of Human Genetics*, **57**, 127-132.

[5] Solano, F., Briganti, S., Picardo, M. and Ghanem, G. (2006) Hypopigmenting Agents: An Updated Review on Biological, Chemical and Clinical Aspects. *Pigment Cell Research*, **19**, 550-571.
http://dx.doi.org/10.1111/j.1600-0749.2006.00334.x

[6] Kim, H., Choi, H.R., Kim, D.S., *et al.* (2012) Topical Hypopigmenting Agents for Pigmentary Disorders and Their Mechanisms of Action. *Annals of Dermatology*, **24**, 1-6. http://dx.doi.org/10.5021/ad.2012.24.1.1

[7] Singh, S.K., Kurfurst, R., Nizard, C., *et al.* (2010) Melanin Transfer in Human Skin Cells Is Mediated by Filopodia—A Model for Homotypic and Heterotypic Lysosome-Related Organelle Transfer. *FASEB Journal*, **24**, 3756-3769.
http://dx.doi.org/10.1096/fj.10-159046

[8] Ando, H., Niki, Y., Yoshida, M., *et al.* (2010) Keratinocytes in Culture Accumulate Phagocytosed Melanosomes in the Perinuclear Area. *Pigment Cell Melanoma Res*, **23**, 129-133. http://dx.doi.org/10.1111/j.1755-148X.2009.00640.x

[9] Chakraborty, A.K., Funasaka, Y., Araki, K., *et al.* (2003) Evidence That the Small GTPase Rab8 Is Involved in Melanosome Traffic and Dendrite Extension in B16 Melanoma Cells. *Cell and Tissue Research*, **314**, 381-388.
http://dx.doi.org/10.1007/s00441-003-0773-6

[10] Ando, H., Niki, Y., Yoshida, M., *et al.* (2011) Involvement of Pigment Globules Containing Multiple Melanosomes in the Transfer of Melanosomes from Melanocytes to Keratinocytes. *Cellular Logistics*, **1**, 12-20.
http://dx.doi.org/10.4161/cl.1.1.13638

[11] Tarafder, A.K., Bolasco, G., Correia, M.S., *et al.* (2014) Rab11b Mediates Melanin Transfer between Donor Melanocytes and Acceptor Keratinocytes via Coupled Exo/Endocytosis. *Journal of Investigative Dermatology*, **134**, 1056-1066. http://dx.doi.org/10.1038/jid.2013.432

[12] Byers, H.R., Maheshwary, S., Amodeo, D.M., *et al.* (2003) Role of Cytoplasmic Dynein in Perinuclear Aggregation of Phagocytosed Melanosomes and Supranuclear Melanin Cap Formation in Human Keratinocytes. *Journal of Investigative Dermatology*, **121**, 813-820. http://dx.doi.org/10.1046/j.1523-1747.2003.12481.x

[13] Yamaguchi, Y., Takahashi, K., Zmudzka, B.Z., *et al.* (2006) Human Skin Responses to UV Radiation: Pigment in the Upper Epidermis Protects against DNA Damage in the Lower Epidermis and Facilitates Apoptosis. *FASEB Journal*, **20**, 1486-1488. http://dx.doi.org/10.1096/fj.06-5725fje

[14] Takeuchi, S., Zhang, W., Wakamatsu, K., *et al.* (2004) Melanin Acts as a Potent UVB Photosensitizer to Cause an Atypical Mode of Cell Death in Murine Skin. *Proceedings of the National Academy of Sciences of the United States of*

*America*, **101**, 15076-15081. http://dx.doi.org/10.1073/pnas.0403994101

[15] Timares, L., Katiyar, S.K. and Elmets, C.A. (2008) DNA Damage, Apoptosis and Langerhans Cells—Activators of UV-Induced Immune Tolerance. *Photochemistry and Photobiology*, **84**, 422-436. http://dx.doi.org/10.1111/j.1751-1097.2007.00284.x

[16] Hsieh, W.L., Lin, Y.K., Tsai, C.N., *et al.* (2012) Indirubin, an Acting Component of Indigo Naturalis, Inhibits EGFR Activation and EGF-Induced CDC25B Gene Expression in Epidermal Keratinocytes. *Journal of Dermatological Science*, **67**, 140-146. http://dx.doi.org/10.1016/j.jdermsci.2012.05.008

[17] Choi, H.-I., Sohn, K.-C., Hong, D.-K., *et al.* (2013) Melanosome Uptake Is Associated with the Proliferation and Differentiation of Keratinocytes. *Archives of Dermatological Research*. [Epub ahead of print]

[18] Denicol, A.C., Dobbs, K.B., McLean, K.M., *et al.* (2013) Canonical WNT Signaling Regulates Development of Bovine Embryos to the Blastocyst Stage. *Scientific Reports*, **3**, 1266. http://dx.doi.org/10.1038/srep01266

[19] Daoussis, D. and Andonopoulos, A.P. (2011) The Emerging role of Dickkopf-1 in Bone Biology: Is It the Main Switch Controlling Bone and Joint Remodeling? *Seminars in Arthritis & Rheumatism*, **41**, 170-177. http://dx.doi.org/10.1016/j.semarthrit.2011.01.006

[20] Zhang, R., Oyajobi, B.O., Harris, S.E., *et al.* (2013) Wnt/β-Catenin Signaling Activates Bone Morphogenetic Protein 2 Expression in Osteoblasts. *Bone*, **52**, 145-156. http://dx.doi.org/10.1016/j.bone.2012.09.029

[21] Miao, C.G., Yang, Y.Y., He, X., *et al.* (2013) Wnt Signaling Pathway in Rheumatoid Arthritis, with Special Emphasis on the Different Roles in Synovial Inflammation and Bone Remodeling. *Cellular Signalling*, **25**, 2069-2078. http://dx.doi.org/10.1016/j.cellsig.2013.04.002

[22] Kocemba, K.A., Groen, R.W., van Andel, H., *et al.* (2012) Transcriptional Silencing of the Wnt-Antagonist DKK1 by Promoter Methylation Is Associated with Enhanced Wnt Signaling in Advanced Multiple Myeloma. *PLoS One*, **7**, e30359. http://dx.doi.org/10.1371/journal.pone.0030359

[23] Yamaguchi, Y., Itami, S., Watabe, H., *et al.* (2004) Mesenchymal-Epithelial Interactions in the Skin: Increased Expression of Dickkopf1 by Palmoplantar Fibroblasts Inhibits Melanocyte Growth and Differentiation. *Journal of Cell Biology*, **165**, 275-285. http://dx.doi.org/10.1083/jcb.200311122

[24] Yamaguchi, Y., Passeron, T., Watabe, H., *et al.* (2007) The Effects of Dickkopf 1 on Gene Expression and Wnt Signaling by Melanocytes: Mechanisms Underlying Its Suppression of Melanocyte Function and Proliferation. *Journal of Investigative Dermatology*, **127**, 1217-1225. http://dx.doi.org/10.1038/sj.jid.5700629

[25] Yamaguchi, Y., Passeron, T., Hoashi, T., *et al.* (2008) Dickkopf 1 (DKK1) Regulates Skin Pigmentation and Thickness by Affecting Wnt/Beta-Catenin Signaling in Keratinocytes. *FASEB Journal*, **22**, 1009-1020. http://dx.doi.org/10.1096/fj.07-9475com

[26] Yamaguchi, Y., Morita, A., Maeda, A., *et al.* (2009) Regulation of Skin Pigmentation and Thickness by Dickkopf 1 (DKK1). *Journal of Investigative Dermatology Symposium Proceedings*, **14**, 73-75. http://dx.doi.org/10.1038/jidsymp.2009.4

# 29

# Scalp Psoriasis: Systematic Review Comparing Topical Treatments and Placebo

Regina Jales[1], Sérgio Hirata[2], Álvaro Attalah[3], Danúbia Sá-Caputo[4], Adriano Arnóbio[5],
Éric Heleno Frederico[5], Mario Bernardo-Filho[5], Humberto Saconato[1]

[1]Departamento de Clínica Médica, Hospital Universitário Onofre Lopes, Universidade Federal do Rio Grande do
Norte, Natal, Brazil
[2]Departamento de Dermatologia, Hospital São Paulo, Universidade Federal de São Paulo, São Paulo, Brazil
[3]Departamento de Medicina Interna, Hospital São Paulo, Universidade Federal de São Paulo, São Paulo, Brazil
[4]Programa de Pós-Graduação em Fisiopatologia Clínica e Experimental, Universidade do Estado do Rio de
Janeiro, Rio de Janeiro, Brazil
[5]Departamento de Biofísica e Biometria, Universidade do Estado do Rio de Janeiro, Rio de Janeiro, Brazil
Email: bernardofilhom@gmail.com

## Abstract

Patients with scalp psoriasis suffered from a lower quality of life relating to the highly visible site
of their psoriatic lesions. In consequence this fact stimulates investigations involving treatments
of this dermatologic disease. The aim of this review is to evaluate the topical treatments for scalp
psoriasis compared with placebos. Methods: A systematic review was performed using searches in
the database LILACS, MEDLINE, Cochrane Library, and Embase. As selection criteria were chosen
eligible publications involving randomized controlled trials, patients with scalp psoriasis diagnosed clinically or by biopsy, interventions with topical treatments for scalp psoriasis compared
with placebo. Outcome related to the reduction in severity of psoriasis of the scalp, assessed by
physicians and patients, and assessment of adverse effects that required discontinuation of treatment. The results have shown that the patients were aged 12 to 97 years, including 3441 patients.
Ten of the fifteen studies included reported gender data. Patients were mostly female. Twelve studies were about psoriasis's severity. These studies in which the severity has been described, the
classification of severity was mild (0 study), mild to moderate (1 study), moderate to severe (11
studies) and severe (0 study). In conclusion, topical corticosteroids, calcipotriol, ciclopirox olamine and associations between them are effective in the treatment of scalp psoriasis. Clobetasol
propionate (0.05%) was the most effective active ingredient in several vehicles in the induction
treatment of scalp psoriasis.

## Keywords

**Scalp Psoriasis, Topical Treatments, Placebo, Topical Corticosteroids**

---

## 1. Introduction

Psoriasis is a hereditary disorder that affects 3% of the population worldwide [1]-[3]. There are two common ages for the onset of psoriasis. The first is around 21 years and the second at approximately 50 years [4] [5]. The most frequent type is psoriasis vulgaris, which appears as chronic, erythematous (reddish), and scaling skin lesions [6]. Clinical presentation varies from those with only a few localized lesions to those with generalized skin involvement [4].

There is evidence indicating that interaction between genes and certain environmental factors is an important cause of this disease [7]. Inflammatory cytokines such as tumor necrosis factor alpha, interferon gamma, and other type 1 cytokines also play an important role in the pathogenesis of psoriasis [8]. Many drugs that are used to treat other clinical conditions have also been reported to be responsible for the onset or exacerbation of psoriasis [9]. Among these drugs are lithium salts, antimalarials, beta-blocking agents, non-steroidal anti-inflammatory drugs (NSAIDS), angiotensin-converting enzyme (ACE) inhibitors, and the withdrawal of corticosteroids [10] [11].

Many clinical variants to the psoriasis are described, such as psoriasis vulgaris, guttate psoriasis (drops psoriasis), erythrodermic psoriasis (red psoriasis) and pustular psoriasis [11] [12]. The scalp is one of the most commonly affected parts of the body in people with psoriasis, and the frequency of involvement increases with the duration of the disease [13]. It may be part of generalized psoriasis or coexist with isolated plaques, or the scalp may be the only site involved. Signs and symptoms of scalp psoriasis vary significantly in different people, but pruritus, scaling and cosmetic embarrassment are often present [14] [15]. Because sensitive facial skin is so near the scalp, the use of potentially irritating topical treatments may be limited. Even so, the specific challenges of scalp psoriasis are often neglected in treatment guidelines [15] [16].

Scalp psoriasis can occasionally be confused with seborrhoeic dermatitis affecting the scalp [17]. Seborrhoeic dermatitis is another inflammatory condition which commonly affects the whole of the scalp resulting in mild inflammation and dandruff [17]. Psoriasis on the other hand is usually well-demarcated and has a coarser scale, but early diffuse psoriasis of the scalp can sometimes look very similar to seborrhoeic dermatitis. Sometimes a scalp biopsy may help [18] [19]. Those with psoriasis may also suffer from psychological distress, especially as a result of stigmatization and self-consciousness, so relatively high rates of depression have been reported [20].

The Psoriasis Area and Severity Index (PASI) is one of the most frequently used instruments to evaluate the severity of the disease and its response to different treatments, and its use is based on the extension and severity of the impact on the skin's surface [21] [22].

Relevant aspects of psoriasis that affect the person with this disease are evaluated using a variety of instruments, including the Psoriasis Disability Index (PDI) [23], Dermatology Quality of Life Index (DLQI) [24], the Psoriasis Symptom Assessment [25], and the Itching Scale [26]. The Physician Global Assessment is a tool to evaluate the psoriatic plaques [27]. This is a seven-point scale, with 7 being clear and 6 almost clear, 5 mild, 4 mild to moderate, 3 moderate, 2 moderately severe and 1 being severe psoriasis.

The aim of this review is to evaluate the topical treatments for scalp psoriasis compared with placebos.

## 2. Material and Methods

### 2.1. Keywords and Searches in the Databases

The keywords, psoriasis, scalp psoriasis and topical treatment were searched. The searches for identification of the publications used in this study were in Pubmed, Embase, The Cochrane Skin Group Specialised Register and in The Cochrane Central Register of Controlled Trials (CENTRAL) in The Cochrane Library. PubMed was searched from 2005 to august 2011. EMBASE, searched from 2010 to August 2011, LILACS (Latin American and Caribbean Health Science Information database, from 1982 to August 2011. The Salford Database of Psoriasis trials was searched up to August 2011.

## 2.2. Inclusion Criteria to Select Publications in This Investigation

Concerning to the types of studies, only randomised controlled trials (RCTs) were included. The Participants of these studies had the diagnosis of scalp psoriasis, according to clinical or biopsy findings used by authors of primary studies, for example: the classical history, symptoms and signs and typical histopathologic features. The types of interventions were any comparisons of local therapies for scalp psoriasis and placebo, such as, Corticosteroids plus calcipotriol versus placebo, Calcipotriol versus placebo, Corticosteroids versus placebo, Ciclopirox olamine versus placebo, among others. In the studies the outcome measures were Primary outcomes (Reduction in clinician-assessed severity, Improvement in quality of life, Adverse events requiring withdrawal of the treatment such as serious allergic reactions) and Secondary outcomes (Subjective reduction in severity of psoriasis, Minor adverse events not requiring withdrawal of the treatment like rash, itching, Time free of disease, duration of response, measured by the proportion of participants relapsing to baseline scores during continued treatment or following discontinuation of treatment.

## 2.3. Exclusion Criteria to Select Publications in This Investigation

Quasi-randomized studies were not considered for inclusion. Papers published in other languages than in English were excluded.

## 2.4. PRISMA Flowchart Involving the Steps in Selecting Full

A flowchart, based in the PRISMA analysis [28], was done to show the steps in the selection of the full papers analyzed in this revision.

## 2.5. Data Analysis

Data was not comparable and therefore statistical pooling not appropriate with the result that the findings of this review were summarized in a narrative form.

## 3. Results

The electronic search found in PubMed 239 articles, in Embase, 39 articles and in the Cochrane Library, 125 articles. No article was found in the search of LILACS. Fifteen placebo-controlled studies were selected. The flowchart used in the selection of the papers discussed in this review is show in **Figure 1**.

The 15 studies included 3441 patients. The patient age was between 12 and 97 years old. Gender data were mentioned in 10 of the 15 studies included (66%). Patients were mostly female (1934 women and 1691 men). Twelve studies have discussed about the severity of psoriasis. In these studies that the severity has been described, the classification of severity was mild (0 study), mild to moderate (one study), moderate to severe (11 studies) and severe (0 trial). However, four studies did not provide sufficient information to assess the clinical severity. The evaluation score most widely used to assess the clinical severity was the GSS-TSS (global-total severity score). Quality of life was also mentioned.

The duration of treatment ranged from two weeks to two months. The evaluation included Individual signs (erythema, scaling, and thickening) and Total score or global severity (TSS or GSS).

Concerning to the randomized controlled trials, among the fifteen selected publications, 8 studies (53%) reported clearly the method used for randomization and 3 studies (20%) used the computer randomization. Related to the anthropometric characteristics of participants used in the studies selected, as the age and gender, six studies (40%) provided data regarding age, gender and characteristics of clinical patients. Eight studies (53%) provided incomplete data. Eight studies were excluded. One study was not considered due to it did not provide data properly. Seven studies were excluded because there was no comparison with placebo.

In **Table 1** are shown the selected publications, the treatments suggested involving medication and placebo, and the conclusion of the studies.

## 4. Discussion

Van Voorhees and Fried, 2009 [44] have pointed out that the involvement of the scalp in patient with psoriasis is frequent. Due to the greater exposure to the environmental, it has a considerable effect on the quality of life of

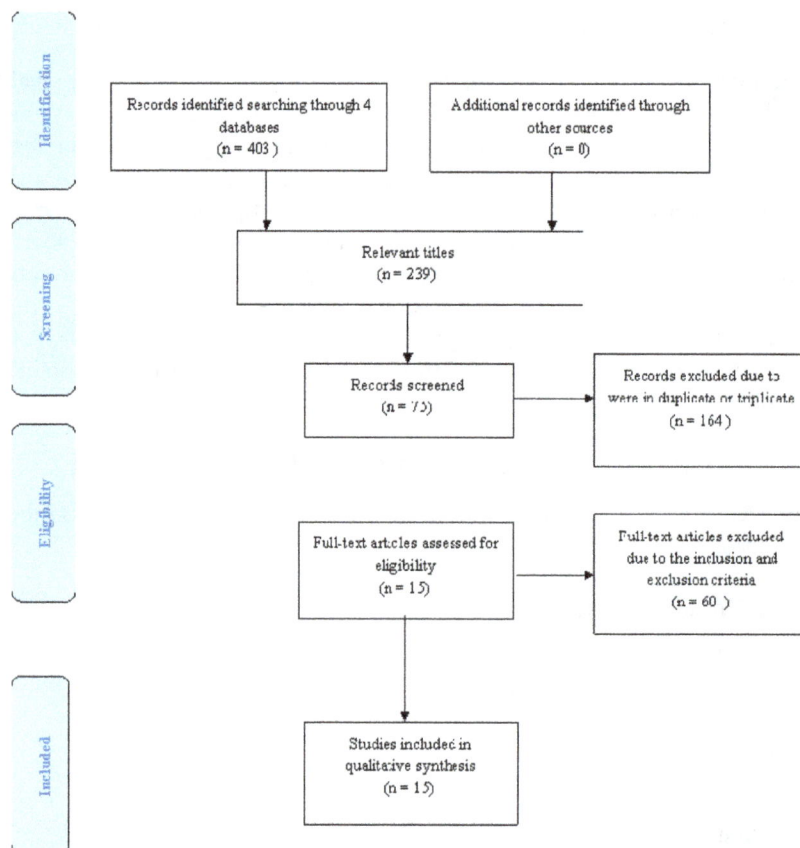

**Figure 1**. Flowchart indicating the steps to select the papers analyzed in this revision.

the patient. In this case, nevertheless, this fact must be discussed, due to the published studies rarely use tools to address these issues. Zampieron *et al.*, 2015 [45] have also reported that patients with scalp psoriasis suffered from a lower quality of life relating to the highly visible site of their psoriatic lesions. In consequence this fact stimulates investigations with this dermatologic disease, as it is presented in our work.

Firstly 403 papers were found in the databases that were searched. However, the analysis of the available papers used in this review included only 15 randomized controlled trials (see flowchart in **Figure 1**) due to the inclusion and exclusion criteria use.

The number of participants with scalp psoriasis with topical treatment in the publications is more than three thousand. The selected papers involve a total of 3 441 patients. Each of the studies utilized a comparison with a placebo, and the results of active ingredients were found to be more statistically significant than the placebos.

Many topical treatments, such as corticosteroids, calcipotriol, coal tar, salicylic acid are used for scalp psoriasis [46]. But, it is necessary to verify that there are few adequately controlled investigations that support the effectiveness of the suggested topical managements.

On the basis of the findings of this review, it was found that the best results were obtained with the use of clobetasol propionate in different vehicles (solution, foam and lotion) [29] [30]. When the placebo was compared to calcipotriol, there were better results with calcipotriol [47]-[49]; however, the magnitude of the effect was lower than in relation to clobetasol and It was similar to other corticosteroids, such as valerate of betamethasone, ancinonide, halcinonide, and fluocinolone acetonide. The opposite was observed for psoriasis on the body, which is described a greater efficiency in the association between calcipotriol and betamethasone dipropionate [50]. This study found no effect in terms of the overall gain in response to treatment in cases of psoriasis of the scalp. In **Table 1**, it is possible finding suitable information about the different formulations used to treat scalp psoriasis and the type of vehicle.

Characteristically, psoriasis is recurrent over years, and maintenance of the controlled disease, is a clinical challenge [51]. This fact is also true for scalp psoriasis. In this study, Meredith and Ormerod, 2012 [51] reported

**Table 1.** Selected publications, the treatments and conclusion of the studies.

| References | Type of application | Treatment | Conclusion |
|---|---|---|---|
| Sofen *et al.*, 2011 [29] | Spray | Clobetasol propionate and placebo | Treatment for up to four weeks is effective and well tolerated for moderate-to-severe plaque psoriasis of the scalp. |
| Olsen *et al.*, 1991 [30] | Ointment | Clobetasol propionate and placebo | Clobetasol propionate 0.05% scalp application appears to be a safe and an effective treatment for scalp psoriasis. |
| Jarratt *et al.*, 2004 [31] | Shampoo | Clobetasol propionate and placebo | The shampoo formulation of clobetasol propionate is convenient and efficacious and minimizes systemic exposure while being efficient, safe and well-tolerated in the treatment of moderate to severe scalp psoriasis. |
| Franz *et al.*, 2000 [32] | Foam | Clobetasol propionate and placebo | The results of the studies demonstrate that the enhancement of absorption induced by the foam vehicle also leads to an increase in efficacy. Data from 188 subjects show that those treated with clobetasol propionate (CP) foam experienced greater psoriatic improvement than subjects treated with a currently marketed solution product. For each of the signs and symptoms of psoriasis, as well as for the investigator's global assessment, CP foam was found to be superior to CP solution. |
| Reygagne *et al.*, 2002 [33] | Shampoo or gel | Clobetasol propionate and placebo | After 4 weeks of treatment, clobetasol proprionate 0.05%, shampoo was at least equivalent to the gel form and superior to its vehicle. The two active treatments were found to be equivalent safe. |
| Franz *et al.*, 1999 [34] | Foam | Betamethasone valerate and placebo | This formulation has increased efficacy in the treatment of scalp psoriasis without an associated increase in toxicity. |
| Medansky and Handler, 1974 [35] | Lotion | Betamethasone valerate and placebo | The lotion with betamethasone was more them the vehicle. |
| Tyring *et al.*, 2010 [36] | Ointment | Betamethasone valerate and placebo Calcipotriol and betamethasone dipropionate with placebo | Calcipotriol and betamethasone dipropionate was significantly superior to placebo. 71.9% of patients had cleared ou minimal disease after 8 weeks of treatment. |
| Harris, 1972 [37] | Lotion (alcoholic) | Valerate betamethasone with placebo | Significant differences were found to exist in favor of betamethasone valerate lotion 0.1% in lichenification, excoriation, inflammation, scaling and pruritus than vehicle group. |
| Jemec *et al.*, 2008 [38] | (*) | Two active ingredients (calcipotriol and betamethasone dipropionate) with each one active ingredients separately and with placebo | The two active ingredients formula was superior to placebo and both of the active ingredients separately. Adverse effects were similar in the two compound group and betamethasone group and significantly smaller than calcipotriol group and placebo group. |
| Green *et al.*, 1994 [39] | Solution | Calcipotriol with placebo | Calcipotriol was significantly superior to placebo in reducing redness, thickness, scaliness and extent of psoriasis, and in the patients' assessment in reducing scalp flaking and itching. No statistically significant changes in blood biochemistry were detected during the study, and the solution was generally well tolerated. |
| Pauporte *et al.*, 2004 [40] | Topical oil | Fluocinolone acetonide with placebo | It is shown that fluocinolone acetonide (FA) in an oil base that aids in the softening of the skin and allows penetration of the steroid into the stratum corneum, is an effective treatment for psoriasis of the scalp. This study also showed that the vehicle alone causes an improvement in the signs of psoriasis, but that the addition of 0.1% of the low potency steroid, FA leads to a significantly better improvement. |

**Continued**

| | | | |
|---|---|---|---|
| Lepaw, 1978 [41] | Solution of edetate disodium, polyethylene glycol 300, purified water and butylated hydroxytoluene. | Halcinonide solution with placebo | The treatment was excellent in sixteen patients treated with halcinonide and in one patient treated with placebo. In the comparative evaluation halcinonide was superior in twenty-two patients, the placebo was superior in four patients, and both drugs were equally effective in one patient. There were no adverse reactions due to halcinonide, but one patient experienced pruritus with the placebo solution. |
| Ellis *et al.*, 1988 [42] | Lotion | Amcinonide with placebo | Among the patients, overall improvements in psoriatic lesions was seen in 78% amcinonide group and 27% of the placebo group. There was no serious side effects attributtabe to this study. |
| Shuttleworth *et al.*, 1998 [43] | Shampoo | Ciclopirox olamine and placebo | For ciclopirox olamine only, there was significant ($P < 0.05$) improvement over baseline for clinical assessment of overall scalp psoriasis (day 29) and degree of scaling (days 8, 15 and 29) and for patients' self-assessments of overall scalp psoriasis (days 15 and 29) and scalp itching (day 15), but differences from placebo were not significant. Ciclopirox olamine tolerability and acceptability were good. |

that it was not possible to assess recurrence rates because there was only a short period of follow up.

It is important to state that is often necessary to combine oral treatments and topicals, especially in severe cases of scalp psoriasis, there are, extensive or resistant to topical treatments. In these cases, some authors have pointed out the importance of medications, such as methotrexate, cyclosporine, acitretin, and treatment involving psoralen plus ultraviolet A (PUVA) [52]-[55].

Vergou *et al.*, 2011 [56] have also suggested immunobiologicals, including infliximab, adalimumab and the etarnecept to be administered. For this class of drugs, a complete healing of the lesions and maintenance of the healing period of three years for adalimumab treatment has been described [57].

Psoriasis of the scalp, especially those cases classified as moderate to severe is associated with emotional and social disorders that affect the well-being of patients [58]. Despite this, few studies evaluate the emotional repercussions of this type of psoriasis patients. The National Psoriasis Foundation 2006 Benchmark Survey estimates that psoriasis has a moderate to large negative impact on quality of life (QoL) in approximately 75% of affected patients [59]. It is also noted that those patients are more likely to commit suicide when compared to those who do not have the disease [20] [60].

Adverse effects were found in 9 of 15 studies. Studies generally omit reporting adverse events. Due to the small sample of studies and the short follow-up period, ranging from two weeks to two months, the possibility of not detecting more serious adverse events or consequence of the chronic use of medications may be higher than they would be under other conditions.

## 5. Conclusion

In conclusion, this investigation demonstrates the efficacy of topical treatments for scalp psoriasis, such as corticosteroids, calcipotriol, ciclopirox olamine, and associations, when compared with placebos. Clobetasol propionate (0.05%) was the most active ingredient, in various vehicles, in terms of the induction treatment of psoriasis of the scalp. However, due to the small clinical follow-up time of the studies, it was not possible to obtain data concerning the maintenance of the outcome or recurrence rates, so more research is needed in this area. It is important to consider that among the active principles used for the topical treatment of scalp psoriasis and compared with placebo, clobetasol propionate was the most effective, in all types of vehicle.

## Acknowledgements

The authors thank the Conselho *Nacional de Desenvolvimento Científico e Tecnológico* (CNPq) (National Counsel of Technological and Scientific Development) for the support.

## Conflict of Interest

There is no conflict of interest in this paper.

# References

[1] Huerta, C., Rivero, E. and Rodriguez, L.A. (2007) Incidence and Risk Factors for Psoriasis in the General Population. *Archives of Dermatology*, **143**, 1559-1565. http://dx.doi.org/10.1001/archderm.143.12.1559

[2] Braathen, L.R., Botten, G. and Bjerkedal, T. (1989) Prevalence of Psoriasis in Norway. *Acta Dermato-Venereologica*, **142**, 5-8.

[3] Nevitt, G.J. and Hutchinson, P.E. (1966) Psoriasis in the Community: Prevalence, Severity and Patients' Beliefs and Attitudes towards the Disease. *British Journal of Dermatology*, **135**, 533-537. http://dx.doi.org/10.1111/j.1365-2133.1996.tb03826.x

[4] Lomholt, G. (1963) Psoriasis: Prevalence, Spontaneous Course and Genetics. A Census Study on the Prevalence of Skin Disease on the Faroe Islands. G.E.C. Gad, Copenhagen.

[5] Zeljko-Penavic, J., Situm, M., Simic, D. and Vurnek-Zivkovic, M. (2010) Quality of Life in Psoriatic Patients and the Relationship between Type I and Type II Psoriasis. *Collegium Antropologicum*, **34**, 195-198.

[6] Kastelan, M., Prpić-Massari, L. and Brajac, I. (2009) Apoptosis in Psoriasis. *Acta Dermatovenerologica Croatica*, **17**, 182-186.

[7] Castelijns, F.A., Gerritsen, M.J., van Erp, P.E. and van de Kerkhof, P.C. (2000) Cell-Kinetic Evidence for Increased Recruitment of Cycling Epidermal Cells in Psoriasis: The Ratio of Histone and Ki-67 Antigen Expression Is Constant. *Dermatology*, **201**, 105-110. http://dx.doi.org/10.1159/000018471

[8] Soler, D.C. and McCormick, T.S. (2011) The Dark Side of Regulatory T Cells in Psoriasis. *Journal of Investigative Dermatolology*, **131**, 1785-1786. http://dx.doi.org/10.1038/jid.2011.200

[9] Chan, C.S., Van Voorhees, A.S., Lebwohl, M.G., Korman, N.J., Young, M., Bebo, B.F., *et al.* (2009) Treatment of Severe Scalp Psoriasis: From the Medical Board of the National Psoriasis Foundation. *Journal of the American Academy of Dermatology*, **60**, 962-971. http://dx.doi.org/10.1016/j.jaad.2008.11.890

[10] Tracey, W. (2010) Psoriasis: Impact and Management of Moderate to Severe Disease. *British Journal of Nursing*, **19**, 10-17. http://dx.doi.org/10.12968/bjon.2010.19.1.45905

[11] Rongioletti, F., Fiorucci, C. and Parodi, A. (2009) Psoriasis Induced or Aggravated by Drugs. *Journal of Rheumatology*, **83**, 59-61. http://dx.doi.org/10.3899/jrheum.090227

[12] Telfer, N.R., Chalmers, R.J., Whale, K. and Colman, G. (1992) The Role of Streptococcal Infection in the Initiation of Guttate Psoriasis. *Archives of Dermatolology*, **128**, 39-42. http://dx.doi.org/10.1001/archderm.1992.01680110049004

[13] Navarini, A.A. and Trueb, R.M. (2010) Psoriasis. *Therapeutische Umschau*, **67**, 153-165. http://dx.doi.org/10.1024/0040-5930/a000029

[14] Van de Kerkhof, P.C., de Hoop, D., de Korte, J. and Kuipers, M.V. (1998) Scalp Psoriasis Clinical Presentations and Therapeutic Management. *Dermatology*, **197**, 326-334. http://dx.doi.org/10.1159/000018026

[15] Farber, E.M. and Nall, M.L. (1974) The Natural History of Psoriasis in 5,600 Patients. *Dermatologica*, **148**, 1-18. http://dx.doi.org/10.1159/000251595

[16] Ortonne, J., Chimenti, S., Luger, T., Puig, L., Reid, F. and Trüeb, R. (2009) Scalp Psoriasis: European Consensus on Grading and Treatment Algorithm. *Journal of the European Academy of Dermatology & Venereology*, **23**, 1435-1444. http://dx.doi.org/10.1111/j.1468-3083.2009.03372.x

[17] Kim, G.W., Jung, H.J., Ko, H.C., Kim, M.B., Lee, W.J., Lee, S.J., Kim, D.W., *et al.* (2011) Dermoscopy Can Be Useful in Differentiating Scalp Psoriasis from Seborrhoeic Dermatitis. *British Journal of Dermatology*, **164**, 652-656. http://dx.doi.org/10.1111/j.1365-2133.2010.10180.x

[18] Mashaly, H.M., Masood, N.A. and Mohamed, A.S. (2011) Classification of Papulo-Squamous Skin Diseases Using Image Analysis. *Skin Research and Technology*, **18**, 36-44. http://dx.doi.org/10.1111/j.1600-0846.2011.00511.x

[19] Del Rosso, J.Q. (2011) Adult Seborrheic Dermatitis: A Status Report on Practical Topical Management. *The Journal of Clinical Aesthetic Dermatology*, **4**, 32-38.

[20] Kimball, A.B., Guerin, A., Tsaneva, M., Yu, A.P., Wu, E.Q., Gupta, S.R., *et al.* (2011) Economic Burden of Comorbidities in Patients with Psoriasis Is Substantial. *Journal of the European Academy of Dermatology & Venereology*, **25**, 157-163. http://dx.doi.org/10.1111/j.1468-3083.2010.03730.x

[21] Antoni, C.E., Kavanaugh, A., Kirkham, B., Tutuncu, Z., Burmester, G.R., Schneider, U., *et al.* (2005) Sustained Benefits of Infliximab Therapy for Dermatologic and Articular Manifestations of Psoriatic Arthritis: Results from the Infliximab Multinational Psoriatic Arthritis Controlled Trial (IMPACT). *Arthritis & Rheumatism*, **52**, 1227-1236. http://dx.doi.org/10.1002/art.20967

[22] Mazzotta, A., Esposito, M., Carboni, I., Schipani, C. and Chimenti, S. (2007) Clobetasol Propionate Foam 0.05% as a Novel Topical Formulation for Plaque-Type and Scalp Psoriasis. *Journal of Dermatological Treatment*, **8**, 84-87. http://dx.doi.org/10.1080/09546630601123835

[23] Spandonaro, F., Altomare, G., Berardesca, E., Calzavara-Pinton, P., Chimenti, S., Girolomoni, G., *et al.* (2011) Health-Related Quality of Life in Psoriasis: An Analysis of Psocare Project Patients. *Giornale Italiano di Dermatologia e Venereologia*, **146**, 169-178.

[24] Basra, M.K., Fenech, R., Gatt, R.M., Salek, M.S. and Finlay, A.Y. (2008) The Dermatology Life Quality Index 1994-2007: A Comprehensive Review of Validation Data and Clinical Results. *British Journal of Dermatology*, **159**, 997-1035. http://dx.doi.org/10.1111/j.1365-2133.2008.08832.x

[25] Shikiar, R., Bresnahan, B.W., Stone, S.P., Thompson, C., Koo, J. and Revicki, D.A. (2003) Validity and Reliability of Patient Reported Outcomes Used in Psoriasis: Results from Two Randomized Clinical Trials. *Health & Quality of Life Outcomes*, **1**, 53. http://dx.doi.org/10.1186/1477-7525-1-53

[26] Menter, A., Gordon, K., Carey, W., Hamilton, T., Glazer, S., Caro, I., *et al.* (2005) Efficacy and Safety Observed during 24 Weeks of Efalizumab Therapy in Patients with Moderate to Severe Plaque Psoriasis. *Archives of Dermatolology*, **141**, 31-38. http://dx.doi.org/10.1001/archderm.141.1.31

[27] Gottlieb, A.B., Chaudhari, U., Baker, D.G., Perate, M. and Dooley, L.T. (2003) The National Psoriasis Foundation Psoriasis Score (NPF-PS) System versus the Psoriasis Area Severity Index (PASI) and Physician's Global Assessment (PGA): A Comparison. *Journal of Drugs in Dermatology*, **2**, 260-266.

[28] Liberati, A., Altman, D.G., Tetzlaff, J., Mulrow, C., Gøtzsche, P.C., Ioannidis, J.P., *et al.* (2009) The PRISMA Statement for Reporting Systematic Reviews and Meta-Analyses of Studies That Evaluate Health Care Interventions: Explanation and Elaboration. *PLoS Medicine*, **6**, e1000100. http://dx.doi.org/10.1371/journal.pmed.1000100

[29] Sofen, H., Hudson, C.P., Cook-Bolden, F.E., Preston, N., Colón, L.E., Colón, L.E, *et al.* (2011) Clobetasol Propionate 0.05% Spray for the Management of Moderate-to-Severe Plaque Psoriasis of the Scalp: Results from a Randomized Controlled Trial. *Journal of Drugs in Dermatology*, **10**, 885-892.

[30] Olsen, E.A., Cram, D.L., Ellis, C.N., Hickman, J.G., Jacobson, C., Jenkins, E.E., *et al.* (1991) A Double-Blind, Vehicle-Controlled Study of Clobetasol Propionate 0.05% (Temovate) Scalp Application in the Treatment of Moderate to Severe Scalp Psoriasis. *Journal of the American Academy of Dermatology*, **24**, 443-447. http://dx.doi.org/10.1016/0190-9622(91)70069-E

[31] Jarratt, M., Breneman, D., Gottlieb, A.B., Poulin, Y., Liu, Y. and Foley, V. (2004) Clobetasol Propionate Shampoo 0.05%: A New Option to Treat Patients with Moderate to Severe Scalp Psoriasis. *Journal of Drugs in Dermatology*, **3**, 367-373.

[32] Franz, T.J., Parsell, D.A., Myers, J.A. and Hannigan, J.F. (2000) Clobetasol Propionate Foam 0.05%: A Novel Vehicle with Enhanced Delivery. *International Journal of Dermatology*, **39**, 535-538. http://dx.doi.org/10.1046/j.1365-4362.2000.00986-4.x

[33] Reygagne, P., Diaconu, J., Pres, H., Ernst, T.M., Meyer, K.G. and Arsonnaud, S. (2002) Efficacy and Safety Comparison of Clobetasol Propionate Shampoo, Gel and Vehicle in Scalp Psoriasis. *European Academy of Dermatology and Venereology*, **16**, 283.

[34] Franz, T.J., Parsell, D.A., Halualani, R.M., Hannigan, J.F., Kalbach, J.P. and Harkonen, W.S. (1999) Betamethasone Valerate Foam 0.12%: A Novel Vehicle with Enhanced Delivery and Efficacy. *International Journal of Dermatolology*, **38**, 628-632. http://dx.doi.org/10.1046/j.1365-4362.1999.00782.x

[35] Medansky, R.S. and Handler, R.M. (1974) Treating Psoriasis of the Scalp with a New Corticosteroid Lotion. *IMJ Illinois Medical Journal*, **145**, 503-504.

[36] Tyring, S., Mendoza, N., Appell, M., Bibby, A., Foster, R., Hamilton, T., *et al.* (2010) A Calcipotriene/Betamethasone Dipropionate Two-Compound Scalp Formulation in the Treatment of Scalp Psoriasis in Hispanic/Latino and Black/African American Patients: Results of the Randomized, 8-Week, Double-Blind Phase of a Clinical Trial. *International Journal of Dermatology*, **49**, 1328-1333. http://dx.doi.org/10.1111/j.1365-4632.2010.04598.x

[37] Harris, J.J. (1972) A National Double-Blind Clinical Trial of a New Corticosteroid Lotion: A 12-Investigator Cooperative Analysis. *Current Therapeutic Research, Clinical and Experimental*, **14**, 638-646.

[38] Jemec, G.B., Ganslandt, C., Ortonne, J.P., Poulin, Y., Burden, A.D., de Unamuno, P., *et al.* (2008) A New Scalp Formulation of Calcipotriene Plus Betamethasone Compared with Its Active Ingredients and the Vehicle in the Treatment of Scalp Psoriasis: A Randomized, Double-Blind, Controlled Trial. *Journal of the American Academy of Dermatology*, **59**, 455-463. http://dx.doi.org/10.1016/j.jaad.2008.04.027

[39] Green, C., Ganpule, M., Harris, D., Kavanagh, G., Kennedy, C., Mallett, R., *et al.* (1994) Comparative Effects of Calcipotriol (MC903) Solution and Placebo (Vehicle of MC903) in the Treatment of Psoriasis of the Scalp. *British Journal of Dermatology*, **130**, 483-487. http://dx.doi.org/10.1111/j.1365-2133.1994.tb03382.x

[40] Pauporte, M., Maibach, H., Lowe, N., Pugliese, M., Friedman, D.J., Mendelsohn, H., *et al.* (2004) Fluocinolone Acetonide Topical Oil for Scalp Psoriasis. *Journal of Dermatological Treatment*, **15**, 360-364. http://dx.doi.org/10.1080/09546630410023566

[41]  Lepaw, M.I. (1978) Double-Blind Comparison of Halcinonide Solution and Placebo Control in Treatment of Psoriasis of the Scalp. *Cutis*, **21**, 571-573.

[42]  Ellis, C.N., Horwitz, S.N. and Mente, A. (1988) Amcinonide Lotion 0.1% in the Treatment of Patients with Psoriasis of the Scalp. *Current Therapeutic Research, Clinical and Experimental*, **44**, 315-324.

[43]  Shuttleworth, D., Galloway, D.B., Boorman, G.C. and Donald, A.E. (1998) A Double-Blind, Placebo-Controlled Study of the Clinical Efficacy of Ciclopirox Olamine (1.5%) Shampoo for the Control of Scalp Psoriasis. *Journal of Dermatological Treatment*, **9**, 163-167. http://dx.doi.org/10.3109/09546639809160548

[44]  Van Voorhees, A.S. and Fried, R. (2009) Depression and Quality of Life in Psoriasis. *Postgraduate Medicine*, **121**, 154-161. http://dx.doi.org/10.3810/pgm.2009.07.2040

[45]  Zampieron, A., Buja, A., Fusco, M., Linder, D., Bortune, M., Piaserico, S., *et al.* (2015) Quality of Life in Patients with Scalp Psoriasis. *Giornale Italiano di Dermatolologia e Venereologia*, **150**, 309-316.

[46]  Mrowietz, U., Macheleidt, O. and Eicke, C. (2011) Effective Treatment and Improvement of Quality of Life in Patients with Scalp Psoriasis by Topical Use of Calcipotriol/Betamethasone (Xamiol®-Gel): Results. *Journal der Deutschen Dermatologischen Gesellschaft*, **9**, 825-831. http://dx.doi.org/10.1111/j.1610-0387.2011.07695.x

[47]  Griffiths, C.E., Finlay, A.Y., Fleming, C.J., Barker, J.N., Mizzi, F. and Arsonnaud, S. (2006) A Randomized, Investigator-Masked Clinical Evaluation of the Efficacy and Safety of Clobetasol Propionate 0.05% Shampoo and Tar Blend 1% Shampoo in the Treatment of Moderate to Severe Scalp Psoriasis. *Journal of Dermatological Treatment*, **17**, 90-95. http://dx.doi.org/10.1080/09546630500515701

[48]  Wauters, O., Roland, I. and De la Brassinne, M. (2007) Corticosteroids and Their Vehicle in the Treatment of Scalp Psoriasis. *Revue Medicale de Liege*, **62**, 196-199.

[49]  Freeman, K. (2010) The Two-Compound Formulation of Calcipotriol and Betamethasone Dipropionate for Treatment of Moderately Severe Body and Scalp Psoriasis—An Introduction. *Current Medical Research Opinion*, **27**, 197-203. http://dx.doi.org/10.1185/03007995.2010.540985

[50]  Menter, A., Abramovits, W., Colón, L.E., Johnson, L.A. and Gottschalk, R.W. (2009) Comparing Clobetasol Propionate 0.05% Spray to Calcipotriene 0.005% Betamethasone Dipropionate 0.064% Ointment for the Treatment of Moderate to Severe Plaque Psoriasis. *Journal of Drugs in Dermatolology*, **8**, 52-57.

[51]  Meredith, F. and Ormerod, A.D. (2012) Patient Preferences for Psoriasis Treatment: Process Characteristics Considered More Important than Outcome Attributes. *Expert Review of Pharmacoeconomics & Outcomes Research*, **12**, 145-147. http://dx.doi.org/10.1586/erp.12.9

[52]  Nast, A., Boehncke, W.H., Mrowietz, U., Ockenfels, H.M., Philipp, S., Reich, K., *et al.* (2012) Deutsche Dermatologische Gesellschaft (DDG); Berufsverband Deutscher Dermatologen (BVDD). S3—Guidelines on the Treatment of Psoriasis Vulgaris (English Version). Update. *Journal der Deutschen Dermatologischen Gesellschaft*, **10**, S1-S95. http://dx.doi.org/10.1111/j.1610-0387.2012.07919.x

[53]  Kortuem, K.R., Davis, M.D., Witman, P.M., McEvoy, M.T. and Farmer, S.A. (2010) Results of Goeckerman Treatment for Psoriasis in Children: A 21-Year Retrospective Review. *Pediatric Dermatology*, **27**, 518-524. http://dx.doi.org/10.1111/j.1525-1470.2010.01124.x

[54]  Carretero, G., Puig, L., Dehesa, L., Carrascosa, J.M., Ribera, M., Sánchez-Regaña, M., *et al.* (2010) Metotrexato: Guía de uso en psoriasis (Guidelines on the Use of Methotrexate in Psoriasis). *Actas Dermo-Sifiliográficas*, **101**, 600-613. http://dx.doi.org/10.1016/j.ad.2010.04.002

[55]  Due, E., Blomberg, M., Skov, L. and Zachariae, C. (2011) Discontinuation of Methotrexate in Psoriasis. *Acta Dermato Venereologica*, **92**, 353-354. http://dx.doi.org/10.2340/00015555-1233

[56]  Vergou, T., Moustou, A.E., Sfikakis, P.P., Antoniou, C. and Stratigos, A.J. (2011) Pharmacodynamics of TNF-α Inhibitors in Psoriasis. *Expert Review of Clinical Pharmacology*, **4**, 515-523. http://dx.doi.org/10.1586/ecp.11.28

[57]  Gordon, K., Papp, K., Poulin, Y., Gu, Y., Rozzo, S. and Sasso, E.H. (2012) Long-Term Efficacy and Safety of Adalimumab in Patients with Moderate to Severe Psoriasis Treated Continuously over 3 Years: Results from an Open-Label Extension Study for Patients from REVEAL. *Journal of the American Academy of Dermatology*, **66**, 241-251. http://dx.doi.org/10.1016/j.jaad.2010.12.005

[58]  Kimball, A.B., Jacobson, C., Weiss, S., Vreeland, M.G. and Wu, Y. (2005) The Psychosocial Burden of Psoriasis. *American Journal of Clinical Dermatology*, **6**, 383-392. http://dx.doi.org/10.2165/00128071-200506060-00005

[59]  Kurd, S.K., Troxel, A.B., Crits-Christoph, P. and Gelfand, J.M. (2010) The Risk of Depression, Anxiety, and Suicidality in Patients with Psoriasis: A Population-Based Cohort Study. *Archives of Dermatology*, **146**, 891-895.

[60]  Gupta, M.A., Schork, N.J., Gupta, A.K., Kirkby, S. and Ellis, C.N. (1993) Suicidal Ideation in Psoriasis. *International Journal of Dermatology*, **32**, 188-190. http://dx.doi.org/10.1111/j.1365-4362.1993.tb02790.x

# Permissions

All chapters in this book were first published in JCDSA, by Scientific Research Publishing; hereby published with permission under the Creative Commons Attribution License or equivalent. Every chapter published in this book has been scrutinized by our experts. Their significance has been extensively debated. The topics covered herein carry significant findings which will fuel the growth of the discipline. They may even be implemented as practical applications or may be referred to as a beginning point for another development.

The contributors of this book come from diverse backgrounds, making this book a truly international effort. This book will bring forth new frontiers with its revolutionizing research information and detailed analysis of the nascent developments around the world.

We would like to thank all the contributing authors for lending their expertise to make the book truly unique. They have played a crucial role in the development of this book. Without their invaluable contributions this book wouldn't have been possible. They have made vital efforts to compile up to date information on the varied aspects of this subject to make this book a valuable addition to the collection of many professionals and students.

This book was conceptualized with the vision of imparting up-to-date information and advanced data in this field. To ensure the same, a matchless editorial board was set up. Every individual on the board went through rigorous rounds of assessment to prove their worth. After which they invested a large part of their time researching and compiling the most relevant data for our readers.

The editorial board has been involved in producing this book since its inception. They have spent rigorous hours researching and exploring the diverse topics which have resulted in the successful publishing of this book. They have passed on their knowledge of decades through this book. To expedite this challenging task, the publisher supported the team at every step. A small team of assistant editors was also appointed to further simplify the editing procedure and attain best results for the readers.

Apart from the editorial board, the designing team has also invested a significant amount of their time in understanding the subject and creating the most relevant covers. They scrutinized every image to scout for the most suitable representation of the subject and create an appropriate cover for the book.

The publishing team has been an ardent support to the editorial, designing and production team. Their endless efforts to recruit the best for this project, has resulted in the accomplishment of this book. They are a veteran in the field of academics and their pool of knowledge is as vast as their experience in printing. Their expertise and guidance has proved useful at every step. Their uncompromising quality standards have made this book an exceptional effort. Their encouragement from time to time has been an inspiration for everyone.

The publisher and the editorial board hope that this book will prove to be a valuable piece of knowledge for researchers, students, practitioners and scholars across the globe.

# List of Contributors

**Hugues Adégbidi, Félix Atadokpèdé, Florencia do Ango-Padonou and Hubert G. Yédomon**
Faculté des Sciences de la Santé de Cotonou, Université d'Abomey-Calavi, Cotonou, Bénin

**Christiane Koudoukpo**
Faculté de Médecine de Parakou, Université de Parakou, Parakou, Bénin

**Asako Ito**
Ookuma Hospital, Nagoya, Japan

**Gabriela Sprada Tavares da Mota and Angela Bonjorno Arantes**
School of Health and Biosciences, Pontifícia Universidade Católica do Paraná, Curitiba, Brasil

**Silvia Vertuani, Stefano Manfredini, Paola Ziosi and Gabriela Sprada Tavares da Mota**
Ambrosialab, University of Ferrara, Ferrara, Italy

**Emanuela Scalambra, Antonella Spagnoletti, Gianni Sacchetti, Silvia Vertuani and Stefano Manfredini**
Department of Life Sciences and Biotechnology, School of Pharmacy and Health Products, University of Ferrara, Ferrara, Italy

**Ahmed Ashour, Asuka Kishikawa, Ryuichiro Kondo and Kuniyoshi Shimizu**
Department of Agro-Environmental Sciences, Faculty of Agriculture, Kyushu University, Fukuoka, Japan

**Saleh El-Sharkawy, Mohamed Amer, Amani Marzouk, Ahmed Zaki and Ahmed Ashour**
Department of Pharmacognosy, Faculty of Pharmacy, Mansoura University, Mansoura, Egypt

**Saleh El-Sharkawy**
Department of Pharmacognosy, Faculty of Pharmacy, Delta University for Science and Technology, Mansoura, Egypt

**Momiji Ohzono**
Zenshin Incorporated, Chikushino City, Japan

**Federica Zanzottera and Emilio Lavezzari**
Hair Transplantation Surgery, Studio Dr. Lavezzari, Como, Italy

**Letizia Trovato, Alessandro Icardi and Antonio Graziano**
HBW Srl, Torino, Italy

**Akihiko Takahashi, Katsura Mori, Takahiro Nishizaka and Hisateru Tanabe**
Kao Corporation, R&D, Skincare Product Research, Tokyo, Japan

**Yoram Harth**
Medical OR Center, Herzlya, Israel

**Einat Ackerman, Ido Frank and Yoram Harth**
EndyMed Medical, Caesarea, Israel

**Monica Elman**
Beit Harofeim, Holon, Israel

**Khalifa E. Sharquie, Adil A. Noaimi and Attaa A. Hajji**
Department of Dermatology and Venereology, Baghdad Teaching Hospital, Baghdad, Iraq

**Yoshinari Taguchi, Mikihiko Aoki and Masato Tanaka**
Graduate School of Science and Technology, Niigata University, Niigata, Japan

**Khalifa E. Sharquie and Adil A. Noaimi**
Department of Dermatology, College of Medicine, University of Baghdad, Baghdad, Iraq
Iraqi and Arab Board for Dermatology and Venereology, Baghdad Teaching Hospital, Medical City, Baghdad, Iraq

**Mohammed N. Almallah**
Department of Dermatology and Venereology, Baghdad Teaching Hospital, Baghdad, Iraq

**Kentaro Ishii, Mayumi Kotani and Akihito Fujita**
Bloom Classic Co., Matsuyama, Japan

**Shinichi Moriwaki**
Department of Dermatology, Osaka Medical College, Takatsuki, Japan

**Sheila M. Maregesi, Godeliver A. Kagashe and Fatuma Felix**
Pharmacognosy Department, School of Pharmacy, Muhimbili University College of Health and Allied Sciences, Dar es Salaam, Tanzania

**John Fleming and Saqib Bashir**
Dermatology Department, King's College Hospital, London, UK

**Maha S. Younis**
Department of Psychiatry, College of Medicine, Baghdad University, Baghdad, Iraq

**Bashar S. Al-Sultani**
Department of Dermatology, Baghdad Teaching Hospital, Medical City, Baghdad, Iraq

**Marline L. Squance, Glenn E. M. Reeves and John Attia**
Faculty of Health and Medicine, University of Newcastle, Callaghan, Australia
Hunter New England Health District, New Lambton Heights, Australia

Hunter Medical Research Institute, New Lambton Heights, Australia

**Marline L. Squance**
Faculty of Science and Information Technology, University of Newcastle, Callaghan, Australia

**Marline L. Squance and Glenn E. M. Reeves**
Autoimmune Resource and Research Centre, New Lambton Heights, Australia

**Yuiko Nagata, Atsushi Tanemura, Emi Ono, Aya Tanaka, Kenichi Kato, Mizuho Yamada and Ichiro Katayama**
Department of Dermatology, Integrated Medicine Osaka University Graduate School of Medicine, Suita, Japan

**Hafida Chérifi, Adrien Naveau, Ludwig Loison Robert and Bruno Gogly**
Dental Department, A. Chenevier-H. Mondor Hospital, Créteil, France
UMR S872, Université Paris Descartes, Sorbonne Paris Cité, France
UMR S872, Centre de Recherche des Cordeliers, Université Pierre et Marie Curie, Paris, France
INSERM U872, Paris, France

**Judith Hellman anf Cielo A. Ramirez**
Mt. Sinai Hospital, New York, USA

**Kasama Vejakupta, Montree Udompataikul**
Skin Centre, Srinakarinwirot University, Bangkok, Thailand

**Khawar Abbas, Drew F. Goettler and Zayd C. Leseman**
Mechanical Engineering Department, University of New Mexico, Albuquerque, USA

**Bruce C. Lamartine**
Los Alamos National Laboratory, Los Alamos, USA

**María Matabuena de Yzaguirre**
Department of Biology, Faculty of Sciences, Universidad Autónoma de Madrid, Madrid, Spain

**Gabriela Bacchini, Emili Gil Luna and Eva Vila-Martínez**
Medical Department, Ferrer Health Care, Barcelona, Spain

**Mika Oshima, Maiko Sogawa, Yoshihiro Matsudate, Nozomi Fukui, Kazutoshi Murao and Yoshiaki Kubo**
Department of Dermatology, Institute of Health Biosciences, The University of Tokushima Graduate School, Tokushima, Japan

**Hiroshi Matsunaka, Yumi Murakami and Yumiko Saya**
Tokiwa Pharmaceutical Co., Ltd., Tokyo, Japan

**Takashi Sugita**
Department of Microbiology, Meiji Pharmaceutical University, Tokyo, Japan

**Roya Sadeghi, Azar Tol and Azita Moradi**
Deptartment of Education and promotion, School of Public Health, Tehran University of Medical Sciences, Tehran, Iran

**Masoud Baikpour**
School of Medicine, Tehran University of Medical Sciences, Tehran, Iran

**Mostafa Hossaini**
Department of Epidemiology and Biostatistics, School of Public Health, Tehran University of Medical Sciences, Tehran, Iran

**María Matabuena-de Yzaguirre and Ángeles Juarranz**
Department of Biology, Faculty of Sciences, Universidad Autónoma de Madrid, Madrid, Spain

**Gabriela Bacchini and Eva Vila-Martínez**
Medical Department, Ferrer Health Care, Barcelona, Spain

**Francesco Scarci and Federico Mailland**
Scientific Department, Polichem S.A., Lugano, Switzerland

**Gaétan Chevalier**
Developmental and Cell Biology Department, University of California at Irvine, Irvine, USA

**Hiroyuki Sato, Yoshinari Taguchi and Masato Tanaka**
Graduate School of Science and Technology, Niigata University, Niigata, Japan

**Xianghong Yan**
P & G Innovation Godo Kaisha, Kobe, Japan

**Ta-Min Wang**
Division of Urology, Department of Surgery, Chang Gung Memorial Hospital, Kwei-Shan, Taiwan

**Yung-Ching Ming**
Department of Pediatric Surgery, Chang Gung Children's Hospital, Chang Gung Memorial Hospital, Taiwan

**Yuan-Ming Yeh**
Molecular Medicine Research Center, Chang Gung University, Taiwan

**Tzu-Ya Chen and Jong-Hwei Su Pang**
Graduate Institute of Clinical Medical Sciences, College of Medicine, Chang Gung University, Taiwan

**Regina Jales and Humberto Saconato**
Departamento de Clínica Médica, Hospital Universitário
Onofre Lopes, Universidade Federal do Rio Grande do
Norte, Natal, Brazil

**Sérgio Hirata**
Departamento de Dermatologia, Hospital São Paulo,
Universidade Federal de São Paulo, São Paulo, Brazil

**Álvaro Attalah**
Departamento de Medicina Interna, Hospital São Paulo,
Universidade Federal de São Paulo, São Paulo, Brazil

**Danúbia Sá-Caputo**
Programa de Pós-Graduação em Fisiopatologia Clínica e
Experimental, Universidade do Estado do Rio de Janeiro,
Rio de Janeiro, Brazil

**Adriano Arnóbio, Éric Heleno Frederico and Mario
Bernardo-Filho**
Departamento de Biofísica e Biometria, Universidade do
Estado do Rio de Janeiro, Rio de Janeiro, Brazil